Serono Symposia Publications from Raven Press
Volume 94

GONADAL DEVELOPMENT AND FUNCTION

Serono Symposia Publications from Raven Press

Vol. 94: Gonadal Development and Function, *S.G. Hillier, editor;* 316 pp. 1993.
Vol. 93: Reproductive Medicine, vol. II, in press.
Vol. 92: New Advances on Cytokines, *S. Romagnani T.R. Mosmann and A.K. Abbas, editors;* 386 pp.1992.
Vol. 91: Implantation in Mammals,in press
Vol. 90: Molecular and Cellular Biology of Reproduction, *G. Spera, A. Fabbrini, L. Gnessi and C.W. Bardin, editors;* 296 pp., 1992.
Vol. 89: Recent Advances on Hypoglycemia, *D. Andreani, P.J. Lefebvre, V. Marks and G. Tamburrano, editors;* 400 pp. 1993
Vol. 88: IL-6: Physiopathology and Clinical Potentials, *M. Revel, editor;* 312 pp. 1992.
Vol. 87: "Redo" Vascular Surgery - Renal, Aorto-Iliac and Infrainguinal Areas, *C. Spartera, R. Courbier, P. Fiorani and A.M. Imparato, editors;* 332 pp., 1992.
Vol. 86: Stress and Reproduction, *K.E. Sheppard, J.H. Boublik and J.W. Funder, editors;* 375 pp., 1992.
Vol. 85: Nutritional Aspects of Osteoporosis, *P. Burckhardt and R.P. Heaney, editors;* 380 pp., 1991.
Vol. 84: Advances in Surgery *F.G. Moody, W. Montorsi and M. Montorsi, editors;* 496 pp., 1991.
Vol. 83: Hereditary Tumors, *M.L. Brandi and R. White, editors;* 220 pp., 1991.
Vol. 82: The Status of Differentiation Therapy of Cancer, vol. II, *S. Waxman, G.B. Rossi and F. Takaku, editors;* 152 pp., 1991.
Vol. 81: Growth Disorders: The State of the Art, *L. Cavallo, J.C. Job and M.I. New, editors;* 372 pp., 1991.
Vol. 80: Ovarian Secretions and Cardiovascular and Neurological Function, *F. Naftolin, J.N. Gutmann, A.H. DeCherney and P.M. Sarrel, editors;* 320 pp., 1990.
Vol. 79: Progress and Perspectives in Chemoprevention of Cancer, *G. De Palo, M. Sporn and U. Veronesi, editors;* 296 pp., 1992
Vol. 78: Papillomaviruses in Human Pathology. Recent Progress in Epidermoid Precancers, *J. Monsonego, editor;* 531 pp., 1990.
Vol. 77: Plasminogen Activators: From Cloning to Therapy, *R. Abbate, T. Barni and A. Tsafriri, editors;* 204 pp., 1991.
Vol. 76: Horizons in Endocrinology, vol. II, *M. Maggi and V. Geenen, editors;* 360 pp., 1991.
Vol. 75: Comparative Spermatology 20 Years After, *B. Baccetti, editor;* 1112 pp., 1991.
Vol. 74: The New Biology of Steroid Hormones, *R.B. Hochberg and F. Naftolin, editors;* 360 pp., 1991.
Vol. 73: Major Advances in Human Female Reproduction, *E.Y. Adashi and S. Mancuso, editors;* 410 pp., 1990.
Vol. 72: Computers in Endocrinology: Recent Advances, *V. Guardabasso, D. Rodbard and G. Forti, editors;* 207 pp., 1990.
Vol. 71: Reproduction, Growth and Development, *A. Negro-Vilar and G. Perez-Palacios, editors;* 439 pp., 1991.
Vol. 70: Hormonal Communicating Events in the Testis, *A. Isidori, A. Fabbri and M.L. Dufau, editors;* 296 pp., 1990.
Vol. 69: Diabetic Complications: Epidemiology and Pathogenetic Mechanisms, *D. Andreani, J.L. Gueriguian and G.E. Striker, editors;* 361 pp., 1991.
Vol. 68: Cytokines: Basic Principles and Clinical Applications, *S. Romagnani and A.K. Abbas, editors;* 370 pp., 1990.
Vol. 67: Developmental Endocrinology, *P.C. Sizonenko and M.L. Aubert, editors;* 252 pp., 1990.
Vol. 66: Establishing a Successful Human Pregnancy, *R.G. Edwards, editor;* 281 pp., 1990.
Vol. 65: Structure-Function Relationship of Gonadotropins, *D. Bellet and J.-M. Bidart, editors;* 328 pp., 1989.
Vol. 64: Membrane Technology, *R. Verna, editor;* 155 pp., 1989.
Vol. 63: GIFT: From Basics to Clinics, *G.L. Capitanio, R.H. Asch, L. De Cecco and S. Croce, editors;* 454 pp., 1989.
Vol. 62: Unexplained Infertility, *G. Spera and L. Gnessi, editors;* 304 pp., 1989.
Vol. 61: Microbiological, Chemotherapeutical and Immunological Problems in High Risk Patients, *E. Garaci, G. Renzini, F. Filadoro, A. Goldstein and J. Verhoef, editors;* 310 pp., 1989.

Vol. 60: General Surgery: Current Status and Future Trends, *T.E. Starzl and W. Montorsi, editors;* 473 pp., 1989.
Vol. 59: Pathogenesis and Control of Viral Infections, *F. Aiuti, editor;* 328 pp., 1989.
Vol. 58: Hormonal Regulation of Growth, *H. Frisch and M.O. Thorner, editors;* 307 pp., 1989.
Vol. 57: The Adrenal and Hypertension: From Cloning to Clinic, *F. Mantero, R. Takeda, B.A. Scoggins, E.G. Biglieri and J.W. Funder, editors;* 480 pp., 1989.
Vol. 56: Growth Abnormalities, *J.R. Bierich, E. Cacciari and S. Raiti, editors;* 476 pp., 1989.
Vol. 55: Hormones and Sport, *Z. Laron and A. Rogol, editors;* 320 pp., 1989.
Vol. 54: Platelets and Vascular Occlusion, *C. Patrono and G.A. FitzGerald, editors;* 303 pp., 1989.
Vol. 53: Perspectives in Andrology, *M. Serio, editor;* 544 pp., 1989.
Vol. 52: Horizons in Endocrinology, *M. Maggi and C.A. Johnston, editors;* 359 pp., 1988.
Vol. 51: Advances in Biotechnology of Membrane Ion Transport, *P.L. Jørgensen and R. Verna, editors;* 259 pp., 1988.
Vol. 50: The Molecular and Cellular Endocrinology of the Testis, *B.A. Cooke and R.M. Sharpe, editors;* 332 pp., 1988.
Vol. 49: Cell to Cell Communication in Endocrinology, *F. Piva, C.W. Bardin, G. Forti and M. Motta, editors;* 297 pp., 1988.
Vol. 48: Preservation of Tubo-Ovarian Function in Gynecologic Benign and Malignant Diseases, *K. Ichinoe, S.J. Segal and L. Mastroianni, editors;* 680 pp., 1988.
Vol. 47: Andrology and Human Reproduction, *A. Negro-Vilar, A. Isidori, J. Paulson, R. Abdelmassih and M.P.P. de Castro, editors;* 344 pp., 1988.
Vol. 46: Herpes and Papilloma Viruses, vol. II, *G. De Palo, F. Rilke and H. zur Hausen, editors;* 264 pp., 1988.
Vol. 45: The Status of Differentiation Therapy of Cancer, *S. Waxman, G.B. Rossi and F. Takaku, editors;* 422 pp., 1988.
Vol. 44: Fundamentals and Clinics in Pineal Research, *G.P. Trentini, C. De Gaetani and P. Pévet, editors;* 392 pp., 1987.
Vol. 43: Liver and Hormones, *A. Francavilla, C. Panella, A. Di Leo and D.H. Van Thiel, editors;* 356 pp., 1987.
Vol. 42: Inhibin-Non-Steroidal Regulation of Follicle Stimulating Hormone Secretion, *H.G. Burger, D.M. de Kretser, J.K. Findlay and M. Igarashi, editors;* 315 pp., 1987.
Vol. 41: Genotypic, Phenotypic and Functional Aspects of Haematopoiesis, *F. Grignani, M.F. Martelli and D.Y. Mason, editors;* 405 pp., 1987.
Vol. 40: Recent Advances in Adrenal Regulation and Function, *R. D'Agata and G.P. Chrousos, editors;* 311 pp., 1987.
Vol. 39: Corticosteroids and Peptide Hormones in Hypertension, *F. Mantero and P. Vecsei, editors;* 307 pp., 1987.
Vol. 38: Hypoglycemia, *D. Andreani, V. Marks and P.J. Lefebvre, editors;* 312 pp., 1987.
Vol. 37: Advanced Models for the Therapy of Insulin-Dependent Diabetes, *P. Brunetti and W.K. Waldhusl, editors;* 403 pp., 1987.
Vol. 36: Fertility Regulation Today and Tomorrow, *E. Diczfalusy and M. Bygdeman, editors;* 317 pp., 1987.
Vol. 35: The Control of Follicle Development, Ovulation and Luteal Function: Lessons from In Vitro Fertilization, *F. Naftolin and A. DeCherney, editors;* 354 pp., 1987.
Vol. 34: Biological Regulation of Cell Proliferation, *R. Baserga, P. Foa, D. Metcalf and E.E. Polli, editors;* 367 pp., 1986.
Vol. 33: Drugs and Kidney, *T. Bertani, G. Remuzzi and S. Garattini, editors;* 312 pp., 1986.
Vol. 32: Acute Brain Ischemia: Medical and Surgical Therapy, *N. Battistini, P. Fiorani, R. Courbier, F. Plum and C. Fieschi; editors;* 368 pp., 1986.
Vol. 31: Herpes and Papilloma Viruses, *G. De Palo, F. Rilke and H. zur Hausen, editors;* 380 pp., 1986.
Vol. 30: Monoclonal Antibodies: Basic Principles, Experimental and Clinical Applications; *G. Forti, M. Serio and M.B. Lipsett, editors;* 325 pp., 1986.
Vol. 29: Reproductive Medicine, *E. Steinberger, G. Frajese and A. Steinberger, editors;* 504 pp., 1986.
Vol. 28: Recent Advances in Primary and Acquired Immunodeficiencies, *F. Aiuti, F. Rosen and M. Cooper, editors;* 434 pp., 1985.

Vol. 27: The Adrenal Gland and Hypertension, *F. Mantero, E.G. Biglieri, J.W. Funder and B.A. Scoggins, editors;* 465 pp., 1985.
Vol. 26: Monoclonal Antibodies in Haematopathology, *F. Grignani, M.F. Martelli and D.Y. Mason, editors;* 383 pp., 1985.
Vol. 25: Mechanism of Menstrual Bleeding, *D.T. Baird and E.A. Michie, editors;* 266 pp., 1985.
Vol. 24: The Interferon System, *F. Dianzani and G.B. Rossi, editors;* 445 pp., 1985.
Vol. 23: Immunopharmacology, *P.A. Miescher, L. Bolis and M. Ghione, editors;* 247 pp., 1985.
Vol. 22: Thyroid Disorders Associated with Iodine Deficiency and Excess, *R. Hall and J. Köbberling, editors;* 453 pp., 1985.
Vol. 21: The Endocrine Physiology of Pregnancy and the Peripartal Period, *R.B. Jaffe and S. Dell'Acqua, editors;* 278 pp., 1985.
Vol. 20: The Cytobiology of Leukaemias and Lymphomas, *D. Quaglino and F.G.J. Hayhoe, editors;* 500 pp., 1985.
Vol. 19: Peptide Hormones as Mediators in Immunology and Oncology, *R.D. Hesch, editor;* 254 pp., 1985.
Vol. 18: Catecholamines as Hormone Regulators, *N. Ben-Jonathan, J.M. Bahr and R.I. Weiner, editors;* 382 pp., 1985.
Vol. 17: Contributions of Modern Biology to Medicine, *U. Bertazzoni, F.J. Bollum and M. Ghione, editors;* 249 pp., 1985.
Vol. 16: Thymic Factor Therapy, *N.A. Byrom and J.R. Hobbs, editors;* 441 pp., 1984.
Vol. 15: Occlusive Arterial Diseases of the Lower Limbs in Young Patients, *P. Fiorani, G.R. Pistolese and C. Spartera, editors;* 312 pp., 1984.
Vol. 14: Computers in Endocrinology, *D. Rodbard and G. Forti, editors;* 349 pp., 1984.
Vol. 13: Metabolism of Hormonal Steroids in the Neuroendocrine Structures, *F. Celotti, F. Naftolin and L. Martini, editors;* 199 pp., 1984.
Vol. 12: Neuroimmunology, *P.O Behan and F. Spreafico, editors;* 484 pp., 1984.
Vol. 11: Sexual Differentiation: Basic and Clinical Aspects, *M. Serio, M. Motta and L. Martini, editors;* 368 pp., 1984.
Vol. 10: Pituitary Hyperfunction: Physiopathology and Clinical Aspects, *F. Camanni and E.E. Müller, editors;* 430 pp., 1984.
Vol. 9: Hormone Receptors in Growth and Reproduction, *B.B. Saxena, K.J. Catt, L. Birnbaumer and L. Martini, editors;* 337 pp., 1984.
Vol. 8: Recent Advances in Obesity and Diabetes Research, *N. Melchionda, D.L. Horwitz and D.S. Schade, editors;* 414 pp., 1984.
Vol. 7: Recent Advances in Male Reproduction: Molecular Basis and Clinical Implications, *R. D'Agata, M.B. Lipsett and H.J. Van Der Molen, editors;* 330 pp., 1983.
Vol. 6: Artificial Systems for Insulin Delivery, *P. Brunetti, K.G.M.M. Alberti, A.M. Albisser, K.D. Hepp and M. Massi Benedetti, editors;* 605 pp., 1983.
Vol. 5: Functional Radionuclide Imaging of the Brain, *P.L. Magistretti, editor;* 368 pp., 1983.
Vol. 4: Recent Progress in Pediatric Endocrinology, *G. Chiumello and M.A. Sperling, editors;* 369 pp., 1983.
Vol. 3: Progestogens in Therapy, *G. Benagiano, P. Zulli and E. Diczfalusy, editors;* 270 pp., 1983.
Vol. 2: Molecular Biology of Parasites, *J. Guardiola, L. Luzzato and W. Trager, editors;* 210 pp., 1983.
Vol. 1: Luminescent Assays: Perspectives in Endocrinology and Clinical Chemistry, *M. Serio and M. Pazzagli, editors;* 286 pp., 1982.

Serono Symposia Publications from Raven Press
Volume 94

Gonadal Development and Function

Editor

S.G. Hillier

Reproductive Endocrinology Laboratory
University of Edinburgh Centre for Reproductive Biology
37 Chalmers Street, Edinburgh, EH3 9EW, UK

Raven Press ■ New York

Raven Press, 1185 Avenue of the Americas, New York, New York 10036

© 1992 by Raven Press Book, Ltd. All rights reserved. This book is protected by copyright. No part of it may be reproduced, stored in a retrieval system or transmitted, in any form or by any means, electronic, mechanical, photocopying, recording, or otherwise, without the prior written permission of the publisher.

GONADAL DEVELOPMENT AND FUNCTION
(Serono Symposia Publications from Raven Press; v. 94)

International Standard Book Number 0-88167-906-2
Library of Congress Catalog Number 91-051155

Papers or parts thereof have been used as camera-ready copy as submitted by the authors whenever possible; when retyped, they have been edited by the editorial staff only to extent considered necessary for the assistance of an international readership. The views expressed and the general style adopted remain, however, the responsibility of the named authors. Great care has been taken to maintain the accuracy of the information contained in the volume. However, neither Raven Press, Serono Symposia, nor the editors can be held responsible for errors or any consequences arising from the use of information contained herein.

The use in this book of particular designations of countries or territories does not imply any judgment by the publisher or editors as to the legal status of such countries or territories, of their authorities or institutions or of the delimitation of their boundaries.

Some of the names of products referred to in this book may be registered trade marks or proprietary names, although specific references to this fact may not be made; however, the use of a name without designation is not to be construed as a representation by the publisher or editors that it is in the public domain. In addition, the mention of specific companies or of their products or proprietary names does not imply any endorsement or recommendation on the part of the publisher or editors.

Authors were themselves responsible for obtaining the necessary permission to reproduce copyright material from other sources. With respect to the publisher's copyright, material appearing in this book prepared by individuals as part of their official duties as government employees is only covered by this copyright to the extent permitted by the appropriate national regulations.

Printed in Rome, Italy
by Christengraf

Preface

The IXth Workshop on the Development and Function of Reproductive Organs, sponsored by Ares-Serono Symposia, was held in Peebles, Scotland, on May 25-27, 1992. The meeting dealt with recent progress in basic research on gonadal physiology with particular relevance to reproductive medicine. Sessions were held on gonadal differentiation, sperm and oocyte biology, control of testicular and ovarian function, transgenics and reproduction, and assisted reproduction in men and women. This volume collates individual chairpersons' and speakers' contributions, affording a tantalising glimpse of the complex and diverse cellular and molecular processes upon which human reproduction depends. I am indebted to the authors for their timely provision of manuscripts. Special thanks are also due to Roberta Cenci, Carla Brown and Patricia Rossi in the editorial office of Ares-Serono, Rome, and Carol Irvine of the Reproductive Endocrinology Laboratory in Edinburgh for essential help in compiling these proceedings.

S.G. HILLIER

Contents

VII Preface

1 Gonadal Differentiation
  A. McLaren

5 Sex Determination, Sex-Reversal and *SRY:* A Review
  P.N. Goodfellow, G. Berkovitz, J.R. Hawkins, V.R. Harley and
  R. Lovell-Badge

17 Cellular Basis of Sex Determination and Sex Reversal in Mammals
  P.S. Burgoyne and S.J. Palmer

31 Hormonal Control of Gonadal Differentiation
  N. Josso, B.Vigier, R.L. Cate, R. Behringer, N. di Clemente and L. Lyet

41 Sperm Biology: An Overview
  S. Fishel

49 Control of Sperm Development by Hormones and Growth Factors:
  Testicular expression of Receptor-Encoding Genes
  J.A. Grootegoed, W.M. Baarends, L.J. Blok, J.P. de Winter, M.van
  Helmond, J.W. Hoogerbrugge, F.H. de Jong and A.P.N. Themmen

63 Epididymal Control of Sperm Maturation in Mammals
  H.D.M. Moore

73 Cell Biology of the Oocyte
  R.J. Aitken

75 Molecular Basis of Sperm-Egg Interaction
  R.J. Aitken

85 Cyclin and p34^{cdc2} Kinase Activity in Pig Oocytes During the G2- to
  M-Phase Transition
  R. Moor, T. Jung, T. Miyano and P. Barker

99 Protein Tyrosine Phosphorylation/Dephosphorylation and Control of Meiosis in Rat Oocytes
   N. Dekel and S. Goren

107 Development-Related Gene expression in Oocytes
   J.J. Eppig

119 Vascular Control of Testicular Function
   A.R.J. Bergh

127 Intratesticular Androgen Action
   R.M. Sharpe

139 Nonsteroidal Regulation of Testicular Function
   M.K. Skinner

145 Paracrine Control of Ovarian Endocrine Function
   C.D. Smyth, P.F. Whitelaw, I.M. Turner, C.M. Howles and S.G. Hillier

149 Granulosa Cell Gene Regulation
   J.S. Richards, J.W. Clemens, S.L. Fitzpatrick and J. Sirois

157 Apoptosis as the Basis of Ovarian Follicular Atresia
   J.L. Tilly and A.J.W. Hsueh

167 The Regulation of Ovarian Proteolysis and its Role in Follicular Rupture
   A. Tsafriri, S.-Y. Chun and R. Reich

179 Luteinization and Luteolysis
   A.J. Zeleznik

189 Transgenic Manipulation of Reproduction
   D.W. Lincoln

195 Transgenesis and Infertility
   R. Al-Shawi, J. Burke, J.O. Bishop, J.J. Mullins, R.M. Sharpe, R. Lathe and L. Mullins

207 Targeting the Expression of Gonadotrophin Genes
   A.J. Clark, P. Brown, J. R. McNeilly, J. Mullins and A.S. McNeilly

217 Dominant Negative Mutants of the Activin A Gene
   A.J. Mason

225 Assisted Reproduction in Women
   D.T. Baird

227 Superovulation Strategy
    S. Franks and E.J. Owen

237 Transplantation of Follicle and Germ Cells
    R.G. Gosden and A.A. Murray

251 Management of Male Infertility
    F.C.W. Wu

257 Treatment of Male Infertility
    E. Nieschlag, H.M. Behre, C. Keck and S. Kliesch

273 Assisted Reproductive Technology in the Treatment of Male Infertility
    P.R. Brinsden and S. Avery

293 Subzonal Insemination
    S. Fishel and J. Timson

309 Subject Index

Contributors

R.J. Aitken
MRC Reproductive Biology Unit
University of Edinburgh Centre for
Reproductive Biology
37 Chalmers Street
Edinburgh EH3 9EW
UK

D.T. Baird
Department of Obstetrics &
Gynaecology
University of Edinburgh Centre for
Reproductive Biology
37 Chalmers Street
Edinburgh EH3 9EW
UK

A.R. J. Bergh
Department of Pathology
University of Umea
S901 87 UMEA
Sweden

P.R. Brinsden
Bourn Hall Clinic
Bourn
Cambridge CB3 7TR
UK

P.S. Burgoyne
MRC Mammalian Development Unit
Wolfson House
4 Stephenson Way
London NW1 2HE
UK

A. J. Clark
AFRC Institute of Animal Physiology
& Genetics Research
Roslin
Midlothian EH25 9PS
UK

N. Dekel
Department of Hormone Research
The Weizmann Institute of Science
PO Box 26
Rehovot 76100, Israel

J.J. Eppig
The Jackson Laboratory
Bar Harbor
Maine ME 04609
USA

S. Franks
Department of Obstetrics &
Gynaecology
St Mary's Hospital Medical School
London
W2 1 PG, UK

S.B. Fishel
Nottingham University Research and
Treatment Unit in Reproduction
(NURTURE)
Department of Obstetrics and
Gynaecology
Floor 'B', East Block
University Hospital
Queen's Medical Centre
Nottingham NG7 2UH, UK

P.N. Goodfellow
Laboratory of Human Molecular
Genetics
Imperial Cancer Research Fund
Lincoln's Inn Fields
London WC2A 3PX, UK

R.G. Gosden
Department of Physiology
University of Edinburgh Medical
School
Teviot Place
Edinburgh EH8 9AG, UK

J. A. Grootegoed
Department of Endocrinology &
Reproduction
Medical Faculty
Erasmus University Rotterdam
PO Box 1738
3000 DR Rotterdam
The Netherlands

S.G. Hillier
Reproductive Endocrinology
Laboratory
University of Edinburgh Centre for
Reproductive Biology
37 Chalmers Street
Edinburgh
EH3 9EW
UK

A.J. W. Hsueh
Department of Gynecology &
Obstetrics
Division of Reproductive Biology
Stanford University School of Medicine
Stanford, CA 94305-5317
USA

N. Josso
Unité de Recherches sur
l'Endocrinologie du Développement
Ecole Normale Supérieure
1 rue Maurice-Arnoux
92120 Montrouge
France

R. Lathe
AFRC Centre for Genome Research
University of Edinburgh
King's Buildings
Mayfield Road
Edinburgh EH9 3JQ
UK

D.W. Lincoln
MRC Reproductive Biology Unit
University of Edinburgh Centre for
Reproductive Biology
37 Chalmers Street
Edinburgh EH3 9EW
UK

A.J. Mason
Genentech Inc
460 Pt San Bruno Blvd
South San Francisco
CA 94080
USA

A. McLaren
MRC Mammalian Development Unit
Wolfson House
4 Stephenson Way
London NW1 2HE
UK

R. Moor
AFRC Insitute of Animal Physiology &
Genetics Research
Department of Molecular
Endocrinology
Babraham
Cambridge CB2 4AT
UK

H.D.M. Moore
Institute of Zoology
Regents Park
London NW1 4RY
UK

E. Nieschlag
Institute of Reproductive Medicine of
the University
University of Münster
Steinfurter Str 107
D-4400 Münster
Germany

J.S. Richards
Department of Cell Biology
Baylor College of Medicine
One Baylor Plaza
Houston, TX 77030
USA

R.M. Sharpe
MRC Reproductive Biology Unit
University of Edinburgh Centre for
Reproductive Biology
37 Chalmers Street
Edinburgh EH3 9EW
UK

M.K. Skinner
Reproductive Endocrinology Center
University of California
San Fransisco
CA 94143-0556
USA

A. Tsafriri
Department of Hormone Research
The Bernard Zondek Hormone
Research Laboratory
The Weizmann Institute of Science
Rehovot 76100
Israel

F.C.W. Wu
Department of Medicine
University of Manchester Medical
School
Hope Hospital
Salford
Greater Manchester, UK

A.J. Zeleznik
Department of Physiology
University of Pittsburgh School of
Medicine
Pittsburgh, PA 15261
USA

Gonadal Differentiation

A. McLaren

MRC Mammalian Development Unit, Wolfson House 4 Stephenson Way London NW1 2HE, UK

INTRODUCTION

In introducing this session on gonadal differentiation, I aim to define certain terms that are likely to be used, and to provide a time frame for the events that we shall be discussing.

The adult gonad, whether male or female, is a complicated organ. The fetal gonad is less complicated than the adult, but quite complicated enough. It contains supporting cells, which differentiate in the testis as Sertoli cells, and in the ovary as granulosa or follicle cells. There is a widespread assumption that both these cell types differentiate from the same cell lineage: I think that we shall be making this assumption today unless someone produces evidence to the contrary. Then there is the interstitial (sometimes called the steroidogenic) cell lineage, which again we assume to give rise to Leydig cells in the testis, theca cells in the ovary. A further postulate that we may perhaps make in considering gonadal differentiation, is that the differentiation of Leydig cells in the fetal testis is somehow dependent on the prior differentiation of Sertoli cells. This is the view which was originally put forward by the late Alfred Jost, and which is strongly supported today by Paul Burgoyne (see page 17).

The fetal gonad of course also contains germ cells, that develop into T-prospermatogonia in the fetal testis, oocytes in the ovary; but these probably play little part in the prenatal development of the gonad, since the virtual absence of germ cells from the gonad in certain mouse mutants seems to have little effect on its early differentiation. More important from the point of view of early gonadal architecture are probably the peritubular myoid cells that surround the testis cords, and of course the blood cells and blood vessels, whose pattern is rather different in the two sexes.

In mice most of the events that concern us today take place within a time span of less than a week. Let us use the convention that say that midday on the day the copulation plug is found is 0.5 days post coitum (pc). In the strain of mice that Paul Burgoyne and Robin Lovell-Badge and their colleagues have used, at $9^1/_2$ days pc there is a mesonephros, but no trace yet of the genital ridge that will develop into the gonad. At $10^1/_2$ days pc there is a thin layer of mesenchymal cells between the mesonephros and the coelomic epithelium, and the primordial germ cells are just beginning to colonize it. At $11^1/_2$ day pc the layer is thicker and the cells are actively proliferating, though they still appear to be undifferentiated, but one day later in the testis, Sertoli cells have differentiated and aggregated together to form testis cords.

At the molecular level, we know that *Sry* (the gene in the sex-determining region of the mouse Y chromosome) is expressed at $10^1/_2$ and $11^1/_2$ days pc, less strongly at $10^1/_2$ days, and not at all during the rest of fetal life. *Amh*, the gene coding for anti-Müllerian hormone, which is sometimes referred to as Müllerian inhibiting substance, starts to be transcribed at $12^1/_2$ days pc, the protein can be detected at $13^1/_2$ days pc and expression continues in the testis till shortly after birth. Testosterone production starts in the testis at about $14^1/_2$ days pc, and continues throughout life.

So which cell population produces which substance? Testosterone is of

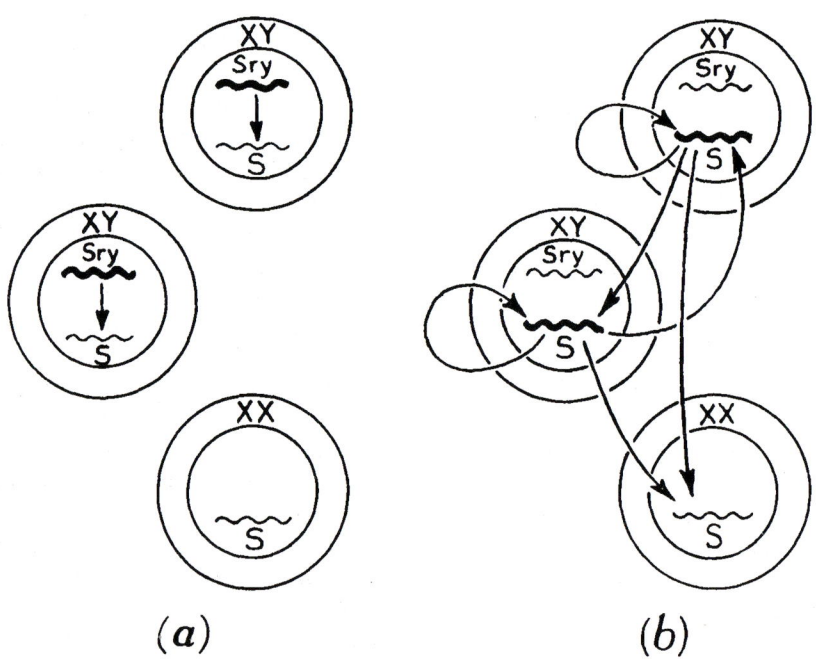

FIG. 1. Molecular control of Sertoli cell differentiation. a) In XY supporting cells, *Sry* switches on S, a cascade or array of non-Y-chromosomal genes that induce Sertoli cell differentiation. b) *Sry* is no longer expressed, but gene products of S continue to act in an autocrine and paracrine manner to maintain the Sertoli cell state.

course produced by Leydig cells, and anti-Müllerian hormone is known to be produced by Sertoli cells. *Sry* is thought to be expressed in the supporting cell lineage. The evidence for this is indirect rather than direct. In mouse aggregation chimeras that contain a mix of XY and XX cells, the Sertoli cells are the only cell lineage in the gonad - indeed, the only cell lineage inthe whole body - that is made up predominantly and disproportionately of XY cells. This is what one would expect if *Sry*, on the Y chromosome, is expressed in the XY cells of the supporting cell lineage, and is responsible for their decision to develop as Sertoli cells rather than as granulosa cells. There must be at least one extra link in the chain (Fig. 1): *Sry* is thought to code for a transcription factor, and that transcription factor must switch on, by directly activating or by inhibiting an inhibitor, a gene or genes whose products induce Sertoli cell differentiation. These genes are probably located on autosomes, or perhaps on the X chromosome. Since a few XX cells are found within the Sertoli cell population in XX/XY chimeras, the inducing factor presumably acts on adjacent cells in a short-range paracrine manner, whether or not they contain a Y chromosome. Indeed, in later development XX granulosa cells may transdifferentiate into Sertoli cells, suggesting that the autosomal inducing factor gene can in certain circumstances be switched on by factors other than the *Sry* transcription factor. Since *Sry* is expressed for a short period only, autoregulation may be required to maintain the differentiated state of Sertoli cells, involving both autocrine and paracrine action.

As well as this brief attempt to provide an orientation in space and time, it is my task to give an introduction to the three papers in this session. Peter Goodfellow's paper (page 5) is concerned with the structure and function of the *Sry/SRY* gene in mouse and man, and pursues the sex determination pathway both upstream and downstream. He describes the exciting new studies that he and his colleauges are carrying out on the DNA binding properties of the *Sry* gene product. He may also discuss the possible involvement of a gene on the short arm of the X chromosome, which when duplicated gives rise to XY women.

It seems likely that this operates downstream of *Sry*, inhibiting in single dose the development of the gonad into a testis. Paul Burgoyne's paper (page 17) discusses in greater depth the factors affecting Sertoli cell determination, and hence the development of a testis rather than an ovary. He stresses the importance of the timing of *Sry* expression, which implies the existence of regulatory factors acting upstream of *Sry*. Finally, Nathalie Josso (page 31) takes us still further downstream of *Sry*, into the realms of *Amh* expression and aromatase inhibitors. This leads on to the control of sex hormone production, which we recognize as one of the two main functions of our gonads. In the testis, the synthesis of testosterone rather than oestrogen is responsible in the male for all the secondary sexual characters associated with maleness.

Sex Determination, Sex-Reversal and *SRY*: A Review

P.N. Goodfellow[1], G. Berkovitz[2], J.R. Hawkins[1], V.R. Harley[1] and R. Lovell-Badge[3]

[1]*Imperial Cancer Research Fund, Lincoln's Inn Fields, London WC2A 3PX, UK*
[2]*Department of Medicine, The Johns Hopkins University School of Medicine, Baltimore, MD 2105, USA*
[3]*National Institute for Medical Research, The Ridgeway, Mill Hill, London NW7 1AA, UK*

ABSTRACT

In mammals, the Y chromosome is a dominant inducer of testis development. By analysis of Y chromosome fragments in the genomes of XX males, it was possible to define a 35 kb minimum sex determining region. The gene *SRY* (sex determining region Y gene, the equivalent mouse gene is *Sry*) is located within this region. De novo mutations in *SRY* are found in about 10% of XY females with gonadal dysgenesis and XX mice transgenic for *Sry* are sex reversed males. Taken together these results demonstrate the essential role played by *SRY* in mammalian sex determination. In this review, we consider the genetic basis of sex reversal in humans and the contribution of *SRY* to this phenomenon. This review has been published in largely the same form in another volume in the Ares Serono Symposia series, under the title: Sex determination, sex reversal and *SRY*.

INTRODUCTION

Sex determination is the process that controls the phenotypic sex of an individual (19,20). In the mammalian embryo, sex is fixed by the antithetical differentiation of either testes or ovaries from undifferentiated genital ridges (32). If testes are formed, subsequent hormonal production induces male sexual differentiation; in the absence of testes female development ensues. Mammalian sex determination is chromosomally based: females have two X chromosomes and males have an X and a Y chromosome. Individuals with a single X chromosome and no Y chromosome are female (17); independent of the number of X chromosomes present, inheritance of a Y chromosome results in male development (27). These observations imply that the Y chromosome is a dominant inducer of testicular development. The responsible Y-located gene(s) has been named the *testis determining factor* in humans (*TDF*); the same gene in mouse is called the *testis determining Y gene* (*Tdy*). Among both humans and mice, there are rare individuals who violate the rule that links the presence of the Y chromosome with testis determination: these exceptions encompass both males without a Y chromosome and females with a Y chromosome. XX males and XY females are described as 'sex-reversed'. Individuals with endocrine defects may present with ambiguous genitalia or inappropriate genitalia for their genotypes; these patients have defects in sexual differentiation and are not 'sex-reversed'.

Molecular analysis of the genomes of sex-reversed patients has been central to unravelling the genetics of sex determination in mammals. The study of Y-sequence positive XX males allowed the construction of maps of the Y chromosome (2,40,59) and these maps defined the minimum region required for male sex determination (46,48). Within the sex determining region is located the gene *SRY* (*sex determining region Y gene*) (53). Several lines of circumstantial evidence suggested that *SRY* is equivalent to *TDF*:

Homologues of *SRY* are present on the Y chromosomes of all eutherian mammals tested (53).

Sry, the mouse homologue of *SRY*, maps to the smallest interval of the mouse Y chromosome that is sex determining (22).

In the mouse embryo, *Sry* expression has been detected only in the somatic tissue of the genital ridge, immediately prior to overt morphological differentiation of the gonads. The precise temporal and tissue specificity implies that several genes are required to regulate *Sry* expression (33).

The conceptual translation of *SRY* indicates the presence of an HMG-box (53), a protein motif associated with DNA binding activity (31). This is consistent with *SRY* encoding a transcription factor that regulates the expression of other genes.

Direct evidence that *SRY/Sry* can be equated with *TDF/Tdy* was obtained from sex-reversed patients (5,28) and by the construction of transgenic mice (34). In about 15 percent of XY females, *de novo* mutations in *SRY* have been found (see below). A 14 kb fragment of the mouse Y chromosome, which includes *Sry*, causes female to male sex reversal in transgenic XX mice (34). We conclude that *SRY* is *TDF* and *Sry* is *Tdy*.

It is a common theme in genetics that unusual phenotypes can be used to identify genes and probes for cloned genes can be used to study unusual phenotypes. In this review we consider the role of *SRY* in patients with sex reversal. More detailed information about the identification, cloning and biology of *SRY/Sry* can be found in several recent reviews (20,21).

XX males:
X-Y interchange XX males.
XX males are similar in phenotype to individuals with Klinefelter syndrome, which is caused by the sex chromosome aneuploidy XXY. Although both sets of patients have testes, these are small and spermatozoa are not produced. The spermatogenic block is caused by the presence of two X chromosomes; the molecular basis for this block is not understood but it has been correlated with failure to inactivate two X chromosomes during spermatogenesis. The small testes can cause endocrine problems due to androgen insufficiency; the problems may be manifest as absence of facial and body hair, reduced libido and gynaecomastia. Klinefelter patients tend to be tall and often suffer from some degree of mental impairment. XX males are usually of normal height and not mentally impaired.

In 1966, Ferguson-Smith proposed that interchange between the X and Y chromosomes might explain the generation of XX males (13). This prescient hypothesis was supported by high resolution karyotypic analysis of patients with an altered appearance of one X chromosome (11,36,37) and was proven when genomic DNA from XX males was hybridised with probes derived from the Y chromosome (23). About 85 percent of XX males have inherited Y-derived sequences and, where tested, these sequences have been found on the paternally-derived X chromosome (3,7). The Y chromosome is composed of two parts. One part, the pseudoautosomal region (PAR), is shared with the X chromosome (8,52) and is thought to be required for sex chromosome pairing and segregation in male meiosis (10,18); the second part is Y-specific and encodes *TDF*. The PAR is terminal on the short arms of the X and Y chromosomes (49,55); *TDF* is present on the short arm of the Y chromosome. In every male meiotic event, a single homologous recombination occurs in the shared region (51). XX males are cause by 'slippage' of the recombination event from the PAR into the sex chromosome specific region resulting in the transfer of *TDF* on to the X chromosome. Theoretically, the breakpoint on the Y chromosome could be anywhere between the position of *TDF* and the Y chromosome centromere. Consistent with this suggestion, different XX males have inherited different fragments of the Y chromosome short arm (2,40,59). By testing the genomes of XX males with multiple probes, deletion maps of the Y chromosome were constructed. A feature of these maps was the distal location of *TDF* (46).

SRY is located immediately adjacent to the boundary of the PAR (47,48,53). Most XX males have inherited *SRY* and a large fragment of the Y chromosome that includes the genes *RPS4Y* and *ZFY* (16,46). A possible contribution to male development from Y-located genes other than *SRY* is considered below.

A minority of XX males have no detectable Y sequences (15,48,50). These males must have inherited 'gain of function' mutations in genes that respond to the presence of *SRY*. The mutated genes may be autosomal or X-linked. The phenotype of XX males without Y sequences overlaps with the Y sequence positive XX males but is more frequently associated with hypospadias and cryptorchidism (1).

XX true hermaphrodites:

True hermaphrodites have both ovarian and testicular material. The most common finding is a testis on one side and an ovary or ovo-testis on the other, however, bilateral ovo-testes and other combinations are also found. The phenotype depends crucially on the amount of testicular material as this affects the level of AMH (anti-Müllerian hormone) and testosterone. In nearly all cases, true hermaphrodites have ambiguous genitalia, often with perineal hypospadias and a vaginal pouch.

Testing for Y-derived sequences has defined three classes of XX true hermaphrodites. Most individuals are Y-sequence negative and have not inherited the Y chromosome pseudoautosomal boundary (4,14,48). By definition, the testicular differentiation in these patients cannot be due to Y-sequences and it is assumed that they have mutations in genes that normally respond to the presence of *SRY*. It seems likely that mutations in genes that can cause testicular development may result in either XX males or XX true hermaphrodites, depending on the gene affected, the specific mutation and interaction with other genes. In support of this hypothesis, rare families with inherited sex reversal, XX males and XX true hermaphrodites can be found in the same kinship (54).

The second class of XX true hermaphrodites have inherited the Y-pseudoautosomal boundary and *SRY* but have not inherited *ZFY*. Two sporadic and one familial case have been reported (29,48). In the familial case, a pair of XX sibs have both inherited 35 kb of Y-derived sequence including *SRY*. One sib is an XX male with cryptorchidism and the other is a true hermaphrodite with bilateral ovotestes. The variability in phenotype, associated with the same Y fragment, emphasises the phenotypic continuum between XX males and XX hermaphrodites. The different phenotypes could be due to:

1. Segregation of a polymorphic gene that interacts with *SRY*.

2. Inherent variability in *SRY* expression due to the absence of other genes on the Y chromosome needed for correct *SRY* expression. Candidate genes would include *ZFY* and *RPS4Y* (16). It is difficult to test this hypothesis, however, it is not consistent with the results from the construction of transgenic sex-reversed XX mice (34).

3. A position effect: either the translocation from the X to the Y chromosome has disrupted sequences required for correct expression of *SRY* or the X-located sequences are now susceptible to X-inactivation. A plausible model would be the sex reversal seen in mice associated with forced X-inactivation of *Sxr* (39).

Recently, a third class of XX true hermaphrodites has been described. A patient was found with ambiguous genitalia, bilateral ovotestes and a cytologically visible deletion of the short arm of the X chromosome. This patient had inherited a large fragment of the Y chromosome short arm, including *SRY*, *RPS4Y* and *ZFY* (4). It is likely that the deleted X chromosome is preferentially inactivated and that X-inactivation spreads into the Y chromosome fragment.

XY females:
The nomenclature describing sex-reversed individuals with an XY karyotype is confusing. In this review we will use the term 'XY female' to describe individuals with an XY karyotype and no testes. Failures in the responses of the soma to the presence of testes also occur, for example, androgen insensitivity. These 'XY females' have testes and will not be considered here.

XY females are caused by mutations in the sex determination pathway and by mutations that disrupt early stages of testis differentiation. Ovarian development would be the expected consequence of failure of male sex determination, however, XY females have dysgenic 'streak' ovaries - similar to those found in Turner Syndrome (XO females) (12). A distinction can be made between patients with 'pure gonadal dysgenesis' (also known as 'complete gonadal dysgenesis') and patients with 'mixed gonadal dysgenesis' (also known as 'partial gonadal dysgenesis'). The former patients have streak gonads identical to those in Turner Syndrome; the latter group have testicular elements, usually including small clusters of Sertoli cells, present in the gonads. Careful histological investigation of gonadal biopsies is needed to distinguish these two phenotypes.

Terminal deletions of the short arm of the Y chromosome, caused by X-Y interchange (35), are associated with deletion of *SRY* and sex reversal (6,9,41). These patients have many of the features of Turner Syndrome, including the streak gonads and mild dysmorphologies, although stature is usually within the normal range. It has been suggested that these results map the stature 'genes' to the proximal part of the Y chromosome short arm (15). An alternative hypothesis is that the stature gene is pseudoautosomal (43).

Page and colleagues have described an XY female with a complex rearrangement of the Y chromosome, which has deleted *SRY* and *ZFY* but not *RPS4Y* (47). This patient is free from the dysmorphologies associated with Turner syndrome and suggests that either *RSP4Y* is the Y-located 'anti-Turner' gene or that this gene maps proximally to *ZFY*.

Mutations in *SRY* can cause the sex-reversal found in XY females. Two groups used PCR to amplify part of the *SRY* gene from XY females. Berta and colleagues (5) screened 11 XY females by 'single strand conformation polymorphism analysis' (SSCP) (45) and found two variants, which were not present in 50 normal controls. The variants were sequenced: in one case,

AA, the sequence change causes a methionine to isoleucine alteration and in the other case, JN, a valine to leucine alteration. In both cases, the change has occured in the HMG-box region of the gene. The *SRY* gene from the fathers of the XY females were also sequenced. The mutation in AA is not present in her father and this *de novo* mutation provides compelling evidence that *SRY* is required for sex determination. A similar conclusion was reached by Jager *et al.* (28) who screened 12 XY females and found one *de novo* mutation. The second variant described by Berta and colleagues is present in the patient's father. The familial variants will be discussed below.

Subsequent studies have confirmed and extended the original observations (25,26,30,38). A total of 10 *SRY* mutations have been reported, all of which are within the region of the gene that encodes the HMG-box (however, in some studies only the 'HMG-box' region has been tested). Six of the mutations are *de novo*, three are familial and one has not been tested (Table 1). All of the mutations have been ascertained in patients with pure gonadal dysgenesis. Combining all the data, between 10 and 20 percent of XY females have changes in the *SRY* sequence. Not all of the patients tested have been subjected to gonadal biopsy and the precise diagnosis in some cases may be in doubt. In a recent series of patients who had been histologically diagnosed as suffering from pure gonadal dysgenesis, three out of five had mutations in *SRY* (26). XY females, without mutations in the *SRY* coding sequence, may have lesions in the undefined regulatory sequences of *SRY* or in genes elsewhere in the sex determining pathway.

Several proteins containing a single 'HMG-box' have been shown to bind to DNA with sequence specificity (44,58,60). In all the published cases, the core sequence recognised is related to the heptamer AACAAAG (Table 2). Recombinant SRY protein, made in *E. coli* also binds to this DNA sequence and some related variants (24). The protein corresponding to the sequence variants found in the XY females has also been tested for DNA binding. In all the cases tested, detectable DNA binding was abolished or greatly reduced. This implies that sequence specific DNA binding is required for sex determination and is consistent with *SRY* exerting its function by controlling the transcription of other genes. In the two familial cases tested, one displayed reduced DNA binding and one negligible binding. The reduced binding provides a simple explanation for the partial penetrance of the mutation. The negligible binding found in the second familial case implies that the *in vitro* conditions of assay are more stringent than the *in vivo* conditions. Possibilities include the existence of other proteins that modify the DNA-binding properties of SRY protein or an alternative DNA target sequence with higher affinity than the test sequence.

Table 1. List of SRY mutations in XY females. The mutations and protein changes are listed as well as the region screened to identify the mutations. Amino acid numbers are based upon the assumtion that the SRY initiator methionine is encoded by the codon at bases 411-413 of the pY53.3 SRY DNA sequence (53). D = deletion; FS = frameshift; * = termination codon. All mutations lie in the DNA-binding HMG-box of SRY, which lies between amino acids 58 and 137. Region screened indicates the region of the gene analysed for mutations; the numbers refer to codon/amino acid numbers. DNA-binding activity is indicated as '-' for drastically reduced or '+/-' for moderately reduced when compared with wild-type SRY (24). N/D indicates not determined.

Reference	Codon change	Amino acid number	Amino acid change	Region screened	DNA-binding (See ref. 23)	Inheritence
5	ATG→ATA	64	M→I	7-189	-	de novo
5	GTG→CTG	60	V→L	7-189	-	familial
27	CCA/TTC (ΔΔTTC)	122	FS	58-137	-	de novo
29	TTC→TCC	109	F→S	58-137	N/D	familial
37	CAG→TAG	93	Q→*	63-185	N/D	de novo
24	GGA→CGA	95	G→R	0-203 (+117bp 5')	-	de novo
24	TGG→TAG	70	W→*	0-203 (+117bp 5')	N/D	de novo
25	AAA→ATA	106	K→I	0-203 (+117bp 5')	-	N/D
25	CCA (ΔA)	109	FS	0-203 (+117bp 5')	N/D	de novo
25	ATC→ATG	90	I→M	0-203 (+117bp 5')	+/-	familial

Table 2. *HMG box proteins with known DNA sequence specificities*

Protein	Target DNA sequence	Reference
Ste11	**AACAAAGAA** "TR boxes" of *matP, matM* and *mei2*	56
TCF-1	**AACAAAG** enhancer of *CD3ε*	58
TCF-1a (or LEF-1)	**CAAAG^G_A** enhancers of *TCR-α, -β, -δ*	57,60
IRE-ABP	**TTCAAAGG** insulin responsive element of *GAPDH*	42
SRY	**AA$_{CT}$CAAA^G_T**	22,42

CONCLUSIONS

The molecular investigation of the genomes of XX males led directly to the identification and cloning of *SRY*. The discovery of *de novo* mutations of *SRY* in XY females proved that *SRY* is required for normal male sex determination. In a reciprocal relationship, knowledge of the structure and biology of *SRY* is revealing the aetiology of XX and XY sex reversal. Identification of those patients that are sex reversed due to causes not related to *SRY* will provide the key to the identification and isolation of other genes in the sex determination pathway.

ACKNOWLEDGEMENTS

We thank all our colleagues past and present at ICRF, NIMR and Johns Hopkins who have contributed to this work over the years.

REFERENCES

1. Abbas, N.E., Toublanc, J.E., Boucekkine, C., Toublanc, M., Affara, N.A., Job, J.C. and Fellous, M. (1989) A possible common origin of "Y" negative human XX males and XX true hermaphrodites. Hum. Genet., 84: 356-360.
2. Affara, N.A., Ferguson-Smith, M.A., Tolmie, J., Kwok, K., Mitchell, M., Jamieson, D., Cooke, A. and Florentin, L. (1986) Variable transfer of Y specific sequences in XX males. Nucl. Acids Res., 14:5375-5387.
3. Andersson, M.M., Page, D.C., and de la Chapelle, A., (1986) Chromosome Y-specific DNA is transferred to the short arm of the X chromosome in human XX males. Science, 233:786-788.
4. Berkovitz, G.D., Fechner, P.Y., Marcantonio, S.M., Bland, G., Stetten, G., Goodfellow,

PN., Smith, K.D. and Midgeon, CJ. (1992) The role of the sex determining region of the Y chromosome (SRY) in the etiology of 46, XX true hermaphroditism. Hum. Genet., 88: 411-416.
5. Berta, P., Hawkins, J.R., Sinclair, A.H., Taylor, A., Griffiths, B.L., Goodfellow, P.N. and Fellous, M. (1990) Genetic evidence equating SRY and the testis determining factor. Nature, 348:448-450.
6. Blagowidow, N., Page, D.C., Huff, D. and Mennuti, M.T. (1989) Ullrich-Turner syndrome in an XY female fetus with deletion of the sex-determining portion of the Y chromosome. Am. J. Med. Genet., 24:159-162.
7. Buckle, V.J., Boyd, Y., Fraser, N., Goodellow, P.N., Goodfellow, P.J., Wolfe, J. and Craig, I.W. (1987) Localisation of Y chromosome sequences in normal and "XX" males. J. Med. Genet., 24:197-203, 1987.
8. Cooke, H.J., Brown, W.R.A. and Rappold, G. (1985) Hypervariable telomeric sequences from the human sex chromosomes are pseudoautosomal. Nature, 317: 688-692.
9. Disteche, C.M., Casanova, M., Saal, H., Freidman, C., Sybert, V., Graham, J., Thuline, H., Page, D.C. and Fellous, M. (1986) Small deletions of the short arm of the Y chromosome in 46, XY females. Proc. Natl. Acad. Sci. USA, 83:7841-7844.
10. Ellis, N.A. and Goodfellow, P.N. (1989) The mammalian pseudoautosomal region. TIGS, 5: 406-410.
11. Evans, H.J., Buckton, K.E., Spowart, G. and Carruthers, D. (1979) Heteromorphic X chromosomes in 46 XX males: evidence for the involvement of X-Y interchange. Hum. Genet, 49:11-31.
12. Ferguson-Smith, M.A. (1965) Karyotype-phenotype correlations in gondal desgenesis and their bearing on the pathogenesis of malformations. J. Med. Genet. 2:142-155.
13. Ferguson-Smith, M.A. (1966) X-Y chromosome interchange in the aetiology of true hermaphroditism and of XX Klinefelter's syndrome. Lancet, ii: 475-476.
14. Ferguson-Smith, M.A., North, M.A., Affara, N.A. and Briggs, H. (1990) The secret of sex. Lancet, 336:809-810.
15. Ferguson-Smith, M.A. (1991) Genotype-phenotype correlations in individuals with disorders of sex determination and development including Turner's syndrome. Seminars Dev. Biol., 2:265-276.
16. Fisher, E.M.C., Beer-Romero, P., Brown, L.G., Ridley, A., McNeil, J.A., Lawrence, J.B., Willard, H.F., Bieber, F.R. and Page, D.C. (1990) Homologous ribosomal protein genes on the human X and Y chromosomes: escape from X-inactivation and possible implictions for Turner syndrome. Cell, 63:1091-1104.
17. Ford, C.E., Miller, O.J., Polani, P.E., de Almeida, J.C. and Briggs, J.H., (1959) A sex-chromosome anomaly in a case of gonadal dysgenesis. Lancet, i: 711.
18 Gabriel-Ropez, O., Rumpler, Y., Ratomponirina, C., Petit, C., Levilliers, J., Croquette, MF. and Couturier, J. (1990) Deletion of the pseudoautosomal region and lack of sex-chromosome pairing at pachytene in two infertile men carrying an X;Y translocation. Cytogenet. Cell Genet., 54:38-42.
19. Goodfellow, P.N. and Darling, S.M., (1988) Genetics of sex determination in man and mouse. Development, 102: 251-258.
20. Goodfellow, P.N. and Lovell-Badge, R. (Eds). (1991) Sex determination and the Y chromosome. Semin. Dev. Biol. 2: 1-291.
21. Goodfellow, P.N., Hawkins, J.R. and Sinclair, A.H. (1991) Cloning the mammalian sex determining gene. In: Genome Analysis: Genes and Phenotypes, editel by Davies, K.E. and Tilghman, S. pp. 105-134. Cold Spring Harbor Press, Cold Spring Harbor.
22. Gubbay, J., Collignon, J., Koopman, P., Capel, B., Economou, A., Munsterberg, A., Vivian, N., Goodfellow, P.N., Lovell-Badge, R. and Goodfellow, P.N. (1990). Nature, 346:245-250.
23. Guellaen, G., Casanova, M., Bishop, C., Geldwerth, D., Audre, G., Fellous, M. and Weissenbach, J. (1984) Human XX males with Y single copy DNA fragments. Nature, 207:172-173.
24. Harley, V.R., Jackson, D.I., Hextall, P.J., Hawkins, J.R., Berkovitz, G.D., Sockanathan, S., Lovell-Badge, R. and Goodfellow, P.N. (1992) DNA binding activity of recombinant SRY from normal males and XY females. Science, 255:453-457.
25. Hawkins, J.R., Taylor, A., Berta, P., Levilliers, J., Van der Auwera, B. and Goodfellow, P.N. (1992) Mutational analysis of SRY: nonsense and missense mutations in XY sex reversal. Hum. Genet., 88:471-474.
26. Hawkins, J.R., Taylor, A., Goodfellow, P.N., Migeon, C.J., Smith, K.D. and Berkovitz, G.D. (1992) Evidence for increased prevalence of SRY mutations in XY females with complete rather than partial gonadal dysgenesis. Submitted for publication

27. Jacobs, P.A. and Strong, J.A., (1959) A case of human intersexuality having apossible XXY sex-determining mechanism. Nature, 183: 302-303.
28. Jager, R.J., Anvret, M., Hall, K. and Scherer, G. (1990) a human XY female with a frame shift mutation in the candidate testis determining gene SRY. Nature, 348:4520454.
29. Jager, R.J., Evensperger, C., Fraccaro, M. and Scherer, G. (1990) A ZFY-negative 46XX true hermaphrodite is positive for the Y pseudoautosomal boundary. Hum. Genet., 85:666-668
30. Jager, R.J., Pfeiffer, R.A. and Scherer, G. (1991) A familial amino-acid substitution in SRY can lead to conditional XY sex inversion. Am. J, Hum. Genet., 49:219
31. Jantzen, H.M., Admon, A., Bell, S.P. and Tjian, R. (1990) Nucleolar transcription factor hUBF contains a DNA-binding motif with homology to HMG proteins. Nature, 344:830-836.
32. Jost, A., Vigier, B., Prepin, J. and PerchelletJ., (1973) Studies on sex differentiation in mammals. Recent Prog. Horm. Res., 29:1-41.
33. Koopman, P., Munsterberg, A., Capel, B., Vivian, N. and Lovell-Badge, R. (1990) Expression of a candidate sex-determining region gene during mouse testis differentiation. Nature, 248:450-452.
34. Koopman, P., Gubbay, J., Vivian, N., Goodfellow, P. and Lovell-Badge, R. (1991) Male development of chromosomally female mice transgenic for Sry. Nature, 351:117-121
35. Levilliers, J., Quack, B., Weissenbach, J. and Petit, C. (1989) Exchange of the terminal poritons of X and Y-chromsomal short arms in human XY females. Proc. Natl. Acad. Sci. USA, 86:2296-2300
36. Madan, K. (1976) Chromosome measurements on an XXp$^+$ male. Hum. Genet., 32:141-142.
37. Magenis, R.E., Webb, M.J., McKean, R.S., Tomar, D., Allen, L.J., Kammer, H., van Dyke, D.L. and Lovrien, E. (1982) Translocation (X;Y) (p22.23;p11.2) in XX males; etiology of male phenotype. Hum. Genet., 62:271-276.
38. McElreavey, K.D., Vilain, E., Boucekkine, C., Vidaud, M., Jaubert, F., Richaud, F. and Fellous, M. (1992) XY sex reversal associated with a nonsense mutation in SRY. Genomics, (In press).
39. McLaren, A. and Monk, (1982) Fertile females produced by inactivation of an X chromosome of sex-reversed mice. Nature, 300:446-448.
40. Muller, U., Donlon, T., Schmid, M., Fitch, N., Richer, C-L., Lalande, M. and Latt, S.A. (1986) Deletion mapping of the testis determining locus with DNA probes in 46, XX males and 46, XY and 46X, dic(YC) females. Nucl. Acids Res., 14:6489-6505.
41. Muller, U., Lalande, M., Donlon, T.A. and Heartlein, M.W. (1989) Breakage of the human Y chromosome short arm between two blocks of tandemly repeated sequences. Genomics, 5:153-156.
42. Nasrin, N., Buggs, C., Kong, X.F., Carnazza, J., Goebl, M. and Alexander-Bridges, M. (1991) DNA-binding properties of the product of the testis-determining gene and a related protein. Nature, 354:317-320.
43. Ogata, T., Goodfellow, P., Petit, C., Aya, M. and Matsuo, N. (1992) Short stature in a girl with a terminal Xp deletion distal to DXYS15: Localisation of a growth gene(s) in the pseudaotosomal region. J. Med. Genet., (In press).
44. Oosterwegel, M., van der Wetering, M., Dooijes, D., klomp, L., Winito, A., Georgopoulos, K., Meijlink, F. and Clevers, H. (1991) Cloning of murine TCF-1, a T cell-specific transcription factor interacting with functional motifs in the CD3-e and T cell receptor a enhancer. J. Exp. Med. 173:1133.
45. Orita, M., Suzuki, Y., Sekiya, T., and Hayashi, K. (1989) Rapid and sensitive detection of point mutations and DNA polymorphisms using the polymerase chain reaction. Genomics, 4:874-879.
46. Page, D.C., Mosher, R., Simpson, E.M., Fisher, E.M.C., Mardon, G., Pollack, J., McGillivray, B., de la Chapelle, A., Brown, L.G. (1987) The sex determining region of the human Y chromosome encodes a finger protein. Cell, 51:1091-1104.
47. Page, D.C., Fisher, E.M.C., McGillivray, B. and Brown, L.G. (1990) Additional deletion in sex-determining region of human Y chromosome resolves paradox of X.t(Y;22) females. Nature, 346:279-281.
48. Palmer, M.S., Sinclair, A.H., Berta, P., Ellis, N.A., Goodfellow, P.N., Abbas, N.E. and Fellous, M. (1990) Genetic evidence that ZFY is not the testis-determining factor. Nature, 342:937-939.
49. Pearson, P.L. and Bobrow, M. (1970) Definitive evidence for the short arm of the Y chromosome associating with the X during meiosis in the human male. Nature, 226:959-961.

50. Petit, C., de la Chapelle, A., Levilliers, J., Castillo, S., Noel, B. and Weissenbach, J. (1987) An abnormal terminal exchange accounts for most but not all cases of human XX maleness. Cell, 49:595-602.
51. Rouyer, F., Simmler, M-C., Johnson, C., Vergnaud, G., Cooke, H.J. and Weissenbach, J. (1986) A gradient of sex linkage in the pseudoautosomal region of the human sex chromosomes. Nature, 319:291-295.
52. Simmler, M.C., Rouyer, F., Vergnaud, G., Nystrom-Lahti, M., Ngo, K.Y., de la Chapelle, A. and Weissenbach, J. (1985) Pseudoautosomal DNA sequences in the pairing region of the human sex chromosomes. Nature, 317:692-697.
53. Sinclair, A.H., Berta, P., Palmer, M.S., Hawkins, J.R., Griffiths, B.L., Smith, M.J., Foster, J.W., Frischauf, A-M., Lovell-Badge, R. and Goodfellow, P.N. A gene from the human sex-determining region encodes a protein with homology to a conserved DNA-bindig motif (1990) Nature, 346:240-244.
54. Skordis, N.A., Stetka, D.G., MacGillivray, M.H. and Greenfield, S.P. (1987) Familial 46, XX males coexisting with familial 46, XX true hermaphrodites in same pedigree. J. Pediatr., 110:244-248.
55. Solari, A.J. (1980) Synaptonemal complexes and associated structures in microspread human speramtocytes. Chromosoma, 81:315-337.
56. Sugimoto, A., Iino, Y., Maeda, T., Watanabe, Y. and Yamamoto, M. (1991) Schizosaccharomyces pombe ste11$^+$ encodes a transcription factor with an HMG motif that is a critical regulatory of sexual development. Genes Dev., 5:1990-1999.
57. Travis, A., Amsterdam, A., Belanger, C. and Grosschedl, R. (1991) Lef-1, a gene encoding a lymphoid-specific protein with HMG domain, regulates T-cell rec eptor a enhancer function. Genes Dev., 5:880-894.
58. Wetering, M. van de., Oosterwegel, M., Dooijes, D. and Clevers, H. (1991) Identification and cloning of TCF-1, a T lymphocyte-specific transcription factor containing a sequence-specific HMG box. EMBO J., 10:123-132.
59. Vergnaud, G., Page, D.C., Simmler, M-C., Brown, L., Rouyer, F., Noel, B., Botstein, D., de la Chapelle, A. and Weissenbach, J. (1986) A deletion map of the human Y chromosome based on DNA hybridization. Am. J. Hum. Genet., 38:109-124.
60. Waterman, M.L., Fischer, W.H. and Jones, K.A. (1991) A thymus-specific member of the HMG protein family regulates the human T cell receptor Ca enhancer. Genes Dev., 5:656-669.

Cellular Basis Of Sex Determination And Sex Reversal In Mammals

P.S. Burgoyne and S.J. Palmer

*MRC Mammalian Development Unit, Wolfson House,
4 Stephenson Way, London NW1 2HE, UK*

SUMMARY

Analysis of the sex chromosome complement of the cell lineages in XX<->XY fetal mouse testes has demonstrated that the only cells showing a bias in favour of XY cells, are the Sertoli cells. This means that the Y-chromosomal testis determining gene *Sry* must act through the 'supporting cell' lineage to divert it from the default ovarian pathway, to form Sertoli cells instead of follicle cells. The diversion of other cell lineages to the testicular pathway must be a consequence of fetal Sertoli cell activity.

It has been assumed that a study of examples of XX and XY gonadal sex reversal will provide pointers to the genes downstream from *Sry* in the testis determining pathway. However, a close examination of a number of examples in the mouse where gonadal sex is at variance with *Sry* status, has shown that this assumption is not always correct.

INTRODUCTION

The recent cloning of the mammalian Y-chromosomal testis-determining gene of mouse (*Sry*) (19) and man (*SRY*) (52), and the demonstration that XX mice transgenic for *Sry* develop as males (30), has moved the molecular focus to the events which follow the expression of *Sry/SRY*. The present review reappraises information (primarily from studies on mice) on the cellular basis of gonadal sex determination in the light of the recent molecular developments, and examines instances of partial or complete sex reversal (where gonadal development is at variance with *Sry* status) to see if they can provide any pointers to the genes downstream from *Sry*.

THE COMPONENTS OF THE 'INDIFFERENT' GONAD

When it first appears as a ridge of tissue on the ventral surface of the mesonephros, the developing gonad ('indifferent' because it is not yet committed to the ovarian or testicular pathway) consists of a number of different somatic cell types together with the primordial germ cells. (See Reference 41 for a recent review describing the formation of the gonadal rudiment in mouse and rat). Thus, in order to divert the developing fetal gonad from the default ovarian pathway to the testicular pathway, *Sry* has to alter the fate of a number of different cell types. These cell types can be categorised as comprising three gonad-specific cell lineages, the supporting cells, steroid cells and germ cells, together with a vascularised connective tissue component (4).

Although there is some debate about the origin of the supporting cells, there is general agreement that they constitute a defined lineage identifiable as an epithelial cell type in the gonadal ridge, from which the follicle cells of the ovary and the Sertoli cells of the testis are derived. The concept of a steroid cell lineage giving rise to Leydig cells in the fetal testis and to thecal cells in the maturing ovary, is less firmly based, but is intellectually attractive since androgen and estrogen synthesis are modulations of the same steroidogenic pathway. The most clearly defined gonad-specific cell lineage is the primordial germ cells. These can be identified as a distinct cell type in the extra-embryonic mesoderm posterior to the primitive streak of egg cylinder stage mouse embryos (18), and subsequently migrate via the hindgut and dorsal mesentery, to the developing gonadal ridge.

The vascularised connective tissue component is derived from mesenchymal and endothelial cells which originate from the adjacent mesonephric region. Very early in testis development these cells invade and surround the mass of epithelial cells and germ cells, delineating the testis cords and forming a layer (the developing tunica albuginea) which separates the cords from the overlying coelomic epithelial cells. The endothelial cells immediately begin to organise into the vascular network necessary for testosterone export; indeed, components of this vasculature are one of the earliest diagnostic features of testicular differentiation. Recent experiments in which isolated 11.5 day post coitum (pc) XY gonadal ridges were reassociated with mesonephroi carrying a cell marker, suggest that the invading cells also include Leydig cell precursors (M. Buehr and A. McLaren, unpublished). In the mouse ovary the equivalent invasion of 'stromal' components into the mass of epithelial cell cords occurs much later (around the time of birth) in conjunction with the formation of individual follicles around the oocytes.

Although there is continuing controversy over the origins of some of the somatic cell types contributing to the gonadal primordium, this fortunately does not prevent us from reaching some firm conclusions about how *Sry* acts to bring about testis determination. The mode of *Sry* action is the subject of the following three sections.

IN WHICH CELL TYPE IS *Sry* EXPRESSED?

An important first step towards understanding how *Sry* diverts all these components of the developing gonad to the testicular pathway, is to establish in which cell type *Sry* is first expressed. The low level of expression of *Sry* in the gonadal ridge has precluded *in situ* hybridization as a means to identify the cell type in which expression occurs. However, expression has been shown to occur in the absence of the germ cells (31). Well before the cloning of *Sry*, we set out to identify the cell type through which the Y-chromosomal testis determinant was expressed, by analysing the sex chromosomal complement of testicular cell types in XX<->XY chimeric testes. It was reasoned that any cell type in which Y chromosome expression had been involved in either *commitment* to the male pathway or in subsequent *differentiation*, must be predominantly or exclusively XY in these chimeric testes. We were aware, that to draw inferences in the opposite direction (from XY predominance/exclusivity to Y expression) it was necessary to rule out the possibility that the selection against XX cells was due to the presence of two X chromosomes, rather than to the absence of a Y. Indeed, selection against cells with two X chromosomes is known to occur in the male germ line (37).

In our initial study we focused on the somatic components of prepubertal and adult XX<->XY testes (6). The choice of stages was originally due to technical constraints and our lack of interest in the germ line was based on earlier studies showing that testis determination does not require the presence of germ cells (42). The results showed that Sertoli cells were the only somatic cell type showing a bias in favour of XY cells and this result is confirmed by two other studies (48,53). It was concluded that the Y-chromosomal testis determinant is expressed in the lineage which gives rise to the Sertoli cells, that is, the supporting cell lineage.

We have substantiated this initial conclusion in three ways. First, we have analysed testicular tissue from three XO/XY/XYY mosaic hermaphrodites. The proportion of Y-bearing cells in the non-testicular tissues analysed (including ovarian tissue) and in testicular interstitial tissue, did not exceed 29%, yet the proportion of Y-bearing Sertoli cells was 84-99% (45). The near exclusion of XO cells from the Sertoli cell population in these mosaics counters the possibility that the selection against XX Sertoli cells in XX<->XY chimeras is due to the presence of two X chromosomes. Secondly, we have analysed fetal XX<->XY chimeric testes and shown that Sertoli cells are the only fetal testicular cell type showing an XY bias (at this stage there is no selection against XX germ cells) (46). This argues that there is a strong bias in favour of XY Sertoli cells at the *commitment* stage, and is not simply a consequence of selection during Sertoli cell differentiation. Finally, we have analysed fetal XY,Sry^+<->XY,Sry^- chimeric testes, in which one XY component carries a 11 kb deletion which has removed *Sry* (19,20). It can be seen from Table 1, that these XY,Sry^- cells, just like XX and XO cells, are rarely recruited to form Sertoli cells. Since *Sry* is the only gene lying within the deletion (8), it must be the absence of *Sry* which is responsible. We therefore conclude that *Sry* expression in the supporting cell lineage is the trigger for Sertoli cell differentiation.

Table 1. *The proportion of XY,Sry⁻ cells in testicular and non-testicular cell lineages from two 14.5 day pc XY<->XY,Sry⁻ chimeras*

	Percentage of XY,Sry⁻ cells (number of cells scored)[a]					
	Non-testicular cells		Testicular cells			
Chimera	Liver	Mesoneph. tubules	Myoid cells	Leydig cells	Prosperm- atogonia	Sertoli cells
1	25(36)	9(554)	9(155)	9(379)	21(492)	2(308)
2	52(50)	42(351)	24(107)	40(366)	27(428)	7(186)

[a]For the liver, counts are based on cytogenetic markers in air-dried mitotic cells. For the other cell types, the estimates are based on *in situ* analysis of a transgenic marker, corrected for the incidence of false negatives as described by Palmer & Burgoyne (46).

Although our initial studies of adult XX<->XY chimeric testes led us to suggest that Sertoli cells were exclusively XY, subsequent studies showed that this was not the case (46,48). The highest proportion of XX Sertoli cells so far reported is 21% in a 15.5 days pc testis from a chimera with an XX contribution of from 60-90% in the other tissues analysed (46). How do we account for the presence of these XX Sertoli cells? Since *Sry* encodes a protein which is thought to be a DNA-binding transcription factor (19,21,52), it seems unlikely that the XX cells are being recruited directly by *Sry* protein coming from neighbouring XY cells. In some situations (see below) XX Sertoli cells can be formed from ovarian supporting cells (this has been termed 'transdifferentiation'); however, the presence of XX Sertoli cells in chimeric testes as early as 13.5 days pc seems to preclude the 'transdifferentiation' route. We therefore favour the view that a gene product in the *Sry*-initiated cascade is responsible for the recruitment of XX cells to form Sertoli cells in these chimeras. Nevertheless, in normal XY testes where all the supporting cells in the gonadal ridge are XY, the diversion of these cells to form Sertoli cells can be viewed as a cell-autonomous consequence of *Sry* activity.

COMMITMENT OF OTHER CELL TYPES TO THE TESTICULAR PATHWAY

The demonstration that XX mice transgenic for *Sry* develop normal testes in fetal life (30) tells us that *Sry* is the only gene on the mouse Y involved in committing the components of the indifferent gonad to the testicular pathway. If we are correct in concluding that *Sry* expression in the indifferent gonad is restricted to the supporting cell lineage, then the diversion of the other cell types to the testicular pathway must be directed by the differentiating Sertoli cells without any further Y chromosome involvement.

An early product of fetal Sertoli cells is the factor responsible for regression of the Müllerian ducts (AMH or MIS) (25,27), for which the human, bovine and mouse genes have been cloned (9,43,49). AMH has been implicated as the causal factor in three instances where Sertoli-like cells are formed from XX ovarian supporting cells; namely, in the bovine freemartin (26), in rat ovaries exposed to AMH *in vitro* (57) and in XX mice carrying an AMH transgene (1). This has led to speculation that AMH may have a role in the normal process of testis determination, in addition to its role in bringing about the regression of the Müllerian ducts. However, the existence of men with persistent Müllerian ducts (due in some cases to a documented AMH gene defect (24) in conjunction with fully-formed (although frequently cryptorchid) testes, clearly shows that AMH is not required for testis determination.

THRESHOLD EFFECTS IN GONADAL SEX DETERMINATION

If you examine adult sex chromosome chimeras or mosaics in mice, it is rare to find true hermaphrodites (38) (individuals with testicular and ovarian tissue), and most of these are found to have an ovary on one side and a testis on the other, rather than ovotestes. From an analysis of the relationship between the proportion of Y-bearing cells and sexual phenotype (38,45), it has been found that true hermaphrodites typically have from 20-30% XY cells; below this range you get two ovaries, and above this range you get two testes. If we accept that gonadal sex is determined by the path of differentiation taken by the supporting cells, and that the fate of individual supporting cells is tightly regulated by the presence or absence of *Sry* in these cells, then we need to explain why ovotestes are so rare.

In fact, if you examine the gonads of fetal sex chromosome mosaics and chimeras, ovotestes are much more common (3,11), so it must be concluded that the majority of fetal ovotestes are subsequently transformed into testes or ovaries. As far as the transformation of fetal ovotestes into testes is concerned, it has been suggested that this is mediated by AMH coming from fetal Sertoli cells (6). Various lines of evidence (reviewed in Reference 40) show that AMH causes the loss of developing oocytes from ovarian tissue, and without oocytes, folliculogenesis and further ovarian development is prevented. In some circumstances (see below) the ovarian supporting cells, when deprived of their interaction with germ cells, may 'transdifferentiate' into Sertoli cells. If this does occur in sex chromosome chimeras and mosaics, the resulting XX Sertoli cells must be at a considerable selective disadvantage, because adult XX<->XY testes have a consistently low proportion of XX Sertoli cells (46,48). Further evidence that the ovarian tissue is being lost rather than being transformed into testicular tissue, is the extremely small size (<15 mg) of some XO/XY mosaic testes (33), which is far smaller than can be explained by the degree of germ cell deficiency.

The transformation of fetal ovotestes into ovaries is less well documented. Prepubertal and adult ovaries from mosaics and chimeras have been shown by *in situ* analysis with Y-specific DNA probes, to have XY follicle cells (45,48); but we do not yet know whether these are derived from XY supporting cells recruited directly to form follicle cells (i.e. the gonads were always ovaries) or whether they were recruited in some way from fetal XY Sertoli cells (i.e. the ovaries were derived from fetal ovotestes). A recent analysis of developing ovotestes in mice with an inherited form of partial or complete XY sex reversal has provided some indirect evidence that ovotestes can transform into ovaries (54), but further studies are required to clarify this.

Whatever the mechanisms involved, this 'canalisation' of gonadal development has the effect of minimising the number of sterile hermaphrodites produced. This may be of much greater significance in non-mammalian groups (including our reptilian ancestors?) where there is a less rigorous genetic control of gonadal sex.

Sry-NEGATIVE XX GONADAL SEX REVERSAL

Under this heading we will discuss examples where XX Sertoli cells are formed in the absence of *Sry*. A much studied example is the bovine freemartin - a genetically female calf with gonads masculinised *in utero* by a factor (almost certainly the anti-Müllerian factor AMH/MIS) originating from a male twin (26,34). An important feature of the freemartin gonad, is that it first develops as an ovary; only after the loss of most of the fetal oocytes do Sertoli-like cells form (26). It is this transformation of ovarian tissue into testicular tissue which has been referred to as 'transdifferentiation'. A number of other possible examples have been reviewed elsewhere (4,5,39,40). Here we will limit ourselves to one particularly compelling example. In this instance early fetal XX mouse ovaries were transplanted under the kidney capsule of adult male and female hosts and the fate of the grafts was followed over a period of weeks (55,56). In a proportion of these ovarian grafts Sertoli-like cells began to appear about two weeks after grafting. As with the freemartin example, ovarian differentiation was well established before any Sertoli cell cords formed and there was an associated loss of oocytes. The importance of this study is that the transition from ovarian supporting cells (pre-granulosa or pre-follicle cells) to Sertoli cells was carefully documented by light and electron microscopy. Furthermore, the ultrastructural evidence that XX Sertoli cells had formed was supported by the documented changes in the stromal components of the graft. These

XX Sertoli cells (just like XY Sertoli cells - see previous section) triggered the differentiation of peritubular myoid cells and of testosterone-secreting Leydig cells (55).

This phenomenon of XX sex-reversal by 'transdifferentiation' is important in two contexts. Firstly, it serves to highlight the fact that the sole function of *Sry* in testis determination is to act as a trigger to set in motion the process of Sertoli cell differentiation. Secondly, it suggests both possibilities and pitfalls for those wishing to identify the genes downstream from *Sry* in the testis determination pathway. The possibilities relate to the changing pattern of gene activity accompanying the transition from ovarian supporting cell to Sertoli cell, which may in part, recapitulate steps downstream from *Sry*. The pitfalls relate to the apparent association between transdifferentiation and the loss of the germ cells. It may be that some mutations interfering with female germ cell development can cause XX sex reversal by the transdifferentiation pathway - a possibility that those investigating examples of *SRY*-negative XX sex reversal in man (2,15,23) should bear in mind.

Sry-POSITIVE XY GONADAL SEX REVERSAL

The most obvious route to XY sex reversal is through loss or inactivation of the testis determining gene *Sry* (19,35). Now that the focus has changed to genes downstream from *Sry* in the process of testis determination, it is examples of *Sry*-positive XY sex reversal (where XY follicle cells form from supporting cells with a functional copy of *Sry*), which are of prime interest.

Establishing that sex reversal in such cases, is due to malfunction of a downstream gene rather than of *Sry* itself, is not an easy task. Let us suppose that we have established that the coding region of *Sry* is intact, with no obvious point mutations which would lead to a non-functional product. Sex reversal may still occur if *Sry* is expressed at too low a level, or if its action is delayed. This is best illustrated by two examples of *Sry*-positive sex reversal in mice.

The first example is a sequel to the exciting report of the production of XX, *Sry* transgenic male mice (30). In some cases *Sry* transgenes transmitted by male carriers failed to generate XX males, even though the XX fetuses carrying the transgene were shown to be expressing *Sry* at the right time in the developing gonad. However, when male carriers of the transgene were mated to female carriers, XX males were now produced; presumably because homozygosity for the transgene had raised the level of expression above some critical threshold level (8).

The second example concerns the partial or complete XY sex reversal which occurs when a 'Poschiavinus' Y chromosome (derived from *Mus m. domesticus* mice originating from the Val Poschiavo, Switzerland) is transferred to a C57BL/6 inbred background (14). When outcrossed to another strain this Y chromosome has been shown to initiate testis development some 14 h later than the BL/6 Y (47). It has therefore been suggested that the Poschiavinus Y carries a late-acting *Sry* allele which fails to pre-empt the C57BL/6 programme of ovary determination (13,47).

When there is genetic proof that an autosomal or X-chromosomal gene is responsible for XY sex reversal, we would seem to be much safer in assuming the gene involved is in the testis determining pathway. However, some further examples of XY sex reversal in mice have called this assumption into question. In 1983 it was reported that the autosomal mutation *T hairpin tail* causes partial or complete sex reversal when placed with an AKR Y onto a C57 BL/6 background (the AKR Y alone does not cause sex reversal). The mutation is due to a deletion on chromosome 17, so it was suggested that a gene in the testis determining pathway lay within this deletion (13,58).

Suspicions are aroused when you consider the parallels with C57BL/6-Y^{POS} XY sex reversal. First, there is the requirement for the BL/6 inbred background. Second, the AKR Y (like Y^{POS}) is of the *domesticus* type and is later acting than the BL/6 Y (Fig. 1).

Furthermore, another unrelated autosomal mutation ($W19$), causing dominant white spotting) which is due to a deletion on chromosome 5, also causes XY sex reversal if transferred with an AKR Y onto a C57/BL6 background (10). We have therefore suggested that these deletions may be exerting their sex-reversing effect by once again creating a 'timing mismatch' in which the process of testis determination fails to pre-empt the process of

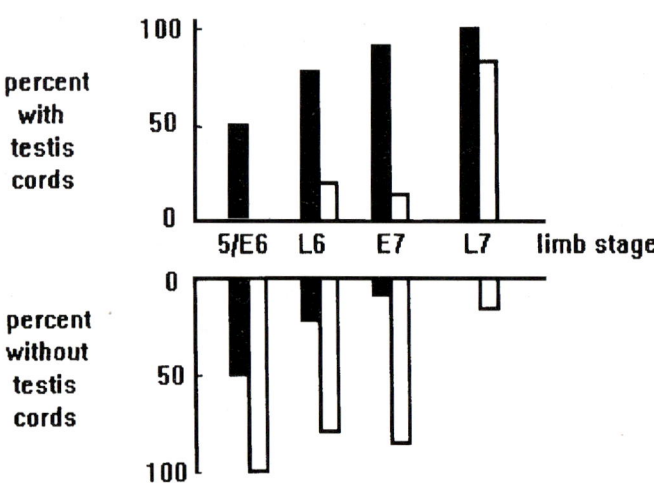

FIG. 1. The percentage of XY fetuses (n=49) with or without visible testis cords at 12 days 15 h *post coitum* plotted against hind limb stage. Solid bars, CXBH x C57BL/6-Y^{C57} F_1; open bars, CXBH x C57BL/6-Y^{AKR}. The fetuses differ only with respect to the source of their Y chromosome. Those with an AKR Y form testis cords later (with respect to limb stage) than those with a C57 Y.

ovary determination. We view the late acting AKR Y and the BL/6 background as predisposing factors; the deletion could then cause XY sex reversal by retarding the onset of testis determination slightly more than ovary determination (7). These observations must call into question the assumption that all mutations causing XY sex reversal in man are affecting genes in the testis determining pathway, especially when the mutations are associated with multiple malformations (50,51).

We have so far avoided commenting on the requirement for a BL/6 genetic background in these examples. From information on the frequency of XY sex reversal during backcrossing the Y^{POS} chromosome to BL/6, Eicher and Washburn have suggested that the C57BL/6 strain carries a recessive allele of an autosomal *testis-determining gene 'Tda-1'*, which fails to interact correctly with the Y^{POS} chromosome (12). We have considered it simpler to view the gene as being in the ovary determining pathway, with the recessive BL/6 allele being an early-acting variant (7). Unfortunately, attempts to map the gene involved have been unsuccessful. A more radical explanation has been put forward by Nallaseth (44) who has suggested that the BL/6 background causes the Y^{POS} to become unstable and lose sequences essential to its testis-determining function. It seems to us that this model would predict that the Y of BL/6 XY^{POS} females has been more substantially altered than the Y of the males and hermaphrodites. We are therefore trying to transmit the Y^{POS} through females to see if this results in a more penetrant form of XY sex reversal among their offspring.

Perhaps the most intriguing example of XY sex reversal in mammals is found in the wood lemming *Myopus schisticolor* (16). These XY females, unlike those of the mouse (36), horse (28,29) and man (51), are fully fertile. They owe their fertility to a novel double non-disjunction mechanism which removes the Y and restores a second X to the developing oocytes (17). Because the females are fertile it has been possible to establish that the sex reversal is due to an X-linked factor. Furthermore the X of these XY females is cytologically distinguishable from that of XY males (22) and carries a variant form of the zinc finger protein gene *Zfx* (32). It has yet to be established that the alterred *Zfx* is the cause of the sex reversal - it may simply be a variant which has become fixed due to the presence of an X chromosome rearrangement. However, the basis for this X-linked XY sex reversal in the wood lemming is certainly worth pursuing, since probable X-linked pedigrees have been reported in the horse (28) and man (51).

CONCLUSIONS

The available evidence leads to the conclusion that the Y-chromosomal testis determining gene *Sry* is expressed in the supporting cell lineage. As a consequence of this expression the supporting cells divert from the default ovarian pathway and differentiate to form fetal Sertoli cells. The differentiating Sertoli cells then direct the other components of the gonad along the testicular pathway. It is argued that the sole function for *Sry* in this process is to act as a cell-autonomous trigger for Sertoli cell differentiation. These conclusions are summarised in Fig 2.

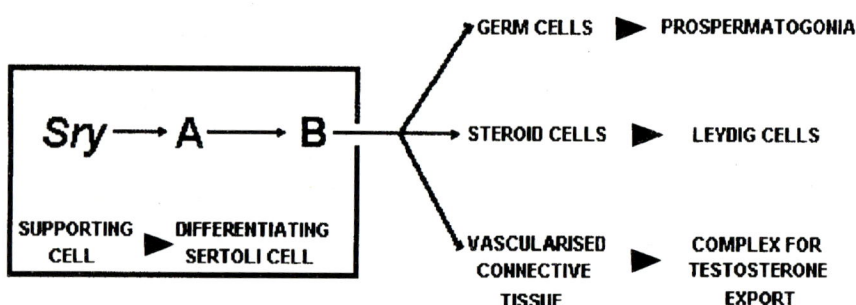

FIG. 2. The role of *Sry* in testis determination. The available evidence suggests that the Y-chromosomal testis determining gene *Sry* is expressed cell-autonomously in the supporting cell lineage. This initiates one or more steps (**A**) which commit the supporting cells to differentiate into Sertoli cells. Evidence from XX<->XY chimeras indicates that one of these steps is not strictly cell-autonomous (i.e. it is able to locally recruit XX cells). The differentiating Sertoli cells then produce one or more signals (**B**) which commit the other gonadal cell types to the testicular pathway. None of these signals are encoded by Y-chromosomal genes.

The model assumes that there is at least one step between *Sry* expression and commitment to Sertoli cell differentiation. It is this step (or steps) which we suggest is not strictly cell limited and is able to recruit a few XX cells to form Sertoli cells in XX<->XY chimeras. Disruption of this step(s) should result in XY sex reversal. Although a number of examples of autosomal or X-linked XY sex reversal have been identified in mice and man, analysis of the mouse examples has raised doubts as to whether they are due to disruption of genes in the testis determining pathway. It is hoped that further analysis of examples of XY sex reversal may eventually lead to the identification of the gene(s) involved.

REFERENCES

1. Behringer, R.R., Cate, R.L., Froelick, G.J., Palmiter, R.D. and Brinster, R.L. (1990) Abnormal sexual development in transgenic mice chronically expressing Mullerian inhibiting substance. Nature, 345:167-170.
2. Berkovitz, G.D., Fechner, P.Y., Marcantonio, S.M., Bland, G., Stetten, G., Goodfellow, P.N., Smith, K.D. and Migeon, C.M. (1992) The role of the sex-determining region of the Y chromosome (SRY) in the etiology of 46,XX true hermaphroditism. Hum. Genet., 88:411-416.
3. Bradbury, M.W. (1987) Testes of XX<->XY chimeric mice develop from fetal ovotestes. Dev. Genet., 8:207-218.

4. Burgoyne, P.S. (1988) Role of mammalian Y chromosome in sex determination. Phil. Trans. Roy. Soc. Lond. B., 322:63-72.
5. Burgoyne, P.S. (1992) Y chromosome function in mammalian development. Adv. Dev. Biol., 1:1-29.
6. Burgoyne, P.S., Buehr, M.,Koopman, P., Rossant, J. and McLaren, A. (1988) Cell-autonomous action of the testis-determining gene: Sertoli cells are exclusively XY in XX<->XY chimaeric mouse testes. Development, 102:443-450.
7. Burgoyne, P.S. and Palmer. S.J. (1991) The genetics of XY sex reversal in the mouse and other mammals. Semin. Dev. Biol., 2:277-284.
8. Capel, B. and Lovell-Badge, R. (1993) The *Sry* gene and sex determination in mammals. Adv. Dev. Biol., (in press)
9. Cate,R.L., Mattaliano, R.J., Hession, C., Tizard, R., Farber, N.M., Cheung, A., Ninfa, E.G., Frey, A.Z., Gash, D. J., Chow, E.P., Fisher, R.A., Bertonis, J.M., Torres, G., Wallner, B.P., Ramachandran, K.L., Ragin, R.C., Manganaro, T.F., MacLaughlin, D.T. and Donahoe, P.K. (1986) Isolation of the bovine and human genes for Mullerian inhibiting substance and expression of the human gene in animal cells. Cell, 45:685-698.
10. Cattanach, B.M. (1987) Sex-reversed mice and sex determination. Ann. N.Y. Acad. Sci., 513:27-29.
11. Eicher, E.M., Beamer, W.G., Washburn, L.L. and Whitten, W.K. (1980) A cytogenetic investigation of inherited true hermaphroditism in Balb/cWt mice. Cytogenet. Cell Genet., 28:104-115.
12. Eicher, E.M. and Washburn, L.L. (1983) Inherited sex reversal in mice: identification of a new primary sex-determining gene. J. Exp. Zool., 228:297-304.
13. Eicher, E.M. and Washburn, L.L. (1986) Genetic control of primary sex determination in mice. Annu. Rev. Genet., 20:327-360.
14. Eicher, E.M., Washburn, L.L., Whitney III, B. and Morrow, K.E. (1982) *Mus poschiavinus* Y chromosome in the C57BL/6J murine genome causes sex reversal. Science, 217:535-537.
15. Ferguson-Smith, M.A., North, M.A., Affara, N.A. and Briggs, J.H. (1990) The secret of sex. Lancet, 336:809-810
16. Fredga, K., Gropp, A., Winking, H. and Frank, F. (1976) Fertile XX- and XY-type females in the wood lemming, *Myopus schisticolor*. Nature, 261:225-227.
17. Fredga, K., Gropp, A., Winking, H. and Frank, F. (1977) A hypothesis explaining the exceptional sex ratio in the wood lemming (*Myopus schisticolor*). Hereditas, 85:101-104.
18. Ginsburg, M., Snow, M.H.L. and McLaren, A. (1990) Primordial germ cells in the mouse embryo during gastrulation. Development, 110:521-528.
19. Gubbay, J., Collignon, J., Koopman, P., Capel, B., Economou, A., Munsterberg, A., Vivian,N., Goodfellow, P. and Lovell-Badge, R. (1990) A member of a novel family of embryonically expressed genes mapping to the sex-determining region of the mouse Y chromosome. Nature, 346:145-150.
20. Gubbay, J., Vivian, N., Economou, A., Jackson, D., Goodfellow, P.N. and Lovell-Badge, R. (1992) Inverted repeat structure of the *Sry* locus in mice. Proc. Natl. Acad. Sci. USA (in press).
21. Harley, V.R., Jackson, D.I., Hextall, P.J., Hawkins, J.R., Berkovitz, G.D., Sockanathan, S., Lovell-Badge, R. and Goodfellow, P.N. (1992) DNA binding activity of recombinant SRY from normal males and XY females. Science, 255: 453-456.
22. Herbst, E.W., Fredga, K., Frank, F., Winking, H. and Gropp, A. (1978) Cytological identification of two X-chromosome types in the wood lemming (*Myopus schisticolor*) Chromosoma, 69:185-189.
23. Jager, R.J., Ebensperger, C., Fraccaro M. and Scherer, G (1990) A ZFY-negative 46,XX true hermaphrodite is positive for the Y pseudoautosomal boundary. Hum. Genet., 85:666-668.
24. Josso, N., Boussin, L., Knebelmann, B., Nihoulfekete, C. and Picard, J.Y. (1991) Anti-Müllerian hormone and intersex states. Trends Endocr. Metab., 2:227-232.
25. Jost, A. (1953) Problems of fetal endocrinology: the gonadal and hypophyseal hormones. Recent Prog. Horm. Res., 8:379-418.
26. Jost, A., Perchellet, J.P., Prepin, J. and Vigier, B. (1975). The prenatal development of bovine freemartins. In: Symposium on intersexuality, edited by Rheinboth, R., pp 392-406. Springer Verlag, Berlin.
27. Jost, A., Vigier, B., Prepin, J. and Perchellet, J.P. (1973) Studies on sex differentiation in mammals. Recent Prog. Horm. Res., 29:1-41.

28. Kent, M.G., Shoffner, R.N., Buoen, L. and Weber, A.F. (1986) XY sex-reversal syndrome in the domestic horse. Cytogenet. Cell Genet., 42:8-18.
29. Kent, M.G., Shoffner, R.N., Hunter, A., Elliston, K.O., Schroder, W., Tolley, E. and Wachtel, S.S. (1988) XY sex reversal syndrome in the mare: clinical and behavioural studies, H-Y phenotype. Hum. Genet., 79:321-328.
30. Koopman, P., Gubbay, J., Vivian, N., Goodfellow, P. and Lovell-Badge, R. (1991) Male development of chromosomally female mice transgenic for *Sry*. Nature, 351:117-121.
31. Koopman, P., Munsterberg, A., Capel, B., Vivian, N. and Lovell-Badge, R. (1990) Expression of a candidate sex-determining gene during mouse testis differentiation. Nature, 348:450-452.
32. Lau, Y-F.C., Yang-Feng, T.L., Elder, B., Chan, K., Fredga, K. and Wiberg, U. (1992) Unusual distribution of *Zfy* and *Zfx* sequences on the sex chromosomes of the wood lemming, a species with XY sex reversal. Genomics, (in press).
33. Levy, E.R. and Burgoyne, P.S. (1986) The fate of XO germ cells in the testes of XO/XY and XO/XY/XYY mouse mosaics: evidence for a spermatogenesis gene on the mouse Y chromosome. Cytogenet. Cell Genet., 42:208-213.
34. Lillie, F.R. (1917) The free-martin; a study of the action of sex hormones in the foetal life of cattle. J. Exp. Zool., 23:371-451.
35. Lovell-Badge, R. and Robertson, E. (1990). XY female mice resulting from a heritable mutation in the murine primary testis determining gene *Tdy*. Development, 109:635-646.
36. Mahadevaiah, S.K., Lovell-Badge, R. and Burgoyne, P.S. (1992) *Tdy*-negative XY, XXY and XYY female mice: breeding data and synatonemal complex analysis. J. Reprod. Fertil., (in press).
37. McLaren, A. (1983) Does the chromosomal sex of a mouse germ cell affect its development? In: Current problems in germ cell differentiation, edited by McLaren, A. and Wylie, C.C., pp 225-240. Cambridge University Press, London.
38. McLaren, A. (1984) Chimeras and sexual differentiation. In: Chimeras in developmental biology, edited by Le Douarin, N., McLaren, A., pp 381-399. Academic Press, New York and London.
39. McLaren, A. (1991a) Sex determination in mammals. In: Oxford reviews of reproductive biology, Vol. 13, edited by Milligan, S.R., pp 1-33. Oxford University Press, Oxford.
40. McLaren, A. (1991b) Development of the mammalian gonad: the fate of the supporting cell lineage. Bioessays, 13:151-156.
41. Merchant-Larios, H. and Taketo, T. (1991) Testicular differentiation in mammals under normal and experimental conditions. J. Electron Microsc. Techn., 19:158-171.
42. Mintz, B. and Russell, E.S. (1957) Gene-induced embryological modifications of primordial germ cells in the mouse. J. Exp. Zool., 134:207-237.
43. Munsterberg, A. and Lovell-Badge, R. (1991) Expression of the mouse anti-Müllerian hormone gene suggests a role in both male and female sexual differentiation. Development, 113:613-624.
44. Nallaseth, F.S. (1992) Sequence instability and functional inactivation of murine Y chromosomes can occur on a specific genetic background. Mol. Biol. Evol., 9:331-365.
45. Palmer, S.J. and Burgoyne, P.S. (1991a) XY follicle cells in the ovaries of XO/XY and XO/XY/XYY mosaic mice. Development, 111:1017-1019.
46. Palmer, S.J. and Burgoyne, P.S. (1991b) *In situ* analysis of fetal, prepuberal and adult XX<->XY chimaeric mouse testes: Sertoli cells are predominantly, but not exclusively, XY. Development, 112:265-268.
47. Palmer, S.J. and Burgoyne, P.S. (1991c) The *Mus musculus domesticus Tdy* allele acts later than the *Mus musculus musculus Tdy* allele: a basis for XY sex-reversal in C57BL/6-Y^{pos} mice. Development, 113:709-714.
48. Patek, C.E., Kerr, J., Gosden, R., Jones, K.W., Hardy,K., Muggleton-Harris, A., Handyside, A., Whittingham, D. and Hooper, M.L. (1991) Sex chimaerism, fertility and sex determination in the mouse. Development, 113:311-325.
49. Picard, J.Y., Benarous, R., Guerrier, D., Josso, N. and Kahn, A. (1986) Cloning and expression of cDNA for anti-Mullerian hormone. Proc. Natl. Acad. Sci. USA, 83:5464-5468.
50. Scherer, G., Schempp, W., Baccichetti, C., Lenzini, E., Bricarelli, F.D., Carbone, L.D.L. and Wolf, U. (1989) Duplication of an Xp segment that includes the ZFX locus causes sex inversion in man. Hum. Genet., 81:291-294.
51. Simpson, J.L. (1989) Genetic heterogeneity in XY sex reversal: potential pitfalls in isolating the testis determining factor (TDF). In: Evolutionary mechanisms in sex determination, edited by Wachtel, S.S., pp 265-277. CRC Press, Boca Raton.

52. Sinclair, A.H., Berta, P., Palmer, M.S., Hawkins, J.R., Griffiths, B.L., Smith, M.J., Foster, J.W., Frischauf, A.M., Lovell-Badge, R. and Goodfellow, P.N. (1989) A gene from the human sex-determining region encodes a protein with homology to a conserved DNA-binding motif. Nature, 346:240-244.
53. Singh, L., Matsukuma, S. and Jones, K.W. (1987) Testis development in a mouse with 10% of XY cells. Dev. Biol. 122:287-290.
54. Taketo, T., Saeed, J., Nishioka, Y. and Donahoe, P.K. (1991) Delay of testicular differentiation in the B6.Y^{DOM} ovotestis demonstrated by immunocytochemical staining for Mullerian inhibiting substance. Dev. Biol., 146:386-395.
55. Taketo-Hosotani, T., Merchant-Larios, H., Thau, R.B. and Koide, S.S. (1985) Testicular cell differentiation in fetal mouse ovaries following transplantation into adult male mice. J. Exp. Zool., 236:229-237.
56. Taketo-Hosotani, T. and Sinclair-Thompson, E. (1987) Influence of the mesonephros on the development of fetal mouse ovaries following transplantation into adult male and female mice. Dev. Biol., 124:423-430.
57. Vigier, B., Watrin, F., Magre, S., Tran, D. and Josso, N. (1987) Purified bovine AMH induces a characteristic freemartin effect in fetal rat prospective ovaries exposed to it *in vitro*. Development, 100:43-55.
58. Washburn, L.L. and Eicher, E.M. (1983) Sex reversal in XY mice caused by dominant mutation on chromosome 17. Nature, 303:338-340.

Hormonal Control of Gonadal Differentiation

N. Josso, B. Vigier, R.L Cate*, R. Behringer**,
N. di Clemente and L. Lyet

*Unité de Recherches sur l'Endocrinologie du Dévelopement
Ecole Normale Supérieure, 1 rue Maurice-Arnoux, 92120 Montrouge, France
*Biogen Research Corporation, Cambridge, Ma 02142, USA
**MD Anderson Cancer Ctr, Dept Molecular Genetics, Houston, Tx 77030, USA*

As discussed by Goodfellow (page 5), gonadal differentiation is the key event of sex determination, the binary switch controlling subsequent steps of sex differentiation. As shown by Jost (6), removal of the gonads from embryos of either sex results in somatic female differentiation, graft of a fetal testicular fragment restores male differentiation. The latter involves Wölffian duct stabilization, virilization of the urogenital sinus and external genitalia and Müllerian duct regression. Insertion of a testosterone crystal instead of fetal testicular tissue results in male differentiation with the exception that Müllerian ducts persist. Two conclusions can be drawn from these experiments. 1) Sex differentiation is an asymmetrical process insofar as the male pathway must be imposed upon a soma which would otherwise differentiate along female lines. 2) The testis produces two discrete hormones, testosterone and a factor inducing Müllerian regression, now known as anti-Müllerian hormone (AMH) or Müllerian-inhibiting substance (MIS) or factor (MIF). AMH has now been isolated (13) and cloned (2), it is a disulfide-bonded glycoprotein dimer, with partial homology to the transforming growth factor-β family and is produced by immature Sertoli and postnatal granulosa cells (12).

Gonadal differentiation in mammals is determined by the presence or absence of a testis-determining gene on the Y chromosome (see page 5). In lower vertebrates, lacking differentiated sex chromosomes, gonadal sex is dependent upon environmental factors, such as incubation temperature (14), but recent experiments (4) suggest that the effects of temperature could be mediated by processes regulating the synthesis or activity of cytochrome-P450 aromatase, an enzyme catalyzing the synthesis of estrogens from androgen precursors. In birds, although gonadal differentiation is normally genetically determined, estrogens exert a feminizing effect on the testis (27). Grafting of fetal testicular tissue into genetically female chick embryos (16) or treatment with an aromatase inhibitor (5) results in bilateral testicular development and a permanent male phenotype. Taken together, these data indicate that gonadal differentiation may be modulated by hormonal manipulation even in species with a genotypic rather than environmental mechanism of sex determination. Does this also apply to mammals?

THE FREEMARTIN MODEL

Freemartins are bovine females resulting from a heterosexual twin pregnancy. In cattle, twin pregnancies are characterized by early placental anastomoses and exchange between the fetal circulations has been held responsible for the masculinization of the freemartin reproductive tract (10). This involves absence of uterus and tubes, a feature which can be ascribed to the effect of AMH synthesized by the testes of the male twin. Müllerian regression occurs simultaneously in twins of both sexes (8), furthermore, AMH concentration in the circulation of both twins are significantly correlated (24).

However, Müllerian regression is not the only reproductive tract abnormality observed in the freemartin. Ovaries are usually absent, or reduced to fibrous streaks, longitudinal studies showed that the gonads cease to grow at the time Müllerian regression becomes apparent, beginning at day 52. At the same period, the number of germ cells, which in normal females increases 90-fold between 50 and 70 days, progressively decreases (7), germ cells are conspicuously absent from the gonads of adult freemartins (18).

Gonadal masculinization, characterized by seminiferous tubule development was observed in approximately 50% of freemartin fetuses but only after 90-100 days of gestation (7). Testosterone-dependent growth of seminal vesicles, epididymes and even prostate may also occur. Thus the freemartin effect involves a constant, early 'inhibitory' phase, marked by Müllerian and ovarian regression, and a later, non-obligatory, masculinizing phase, characterized by seminiferous tubule formation and masculinization of the internal genital tract. Functional masculinization can also be detected: the seminiferous tubules produce immunoreactive AMH (24) and both fetal (17) and adult (18) freemartin gonads produce testosterone.

While the hormonal cause of the freemartin reproductive lesions was recognized as early as 1917 (10), the nature of the endocrine factor has been recognized only recently. Struck by the chronological correlation between the inhibition of the freemartin gonad and that of the Müllerian ducts in both the male and the freemartin, Jost and his colleagues (8) suggested that both effects might be mediated by the same factor, originating at first in the testis of the male partner and later in the freemartin gonad itself. This view has now been confirmed by experimental data.

MORPHOLOGICAL EFFECT OF AMH UPON THE FETAL OVARY

The effect of AMH upon the morphology of the fetal ovary has been tested both *in vivo* and *in vitro*. The first experiments were performed by Vigier *et al.* (25) using rat fetal ovaries explanted at various ages in the presence or absence of purified bovine AMH. In cultures initiated at 14 days post coitum (pc) and maintained in culture 3 to 10 days, AMH consistently induced a characteristic freemartin effect, namely reduction of gonadal volume, germ cell depletion and differentiation, in the gonadal blastema, of epithelial cells with large, clear cytoplasm linked by interdigitations, resembling rat fetal Sertoli cells. After a prolonged period of culture, cords became delineated by a continuous basal membrane. The decrease of germ cell population in AMH-treated ovaries is detectable already 3 days after explantation, at a time when active oogonial proliferation is observed in controls, thus AMH appears to affect mitotic division of female germ cells rather than entry into meiotic prophase. Like Müllerian ducts, fetal ovaries respond to AMH only during a limited 'window' of sensitivity and are not affected by AMH treatment at 20 days pc.

Both the inhibitory and masculinizing effect of AMH upon fetal ovarian development can be obtained *in vivo*. Behringer *et al.* (1) generated a line of transgenic mice carrying a metallothionein-1 (MT)-AMH fusion gene. The MT promoter can direct expression of heterologous genes to a variety of

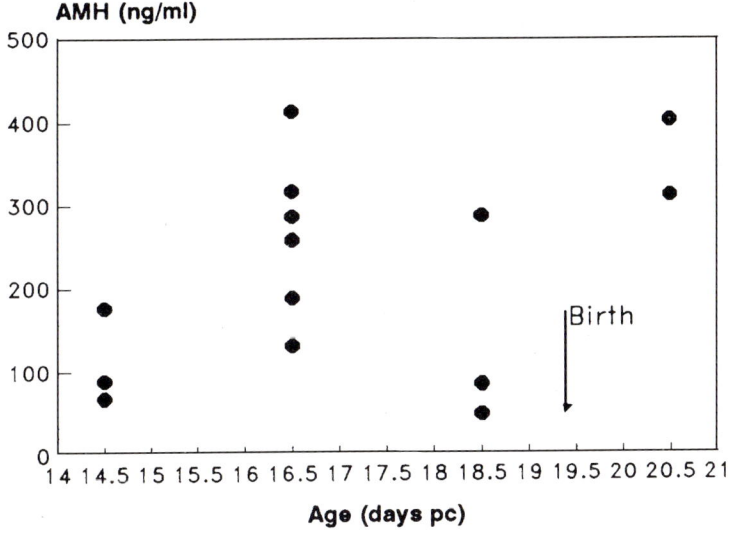

FIG. 1. AMH serum concentration in MT-hAMH transgenic female fetuses, measured by ELISA, using a monoclonal antibody specific for hAMH.

fetal and adult tissues in transgenic mice. Nearly all female progeny inheriting the transgene had a blind vagina and lacked uterus, oviducts and ovaries. Histological examination of the ovaries that persisted in transgenic females showed a range of ovarian morphology from normal to germ-cell deficient. When ovaries were examined 16 days after birth, cord-like structures bearing a striking resemblance to seminiferous tubules were observed.

Preliminary studies of prenatal development of this line of transgenic mice indicate that Müllerian regression is detectable as early as 14.5 pc, and is roughly correlated with the concentration of AMH measured by ELISA in fetal serum (Figs. 1 and 2). In contrast, ovarian stunting and germ cell depletion are noticeable only at 18.5 days pc, whereas in bovine freemartin fetuses, ovarian and Müllerian inhibition occur at the same time (8). A higher level of AMH is apparently needed to produce the ovarian effect than is required for Müllerian duct regression (1), therefore the discrepancy could be due to differences in AMH concentrations during fetal development. In bovine fetuses, serum AMH concentration peaks at the time of Müllerian regression (23), a situation not necessarily duplicated when the AMH gene is driven by a heterologous promoter.

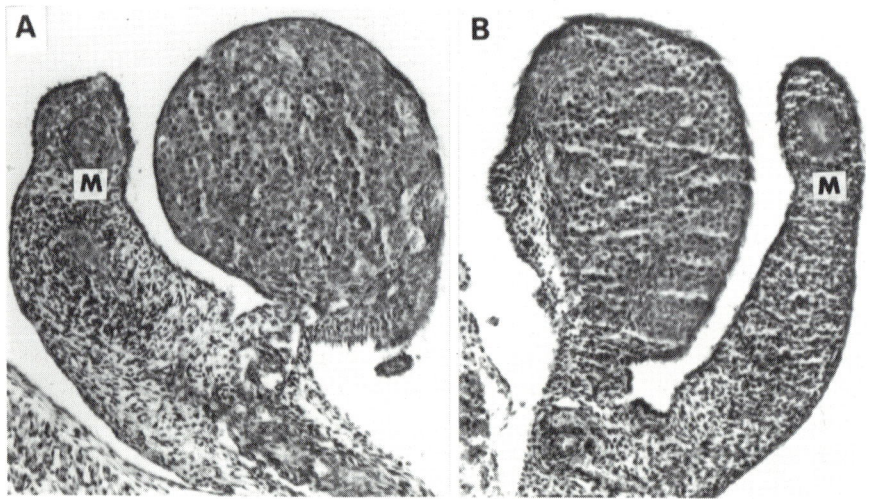

FIG. 2. Müllerian regression in a 14.5-day old female MT-hAMH mouse fetus (A), and normal control (B).

EFFECT OF AMH UPON THE FUNCTIONAL ACTIVITY OF THE FETAL OVARY

The seminiferous tubules induced in fetal ovaries by AMH treatment contain elements which resemble Sertoli cells from both a morphological and a functional viewpoint. Prolonged exposure of rat fetal ovaries to

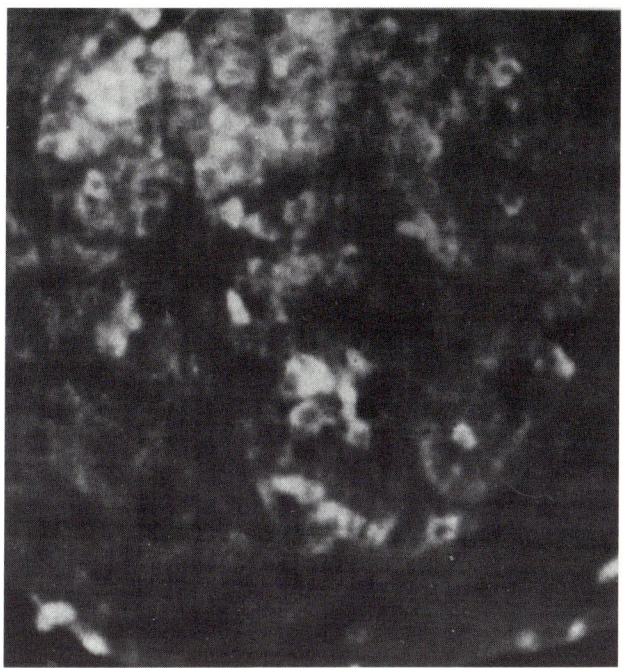

FIG. 3. Immunocytochemical detection of AMH secretion in seminiferous tubules induced in a fetal ovary of a 14.5-day old rat fetus by culture in the presence of hAMH (10 µg/ml during 10 days. Courtesy of Dr. S. Magre (unpublished).

recombinant AMH induces them to produce AMH (Fig. 3), as do fetal freemartin ovaries (24).

AMH can also reproduce *in vitro* the endocrine sex reversal which leads freemartin ovaries to produce testosterone. Ovine fetal ovaries exposed to AMH release testosterone instead of estradiol, due to decrease of aromatase activity (22). This observation has led to the development of a quantitative and interspecific test for the bioactivity of AMH: the fetal ovary aromatase assay (3) (Fig. 4). Linear responses as a function of the logarithm of AMH concentration were observed over ranges of 0.2-7.5 µg/ml for the bovine protein and 0.15-2.0 µg/ml for the human recombinant protein (26), monoclonal antibodies to either bovine or human recombinant AMH decreased hormone bioactivity in this system. Analysis of the species specificity of the fetal ovary aromatase assay indicated that turtle and rat fetal ovaries responded to AMH of other vertebrate classes, whereas aromatase activity of chick embryo ovaries could be repressed only by the homospecific hormone, partially purified from embryonic chick testes (Fig. 5). These findings are in keeping with previously reported data (20) which indicated that rat fetal Müllerian ducts regress when co-cultured with chick testes, but not the opposite.

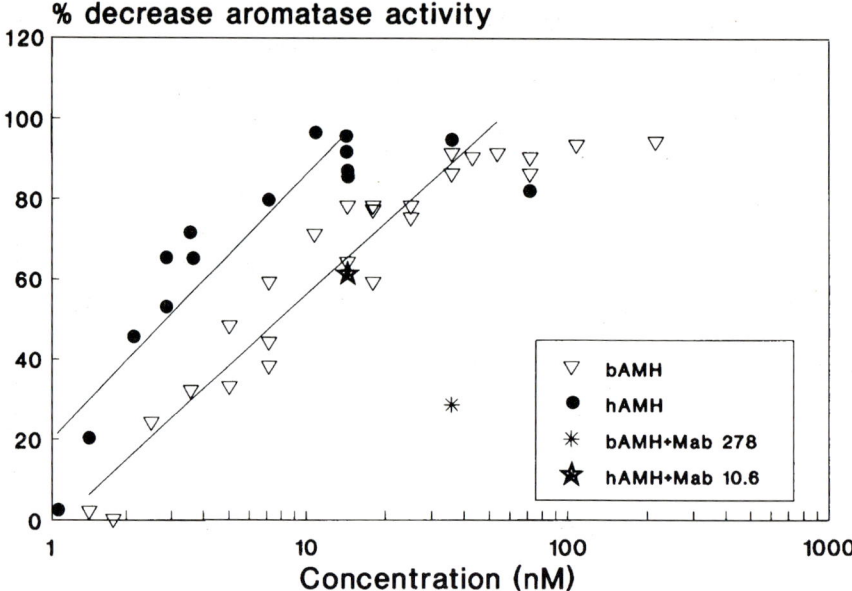

FIG. 4. Validation of a quantitative bioassay for AMH based upon the inhibition of aromatase activity of dibutyryl cyclic AMP-stimulated 16-day-old rat fetal ovaries. Each point represents the mean of triplicate experiments. See Reference 3 for details. Reproduced from Reference 3 with permission.

MECHANISM OF AMH-INDUCED OVARIAN LESIONS: RELATIONSHIP TO TESTICULAR DIFFERENTIATION

In the normal ovary, oocytes induce the supporting cell lineage to develop as follicle cells, and it is the continued presence of oocytes that maintains follicles (11). Ovaries without germ cells, as for instance those of human 45X females, degenerate. It follows that the ovarian aplasia observed in freemartins and in female AMH transgenic mice is probably a consequence of the deleterious effect of AMH upon XX germ cells. Whether AMH-induced virilization of the fetal ovary is a consequence of non-specific germ cell degeneration due to prolonged culture has been debated. Conflicting data have been reported. Taketo *et al.* (19) obtained development of seminiferous tubules by transplantation of fetal ovaries under the kidney capsule of male mice, and concluded that fetal ovaries at early stages of development can form testicular structures, even in the absence of any male-specific factors. Prépin and Hida (15) have reported that fetal rat ovaries maintained 16 days in organ culture lose their germ cell population and develop cord-like structures with anti-Müllerian activity. However at the developmental period tested by these authors, normal ovaries already produce

AMH (21). Since, within the experimental conditions used in the reported studies (1,25), no masculinization occured in control ovaries not exposed to AMH, the virilizing effect of AMH does appear specific.

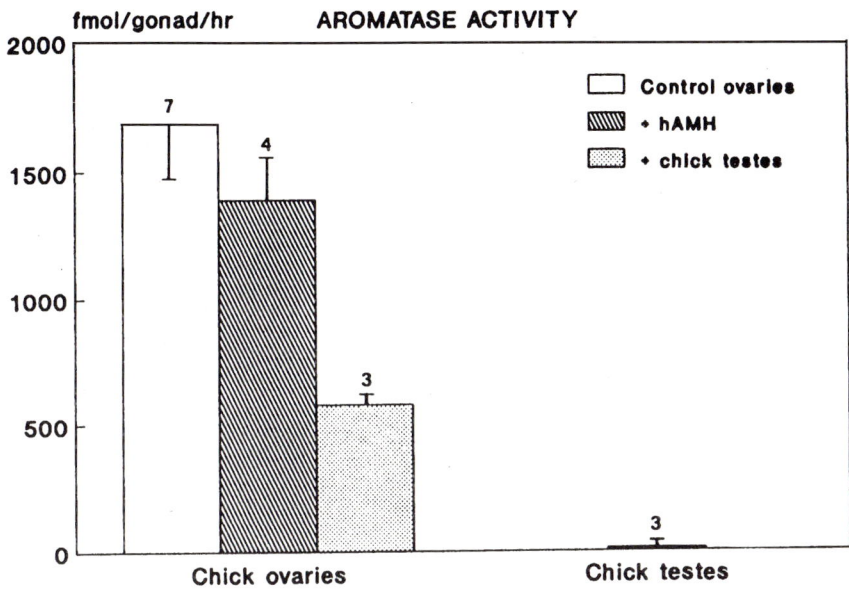

FIG. 5. Species-specificity of AMH effect upon aromatase activity of chick embryonic ovaries. One, quartered, 17-day-old chick embryo ovary was cultured either in control medium or in the presence of 10 μg/ml hAMH, or in association with two halved chick embryonic testes of the same age. Chick testes were cultured in control medium. Chick ovary aromatase activity is significantly ($P<0.01$) inhibited inhibited by co-culture with chick testes, but not by treatment with hAMH. From Reference 3 with permission.

The masculinizing effect of AMH on gonadal differentiation, hitherto reported only in fetal ovaries, warrants a discussion of the possibility that AMH may also be a paracrine factor acting during normal testicular differentiation. The testis-determining gene, by triggering Sertoli cell differentiation, also activates AMH gene expression. AMH decreases aromatase activity in the fetal ovary, and could conceivably have the same effect in the developing testis, although this has not been experimentally demonstrated. The effect of an aromatase inhibitor upon chick gonadal differentiation (5) could be interpreted as support for the hypothesis that AMH, by decreasing aromatase activity, plays an auxiliary role during testicular differentiation. However, the fact that testes differentiate normally in patients unable to produce AMH because of gene mutations (9) indicates that, at least in humans, AMH is not necessary for normal testicular organogenesis.

REFERENCES

1. Behringer R.R., Cate R.L., Froelick G.J., Palmiter R.D. and Brinster R.L. (1990) Abnormal sexual development in transgenic mice chronically expressing Müllerian inhibiting substance. Nature, 345:167-170.
2. Cate R.L., Mattaliano R.J., Hession C., Tizard R., Farber N.M., Cheung A., Ninfa E.G., Frey A.Z., Gash D.J., Chow E.P., Fisher R.A., Bertonis J.M., Torres G., Wallner B.P., Ramachandran K.L., Ragin R.C., Manganaro T.F., MacLaughlin D.T. and Donahoe P.K. (1986) Isolation of the bovine and human genes for müllerian inhibiting substance and expression of the human gene in animal cells. Cell, 45:685-698.
3. di Clemente N., Ghaffari S., Pepinsky R.B., Pieau C., Josso N., Cate R.L. and Vigier B. (1992) A quantitative and interspecific test for biological activity of anti-Müllerian hormone: the fetal ovary aromatase assay. Development, 114:721-727.
4. Dorizzi M., Mignot T.M., Guichard A., Desvages G. and Pieau C. (1991) Involvement of oestrogens in sexual differentiation of gonads as a function of temperature in turtles. Differentiation, 47:9-17.
5. Elbrecht A. and Smith R.G. (1992) Aromatase Enzyme activity and sex determination in chickens. Science, 255:467-470.
6. Jost A. (1953) Problems of fetal endocrinology: the gonadal and hypophyseal hormones. Recent Prog. Horm. Res., 8:379-418.
7. Jost A., Perchellet J.P., Prépin J., and Vigier B. (1975) The prenatal development of bovine freemartins. Symposium on Intersexuality, R. Reinborn ed, Springer Verlag, Berlin, 392-406.
8. Jost A., Vigier B., and Prépin J. (1972) Freemartins in cattle: the first steps of sexual organogenesis. J. Reprod. Fertil., 29:349-379.
9. Knebelmann B., Boussin L., Guerrier D., Legeai L., Kahn A., Josso N., and Picard J.Y. (1991) Anti-Müllerian hormone Bruxelles: a nonsense mutation associated with the persistent Müllerian duct syndrome. Proc. Natl. Acad. Sci. USA, 88:3767-3771.
10. Lillie F.R. (1917) The freemartin, a study of the action of sex hormones in foetal life of cattle. J. Exp. Zool., 23:371-452.
11. McLaren A. (1990) Of MIS and the mouse. Nature, 345:111-112.
12. Münsterberg A., and Lovell-Badge R. (1991) Expression of the mouse anti-Müllerian hormone gene suggests a role in both male and female sex differentiation. Development, 113:613-624.
13. Picard J.Y., and Josso N. (1984) Purification of testicular anti-Müllerian hormone allowing direct visualization of the pure glycoprotein and determination of yield and purification factor. Mol. Cell. Endocrinol., 34:23-29.
14. Pieau C. (1974) Différenciation du sexe en fonction de la température chez les embryons d'Emys orbicularis L. (Chélonien): effets des hormones sexuelles. Ann. Embryol. Morphol., 7:365-394.
15. Prépin J. and Hida N. (1989) Influence of age and medium on formation of epithelial cords in the rat fetal ovary in vitro. J. Reprod. Fertil., 87, 375-382.
16. Rashedi M., Maraud R. and Stoll R. (1983) Development of the testes in female domestic fowls submitted to an experimental sex reversal during embryonic life. Biol. Reprod., 29:1221-1228.
17. Shore L. and Shemesh M. (1981) Altered steroidogenesis by the fetal bovine freemartin ovary. J. Reprod. Fertil., 63:309-314.
18. Short R. V., Smith J., Mann T., Evans E.P., Hallett J., Fryer A. and Hamerton J.L. (1969) Cytogenetic and endocrine studies of a freemartin heifer and its bull co-twin. Cytogenetics, 8:369-388.
19. Taketo T., Koide S.S. and Merchant-Larios H. (1985) Gonadal sex differentiation in mammals. In: Origin and Evolution of Sex Halvorson H.O., Monroy A., eds. New-York: Alan R Liss,:271-288.
20. Tran D. and Josso N. (1977) Relationship between avian and mammalian anti-Müllerian hormone. Biol. Reprod., 16:267-273.
21. Ueno S., Takahashi M., Manganaro T.F., Ragin R.C., and Donahoe P.K. (1989) Cellular localization of mullerian inhibiting substance in the developing rat ovary. Endocrinology, 124:1000-1006.
22. Vigier B., Forest M.G., Eychenne B., Bézard J., Garrigou O., Robel P. and Josso N.

(1989) Anti-Müllerian hormone produces endocrine sex-reversal of fetal ovaries. Proc. Natl. Acad. Sci. USA, 86:3684-3688.
23. Vigier B., Tran D., Du Mesnil du Buisson F., Heyman Y. and Josso N. (1983) Use of monoclonal antibody techniques to study the ontogeny of bovine anti-Müllerian hormone. J. Reprod. Fertil., 69:207-214.
24. Vigier B., Tran D., Legeai L., Bézard J., and Josso N. (1984) Origin of anti-Müllerian hormone in bovine freemartin fetuses. J Reprod Fertil, 70:473-479.
25. Vigier B., Watrin F., Magre S., Tran D. and Josso N. (1987) Purified bovine AMH induces a characteristic freemartin effect in fetal rat prospective ovaries exposed to it in vitro. Development, 100:43-55.
26. Wallen J., Cate R.L., Kiefer D.M., Riemen M.W., Martinez D., Hoffman R.M., Donahoe P.K., Von Hoff D.D., Pepinsky B. and Oliff A. (1989) Minimal anti-proliferative effect of recombinant Müllerian inhibiting substance on gynecological tumor cell lines and tumor explants. Cancer Res., 49:2005-2011.
27. Wolff E., and Haffen K. (1952) Sur le développement et la différenciation sexuelle des gonades embryonnaires d'oiseau en culture in vitro. J. Exp. Zool., 119:381-399.

Sperm Biology: An Overview

S. Fishel

*NURTURE (Nottingham University Research & Treatment Unit in Reproduction),
Department of Obstetrics & Gynaecology,
University Hospital, Queen's Medical Centre,
Nottingham, NG7 2UH, UK*

First serious studies of sperm biology were reported in the 19th Century (19) with the discovery by Von Kolliker (1841) that the testis was the site of sperm formation. Von Leydig (21) published on the structure and characterisation of the Leydig cells in 1857, and Sertoli on the cells which were to bear his name 8 years later. (15) The structure and classification of germ cells in the seminiferous epithelium was elucidated by Von La Vallette in 1876 (20). For the next 30 years, into the beginning of this century, largely as a result of the work of Von Ebner (18), and also Benda (1), and Regaud, the process of spermatogenesis and the spermatogenic cycle were being uncovered.

Today we still marvel at the regulatory processes that take some of the stem cell spermatogonia, which replicate themselves continuously by mitosis, through to primary spermatocytes and then, by meiosis to the spherical shaped haploid spermatids, through spermiogenesis to generate the spermatozoa as we know them. These processes, spermatocytogenesis, meiosis and spermiogenesis take roughly a third each of the time of the spermatogenic cycle.

A morphological appraisal of spermiogenesis provides us with one of the most wondrous events in the cycle of any cell. Its metamorphosis, which can take 13.5 days in mice and 22 days in man, from the round spermatid to the spermatozoon, has three major stages - the Golgi/acrosomal phase, the formation of the sperm tail and mitochondrial migration. During the Golgi/acrosomal phase the Golgi apparatus-lysosomal complex begins to form vesicles which coalesce above one pole of the nucleus to form the acrosomal vesicle, and at some indeterminate time the membrane of these vesicles attaches to the nuclear envelope. Mechanisms which determine these events are unknown to us. At a similar time to acrosome vesicle development the centrioles translocate to the pole opposite the developing acrosome thus establishing a longitudinal polarity. The distal centriole will elaborate the flagellus and itself gradually disappear while the proximal centriole attaches to the nuclear envelope in what is called the implantation fossa. This gives rise to the connecting piece in the neck region; again the regulatory events associated with this process are unknown - although defects can lead to infertility.

At the start of spermiogenesis mitochondria are grouped around the nucleus of the spermatid; in an unknown non-random distribution these migrate to lie at the periphery of the cell just deep to the plasma membrane before a further mysterious migration to positions around the newly formed flagellum.

Eventually the whole shape of this cell changes as the acrosomal vesicle attaches to the nuclear envelope and the acrosomal cap balloons out to cover almost half the nuclear surface; the nucleus condenses and the spermatid assumes the characteristic elongated shape with a remainder of its original cytoplasm protruding partway down the flagellum. During this period other significant events occur, these include the development of the annulus which is associated with the mitochondrial movement towards the developing axoneme and will eventually delineate the lower border of the mitochondrial sheath. This latter structure in itself is a result of structural bonding occurring amongst the mitochondria as they are arranged very precisely in a helix around the axoneme, and the number of mitochondria in the sheath being genetically determined. This brief and incomplete view of the processes of spermiogenesis only hints at the degree of internal, local and peripheral regulation that occurs.

HORMONAL REGULATION OF SPERM DEVELOPMENT

Testicular function is controlled through the secretion of FSH and LH via the hypothalamo-hypophyseal complex. Lostroh, in 1969, demonstrated the need for FSH and LH for spermatogenesis after hypophysectomy. Since the finding, about 15-16 years ago, of receptors for FSH only in the seminiferous tubules there has been considerable debate as to the need for FSH for the maintenance of spermatogenesis.

That LH exerts its action through the stimulation of testosterone production by the Leydig cells, which carry receptors for LH, has been a view supported by much experimental evidence. That testosterone in high doses could maintain spermatogenesis at a level of greater than 85% after hypophysectomy and the report of Raj and Dym (12) demonstrating a failure of passive immunisation against FSH to markedly influence spermatogenesis, threw into question the role of FSH. More recent studies, notably those of Parvinen (10,11) suggested that the action of FSH varied according to the stage of the seminiferous cycle. The most clear (or complex!) lesson from the research of the last decade is that the testis is not an homogenous entity in terms of its biochemistry and physiology. In addition, local factors play an important role in modulating peripheral, especially FSH/LH, stimuli. Biochemical evidence now exists to align with specific cell association of the spermatogenic cycle wave. Each segment of seminiferous tubule is therefore a biochemical microcosm affecting physiological regulation.

For example: it is known that Sertoli cells provide numerous functions and these vary according to the stage of the spermatogenic cycle, and, furthermore, this in turn may be regulated by the particular population of germ cells surrounding the Sertoli cells. Parvinen and colleagues demonstrated that the number of FSH receptors is greatest at stages I and II of the spermatogenic cycle, peak secretion of androgen binding protein and plasminogen activator by the Sertoli cells occurs at stages VII and VIII (4) compared to peak transferrin secretion at stages IX to XIV. Plasminogen activator, which apparently reaches maximal secretion by the Sertoli cells at stages VII and VIII, has been suggested to be involved in opening up the inter-Sertoli cell junctions. This allows passage of the preleptotene spermatocytes from the basal to the luminal compartment. This movement also occurs at stages VII and VIII (13).

As a tool to try to comprehend and study the nature of the mechanisms that control the regulation of sperm development, two major sub-divisions have been considered: Leydig Cell Dependent Mechanisms and Sertoli Cell Dependent Mechanisms.

LEYDIG-CELL DEPENDENT MECHANISMS

Assuming as fact that the maintenance of spermatogenesis requires testosterone, this will be required from the Leydig cell as a result of Leydig cell steroidogenesis. Both peripheral and local mechanisms appear to regulate testosterone secretion by the Leydig cells.

A proteinaceous non-gonadotrophic secretion from the seminiferous tubules, probably from the Sertoli cells, may stimulate both basal and HCG-induced testosterone production by the Leydig cell. Production of this substance may be linked to the presence of specific germ cells within the epithelium, perhaps at stages VII and VIII of the cycle: the stage of maximal dependence upon testosterone. In turn, the production of testosterone by the Leydig cells will influence the seminiferous epithelium. Receptors for testosterone have been found on the peri-tubular myoid cells and the Sertoli cells (although not yet convincingly on germ cells). The presence of FSH and androgen will increase the number of androgen receptors (AR) on the Sertoli cells.

It is not yet clear whether the principal action of testosterone is exerted indirectly through the peri-tubular cells by the production of a protein (or proteins) that modulates Sertoli cell function and/or directly on Sertoli cells. In addition to androgen production, Leydig cells may influence sperm development by the latter being able to effect the capacity of the Sertoli cells to secrete inhibin. Recently Le Gac and de Kretser (5) have shown that HCG activity on the Leydig cells results in an increase in serum inhibin - an action not mediated through testosterone. Inhibin may have a local regulatory action on spermatogenesis.

SERTOLI-CELL DEPENDENT MECHANISMS

Structurally, Sertoli cells tenaciously exclude all germ cells - other than spermatogonia - from contact with the extracellular environment, principally as a result of their tight junctions. This blood-testis barrier, preventing intercellular transport of substrate/metabolites effectively makes the centrally-placed germ cells dependent solely on Sertoli cells, either for the transport of substrates or on the direct synthesis of them; for example, germ cells require lactate for glycolysis and depend upon Sertoli cells to convert glucose to lactate. Similarly, for their iron, germ cells depend upon the synthesis of transferrin by the Sertoli cells. As mentioned earlier, there therefore exists a complex of local control systems, at different stages of the seminiferous cycle - much of which is little understood. Sertoli cell activities include androgen binding protein (ABP) production, aromatase activity, and inhibin secretion. These products are released cyclically and possibly as a result of regulation by specific germ cell types. For example, the recent work of Le Maguresse and Jegou (6,7) suggest that germ cells may secrete a proteinaceous material which can positively influence Sertoli cell ABP and transferrin secretion, but inhibit oestradiol production.

The hormone regulation of sperm development and the stimulation of androgen receptor and activin receptor II gene expression will be considered in the following chapter (page 49).

Spermatogenesis and spermiogenesis, however wonderful and complex their control is, still represent only the initiation of a series of changes and functions occurring throughout both the male and female reproductive tracts before the primary function of the spermatozoon - its competence to fertilise an egg - is completed. The second chapter in this section (page 63) will consider further this biological maze - the control of sperm maturation in the epididymis. This important and vital part of the male reproductive tract has only found the limelight this past quarter of a century.

The epididymis is part of the excurrent duct system including the efferent ducts, the epididymis itself and the vas deferens. Throughout this ductal system the epithelium and lumen lend themselves to the necessary processes of absorption, secretion, metabolism, spermiophagy, sperm transport, provision of sperm fertilising ability (maturation) and sperm storage.

The epididymis comprises the initial segment (being joined to the testes by the ductuli efferentes), the head (Caput), the body (Corpus), the tail (Cauda) which itself is sub-divided into the proximal and distal regions - the latter extending to the vas deferens.

Given that the blood-testis barrier has been established anatomically and functionally for some considerable time, the existence of a blood-epididymis barrier has been mooted only since 1976 and recently demonstrated in the rat and hamster: although its existence is yet to be confirmed in man.

Three major spermatozoa-related functions can be attributed to the epididymis:

1) Conduit for transporting sperm from the ductuli efferentes to the vas deferens. The mechanisms responsible for this include - hydrostatic pressure, muscular constrictions and the action of cilia.

2) Storage of sperm. The major site is the cauda. Normal transit time is 3-10 days, but storage can be up to 30 days (many months in bats and they can still remain functional). Prolonged storage can lead to a decrease in fertilisation ability before loss in motility. A study published nearly 20 years ago by Martin-De Leon *et al.* (8) showed that fertisation using rabbit sperm aged in the cauda epididymis induced a tenfold increase in the incidence of chromosomal abnormalities in resulting blastocysts compared with their fresh counterparts.

3) The site of the maturation of sperm. One of the most consistent morphological changes noted in different species during its passage through the epididymis, is the migration of the cytoplasmic droplet from the region of the neck of the flagellum of the spermatozoon to the end of its midpiece (the mitochondrial sheath). The clear cells, identified only in the epididymis of some species, apparently internalise the remnants of the cytoplasmic droplets. In addition, spermatozoa from a number of species undergo a change in shape, size and/or internal structure of the acrosome, although the latter seems not to occur in man.

An array of biochemical alterations have been reported to occur during the traverse of spermatozoa through the excurrent ducts. Among which are, for example, an increase in the anionic charge on spermatozoa, an increase in the number of concanavalin A binding sites as well as a decreased ability toactivate complement. The lipid composition and the sperm plasma membrane in particular change dramatically during transit.

Although spermatozoa acquire the ability to fertilise only after leaving the testes and passing through the epididymis, it is now clear that the epididymis plays an active rather than passive role in sperm maturation. There is also species variation as to in which segment of the epididymis particular aspects of maturation occur. In addition, the sperm acquire motility during their passage. The underlying cellular and molecular mechanisms for acquiring motility are unclear, but, for example, the following compounds have been proposed - a forward-motility protein, acidic epididymal glycoprotein and albumin, carnitine, cAMP, sperm motility inhibitory factor - etc. Recent data demonstrate that in laboratory animals, specific epitopes present on epididymal principal cells can be transferred to particular domains of the sperm surface. This transfer of material is associated with fertilising competence.

The changes occurring in the epididymis are vital for the molecular interactions between a spermatozoon and egg. The work of Fournies-Delpech and colleagues in 1983 (2) and 1987 (3) showed that the capacity of spermatozoa to bind to the zona pellucida is dependent upon androgen which in turn is dependent upon protein synthesis occurring in the epididymis. The elucidation of the molecular basis of sperm-oocyte interaction is a vitally important area of research, central to the development of contraceptive techniques, and overcoming male infertility.

The zona pellucida is a sulfated glycoprotein, and several different families of glycoproteins have been identified in the zonae of various species. How these glycoproteins are distributed in the zona pellucida is not accurately known. For example, the zona pellucida glycoprotein 2 (ZP2) of mouse zona is distributed throughout the thickness of the zona; whereas in the pig, ZP1, ZP2 and ZP3 glycoproteins are all present on the external surface of the zona. The fertilising spermatozoon binds to the surface of the zona pellucida before penetrating it. It is a reasonable assumption that the surface of the spermatozoon carries receptors for recognising particular zona molecules. Sperm membrane proteins have been shown to have a strong affinity for zona molecules (9,14). The primary sperm receptor on the zona pellucida of mice has been characterised as ZP3, to which a spermatozoon binds before the acrosome reaction. Binding then occurs at the 'secondary' sperm receptor, ZP2, after the acrosome reaction has occurred (16,17).

A number of studies have been concerned with sequencing the primary amino acid structure of ZP3, and this has been determined for a number of mammalian species. It is a highly conserved molecule with approximately 80% sequence homology. The chapter by Professor Aitken (page 75) considers the molecular basis of sperm-oocyte interaction, the crucial event in the procreation of each and every animal species.

REFERENCES

1. Benda, C. (1887) Utersuchungen uber den Bau des funktionierenden samenkanalchens einiger saugetiere and Folgerungen fur die spermatogenese dieser wirbeltierklasse. Arch. Microscope. Anat., 30:49-110.
2. Fournier-Delpech, S., Hamamah S., Colas G. and Courot, M. (1983) Acquisition of zona binding structures by ram spermatozoa during epidiymal passage. In: The sperm cell, edited by Andre, J., pp 103-110. M. Nijhoff, The Hague.
3. Fournier-Delpech S. and Courot M. (1987) Sperm-zona pellucida binding activity. Oxford. Rev. Reprod. Biol., 9:294-321.
4. Lacroix, M., Parvinen, M. and Fritz I.B. (1981) Localization of testicular plasminogen activator in discrete portions (stages VII and VIII) of the seminiferous tubule. Biol. Reprod., 25:143-146.
5. Le Gac F. and de Kretser D.M. (1982) Inhibin production by Sertoli cells. Mol. Cell. Endocrinol., 28:487-498.
6. Le Maguresse B. and Jegou B. (1988) In vitro effects of germ cells on the secretory activity of Sertoli cells recovered from rats of different ages. Endocrinology, 22:1672-1680.
7. Le Maguresse B. and Jegou B. (1988) Paracrine control of immature Sertoli cells by adult germ cells in the rat (an in vitro study). Cell-cell interactions within the testis. Mol. Cell. Endocrinol., 58:65-72.
8. Martin-De Leon, P.A., Shaver, E.L. and Gammal, E.B. (1973) Chromosome abnormalities in rabbit blastocytes resulting from spermatozoa aged in the male tract. Fertil. Steril., 24:212-219.

9. O'Rand, M.G., Matthews, J.E., Welch, J.E. and Fishel, S.J. (1985) Identification of zona binding sites on rabbit spermatozoa and induction of the acrosome reaction by solubilized zonae. Dev. Biol., 119:551-559.
10. Parvinen, M. (1982) Regulation of the seminiferous epithelium. Endocr. Rev., 3:404-417.
11. Parvinen, M., Vihko, K.K. and Topapri, J. Cell interactions during the seminiferous epithelial cycle. Int. Rev. Cytology, 104:115-151.
12. Raj, H.J.M. and Dym, M. (1976) The effects of selective withdrawal of FSH or LH on spermatogenesis in the immature rat. Biol. Reprod., 14:489-494.
13. Russell, L.D. (1977) Movement of spermatocytes from the basal to the adluminal compartments of the rat testis. Am. J. Anat., 148:313-328.
14. Sullivan, R. and Bleau, G. (1985) Interaction of isolated components from mammalian sperm and egg. Gamete Research, 12:101-116.
15. Sertoli, E. (1865) Dell'esistenzia di particolari cellule ramificate nei canalicoli seminiferi del testiculo humano. Il Morgagni, 7:31-39.
16. Wassarman, P.M., Florman, H.M. and Greve, J.M. (1985) Receptor-mediated sperm-egg interactions in mammals. In: Fertilization, Vol. 2, edited by Metz, C.B., Monroy, A., pp 341-360. Academic Press, New York.
17. Watson, P.F. and Plummer J.M. (1986) Relationship between calcium binding sites and membrane fusing during the acrosome reaction induced by ionophore in ram spermatozoa. J. Exp. Zool., 238:113-118.
18. Von Ebner, V. (1871) Untersuchungen uber den Bau der Samenkanalchen und die Entwicklung der spermatozoiden bei den Saugenticren und beim Menschen. Leipzig: Rollets Untersuchungen aus dem Institut fur Physiologie und Histologie in Graz, p2 00.
19. Von Kolliker, R.A. (1841) Beitrage zur Kenntnis der Geschlechts-verhaltnisse und der Samenflussigkeit wirbelloser Tiere. Berlin.
20. Von La Vallette St. G. (1876) Uber die Genese der Samenkorper. Arch. Mikroscop. Anat., 12:797-822.
21. Von Leydig, F. (1857) Lehrbuch der Histologie des Menschen und der Tiere. Frankfurt am Main.

Control of Sperm Development by Hormones and Growth Factors: Testicular Expression of Receptor-Encoding Genes

J.A. Grootegoed, W.M. Baarends, L.J. Blok,
J.P. de Winter, M. van Helmond, J.W. Hoogerbrugge,
F.H. de Jong and A.P.N. Themmen

Department of Endocrinology & Reproduction, Medical Faculty, Erasmus University Rotterdam, P.O. Box 1738, 3000 DR Rotterdam, The Netherlands

INTRODUCTION

In this chapter, we will discuss sperm development from the primordial germ cell stage up to spermiation, in relation to actions of hormones and growth factors.

One of the first steps in gametogenesis involves the migration of primordial germ cells into the developing gonads during embryogenesis. The primordial germ cells are closely associated with the cells over which they migrate, moving by extending filopodia. In recent years, it has become clear that one aspect of the embryonic migration of primordial germ cells involves a mechanism of ligand-receptor interaction. The receptor is encoded by the proto-oncogene *c-kit*, and is a cell surface receptor of the tyrosine kinase family. The proto-oncogene *c-kit* is allelic with the murine *dominant white spotting* (W) locus. Mutations at the W locus cause sterility, due to migration failure of the primordial germ cells. In addition, migration of mast cells, hemopoietic stem cells and melanocytes is affected. Sterility and other cell migration related defects are also caused by mutation of the murine Steel (Sl) locus, and it is now known that the *Steel* gene product is the ligand for *c-kit*. This ligand is a peptide growth factor, called mast cell growth factor (MGF) or stem cell factor (SCF), and is produced in both soluble and plasma membrane-bound forms (see Reference 23 for a review).

SCF mRNA is expressed in many regions of the early mouse embryo, including the areas of migration of the primordial germ cells. It is unlikely that the SCF/*c-kit* interaction guides the primordial germ cells to the genital ridges, but it has been shown that this interaction generates a cell survival signal (15,17,36).

The role of the Sl and W products is not limited to the embryo. There is evidence that this ligand-receptor interaction is involved later in spermatogenesis, because differentiated A spermatogonia express *c-kit* mRNA whereas Sertoli cells express SCF mRNA (37,43,52).

This illustrates that the embryonic and postnatal parts of the life-history of spermatozoa should be regarded as serial events.

Shortly after birth, in the rat (which is the animal of choice in many studies concerning endocrine control of spermatogenesis), undifferentiated A spermatogonia that have evolved from the primordial germ cells develop into differentiating A_1 spermatogonia. This step is controlled by retinoic acid (33), a vitamin A metabolite that interacts with nuclear retinoic acid receptors (RAR) and regulates gene expression through similar mechanisms as the steroid hormones. The RA/RAR signal might act directly on A spermatogonia, but it is also possible that the retinoic acid-induced differentiation and proliferation of A spermatogonia involves the action of retinoic acid on Sertoli cells. The formation of A_1 spermatogonia can be viewed as a point of no return in spermatogenesis. Once the developing germ cells have passed this point, spermatogenesis proceeds according to a precise and well-defined schedule.

The initiation and maintenance of spermatogenesis during postnatal life requires testicular actions of the gonadotropic hormones LH (luteinizing hormone or lutropin) and FSH (follicle-stimulating hormone or follitropin). The LH signal is translated into an androgenic signal, through actions of LH on Leydig cell development and steroidogenesis. Several products from Leydig cells may exert effects on testicular tubules, but within the context of the present chapter the role of Leydig cells will be viewed as being confined to the production of testosterone.

The cellular target of FSH action in the testis is well defined, since Sertoli cells seem to be the only cell type that expresses the FSH receptor. Testosterone action, however, is considerably more complex. In addition to Sertoli cells, the peritubular myoid cells are involved in androgen action on the testicular tubules (42). Classical ligand binding studies (18), as well as studies on mRNA and protein expression that make use of specific cDNA probes and antibodies which have become available after the molecular cloning of the androgen receptor (47), have shown the presence of the androgen receptor in peritubular myoid cells and Sertoli cells, but not in the developing germ cells. There is good evidence that androgen action on peritubular myoid cells induces the production of a peptide growth factor that exerts a major stimulatory role on Sertoli cell function (42). This interaction between peritubular myoid cells and Sertoli cells may be of the same kind as the mesenchymal-epithelial cell interaction that plays a role in prostate development (14). Observations that FSH stimulates the differentiation of peritubular myoid cells (39) indicate that there is a reciprocal interaction between Sertoli cells and peritubular myoid cells.

ACTIONS OF FSH AND ANDROGEN

Testicular non-steroidal factors, produced locally by interstitial and peritubular cells, may play various roles in the regulatory network that controls Sertoli cell activities. However, it is also true that direct actions of testosterone and FSH on Sertoli cells must be of crucial importance in the hormonal control of spermatogenesis. With this in mind, we have carried out experiments to study these direct actions, using isolated Sertoli cells that were cultured on a plastic substratum in the absence of added extracellular matrix components or other cell types. These studies aimed at obtaining biochemical information and molecular tools, that can be used to tackle physiological questions.

One such a physiological question concerns the apparent co-operativity between androgens and FSH in the initiation and maintenance of spermatogenesis (5,24). Studies on protein synthesis by cultured rat Sertoli cells have indicated that either of these two hormones, acting through vastly different mechanisms, stimulates the synthesis of the same proteins, in addition to hormone-specific regulation of the synthesis of several proteins (4). The latter may offer a biochemical explanation for co-operativity.

With respect to FSH action, the transcription of a number of genes is rapidly activated. One example is the inhibin α-subunit gene (25,46). The promoter of this gene contains a cyclic AMP response element (CRE), that most likely is responsible for an increased rate of gene transcription following FSH-induced activation of adenylyl cyclase. Recently, we have investigated whether FSH might exert an effect on the transcription of the gene that encodes the androgen receptor (AR).

In the course of these studies, we were surprised to find that stimulation of cultured Sertoli cells with FSH resulted in rapid down-regulation of AR mRNA expression (9). Further experiments showed that this down-regulation was probably caused by AR mRNA destabilization, because no effect of FSH was observed when the rate of gene transcription was measured using a nuclear run-on assay (9). FSH-induced down-regulation of AR mRNA expression is not an artefact of the cell isolation and culture procedures, because a single injection of FSH (1 µg/g body weight) in intact immature rats resulted in a comparable effect (Fig. 1).

Furthermore, the expression of mRNA encoding the FSH receptor was also down-regulated by FSH (45), in cultured Sertoli cells and in whole testes from immature rats. This effect on FSH receptor mRNA expression is comparable to ligand-induced down-regulation of LH receptor mRNA expression in the ovary (13,34) and may serve a physiological function related to the control of FSH sensitivity of Sertoli cells.

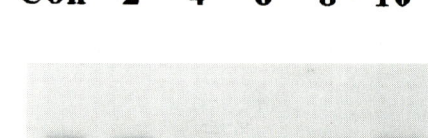

FIG. 1. Effect of FSH on testicular androgen receptor mRNA exspression. Intact 3-week-old rats were injected i.p. with 1 µg/g ovine FSH-S16 and sacrificed 2,4,6,8 or 10 h after injection (Con = 4 h control injected with saline). For Northern analysis, 20 µg of total RNA from whole testes was applied per lane and hybridized to a human androgen receptor cDNA probe (from Reference 9).

The function for FSH-induced down-regulation of testicular AR mRNA expression, however, is not obvious. Also, it was found that this down-regulation was transient, so that 8 h after addition of FSH the AR mRNA had returned to the starting level. Within this 8 h period of FSH treatment, the AR protein level (estimated by Schatchard analysis of the binding of the synthetic androgen R1881) had not significantly decreased (9).

In the cultured Sertoli cells, the transient FSH-induced loss of AR mRNA was followed by an increased expression, during 24-72 h of incubation of the cells in the presence of FSH (9), confirming earlier findings (7,48). In Sertoli cells isolated from 15-day-old rats, this effect was more pronounced than in Sertoli cells from 25-day-old donors, as was also reflected by the magnitude of the effect of FSH on ^{3}H-R1881 binding (Fig. 2).

This long-term stimulatory effect of FSH might play a role in regulating the responsiveness of Sertoli cells to androgens during testis development, and therefore this stimulation was investigated in more detail. The question was asked whether or not FSH-activated signal transduction pathways could stimulate AR gene transcription. Analysis of the AR gene promoter had not revealed the presence of a CRE or any other consensus hormone response element (2), but this does not exclude that FSH can stimulate transcription of this gene. Promoter and leader sequences of the androgen receptor gene were cloned in front of a luciferase reporter gene, and the constructs were transiently transfected into freshly isolated clusters of Sertoli cells. It was then found that treatment of the transfected cells with dibutyryl cAMP resulted in approximately 2-fold stimulation of the transcription of constructs that contained 1.5 kb or more of the sequences 5′ of the transcription start site (10). The DNA sequences that are responsible for this effect have not yet been identified, but the results indicate that FSH may regulate AR gene expression in Sertoli cells through an effect on gene transcription.

The expression of the androgen receptor gene in several androgen-dependent tissues is dependent on the presence of ligand (35). In the prostate,

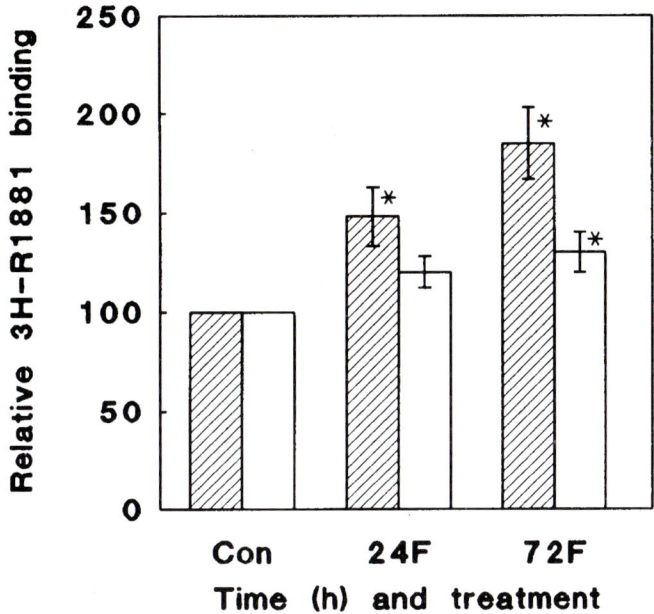

FIG. 2. Effect of FSH on ^{3}H-R1881 binding to Sertoli cells. The cells were isolated from 15-day-old (hatched bars) or 25-day-old (open bars) rats, and cultured for 24 h and 72 h in the presence of 500 ng/ml ovine FSH-S16 (Con = control). The experiment was repeated 4 times (the bars represent the mean ± SD); * significantly different from control ($P<0.01$) (from Reference 9).

this regulation involves a down-regulatory effect of androgens on AR mRNA expression, and a stabilizing effect of androgens on the receptor protein. In the testis and in cultured Sertoli cells, however, androgens do not exert a down-regulatory effect on AR mRNA expression (8).

The high local testosterone concentration in the testis from intact animals, causes complete transformation of all available ARs to a tight nuclear binding form (8). AR transformation and spermatogenesis are maintained when the testicular testosterone concentration is reduced to approximately 20%, using experimental protocols that will not be discussed herein (8,41). The testicular testosterone concentration that is required to maintain spermatogenesis, however, seems to be much higher than the normal circulating level (41,53).

The precise relationship between AR transformation (and activation of its activity as a transcription factor) and the testosterone concentration in Sertoli cells, at relatively low testicular testosterone concentrations (below the 20% level indicated above), is not known. To be able to study this relationship, we have started a search for primary response genes that are under direct regulatory control of androgens in Sertoli cells, using a subtraction hybridization strategy (3).

In the absence of data on androgen receptor transformation and regulation of gene expression at different testicular testosterone concentrations, it can only be speculated why a relatively high concentration seems to be necessary to maintain spermatogenesis. Possibly, not all testicular testosterone is available to the androgen receptors in Sertoli cells and peritubular myoid cells. Another possibility concerns an effect of androgens at the level of the cell surface of Sertoli cells and/or germ cells, through a mechanism comparable to that of progesterone action on spermatozoa or other steroid-mediated effects on various cell types (30).

SERTOLI CELL-GERM CELL INTERACTIONS

One important aspect of the concerted actions of testosterone and FSH on spermatogenesis is that these hormones stimulate and maintain Sertoli cell maturation and activities. Mature Sertoli cells are faced with the difficulty to support a large population of developing germ cells that requires a great variety of supportive actions. This high and complex work load, and the changes in cyto-architecture that are imposed upon Sertoli cells, may have a major effect on biochemical processes. This is reflected by the many changes in Sertoli cell activities and properties during the cycle of the spermatogenic epithelium (22,32).

The Sertoli cell barrier, constructed of tight junctional complexes between neighbouring Sertoli cells, is formed shortly before the first spermatocytes give rise to the haploid spermatids through meiotic divisions. From that time on, the transport of spermatocytes in early meiotic prophase across the Sertoli cell barrier brings new germ cells into the adluminal compartment of the testicular tubules, where the germ cells complete their development in close association with the Sertoli cells. This sets Sertoli cells the task to maintain a microenvironment with the proper physiological conditions, containing the required ion concentrations, substrates and proteins.

Relatively little is known about the biochemistry of cell-cell interactions in the spermatogenic epithelium. It is clear that Sertoli cells and germ cells have very different biochemical properties. Sertoli cells show remarkable flexibility and can perform many metabolic pathways at a high rate. Spermatocytes and spermatids apparently are much more constrained and specialized. One example concerns the metabolism of branched-chain amino acids. We have shown that Sertoli cells, like many other cell types, contain a high activity of branched-chain amino acid transferase and convert leucine to α-ketoisocaproate. Isolated spermatocytes and spermatids do not execute this transamination, but reduce α-ketoisocaproate to α-hydroxyisocaproate. This NADH-dependent reduction, catalyzed by the testis-specific lactate dehydrogenase isoenzyme LDH-C_4, might serve as an alternative mechanism for reoxidation of cytosolic NADH (19). Other examples concern the metabolism of carbohydrates and glutathione (11,12,20).

Structural interactions between Sertoli cells and spermatogenic cells have been described in much detail (38). Desmosomes and gap junctions are present between Sertoli cells and round germ cells, but are small in number. During late spermiogenesis the Sertoli cell-germ cell relation is intensified. A marked interaction between Sertoli and germ cells at this stage of spermatogenesis is evident from morphological observations on so-called ectoplasmic specializations and tubulobulbar complexes, and the spermiation process (38).

A NOVEL GROWTH FACTOR RECEPTOR

There is growing evidence that Sertoli cell-germ cell communication involves non-steroidal paracrine ligand-receptor systems (27,42). As described above, the expression of the SCF/*c-kit* system in the testis is one example of this type of communication. Other possible interactions include the actions of nerve growth factor (40) and members of the TGF-β superfamily of peptide growth factors (27). TGF-β is prototypic of a superfamily of growth, differentiation, and morphogenesis factors that includes in addition to five different TGF-βs, the activins, inhibins, anti-Müllerian hormone, bone morphogenic factors, and at least two other proteins from non-mammalian species. These different growth factors and their receptors are expressed in many cell types and tissues, eliciting a great variety of responses. In the testicular tubules, there is evidence for the production of ligands by Sertoli cells (TGF-βs, activin, inhibin, anti-Müllerian hormone) and germ cells (TGF-βs) (21,27,44).

The recent cloning of activin receptors II and IIB and the TGF-β type II receptor showed that these receptors belong to a new family of cell surface receptors, with a single hydrophobic transmembrane domain and a cytoplasmic serine/threonine kinase domain (1,26,28). This family also includes the *Caenorhabditis elegans* gene product daf-1 which controls certain aspects of larval development in response to an as yet unknown ligand (16). The activin IIB receptor gene generates four receptor isoforms through alternative splicing (1). The mechanism of action of TGF-βs is complex, and also involves type I and type III receptors (26). How the receptors interact with each other is not known, but the serine/threonine kinase domain of the type II receptors is probably a functional kinase in signal transduction.

We have shown, restricting the discussion here to rat testicular tubules, that activin receptor (ActR-II) mRNA is expressed in Sertoli cells (4 and 6 kb mRNAs) and in spermatocytes and round spermatids (4 kb mRNA) (49,50). Germ cells do employ translational control as an important mechanism for control of gene expression, and some expressed mRNAs may not be translated at all. However, the 4 kb mRNA in spermatids was found to be partly polysomal (50), and also binding of activin to spermatocytes and spermatids has been shown (51). There is no evidence that this binding originates from ActR-II mRNA, rather than from transcription of the ActR-IIB gene, but it is clear that spermatocytes and spermatids, in addition to Sertoli cells, are candidate activin target cells.

In the process of our attempts to clone new Sertoli cell-specific and/or hormonally regulated genes (3), we have recently obtained a cDNA clone encoding a new member of the TGF-β/activin receptor superfamily. Using an RNAse protection assay, it was found that this cDNA clone (called C14), hybridizes to a mRNA species that is highly expressed in ovaries and testes, whereas only a very low level of expression was detected in a few other

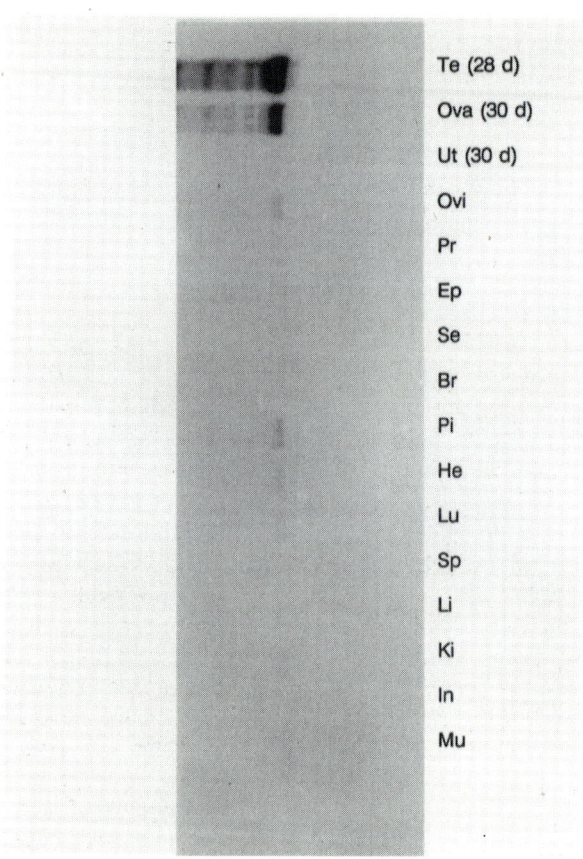

FIG. 3. Expression of clone C14 mRNA in various tissues. The amount of C14 mRNA was estimated using an RNAse protection assay. 10 µg total RNA was used, and the protected fragment has a length of 400 bp. RNA was isolated from testis (Te), ovary (Ova) and uterus (Ut) from 28/30-day-old rats, and from oviduct (Ovi) prostate (Pr), epididymis (Ep), seminal vesicle (Se), brain (Br), pituitary gland (Pi), heart (He), lung (Lu), spleen (Sp), liver (Li), kidney (Ki), intestine (In), and muscle (Mu) from adult rats.

tissues (Fig. 3). In the testis, mRNA expression was found in Sertoli cells, but not in other cell types.

Clone C14 shows a relatively low level of identity with the serine/threonine kinase domain of the other known receptors of the TGF-β receptor family (Fig. 4), but the kinase subdomains are present. The ligand and its source have not yet been identified.

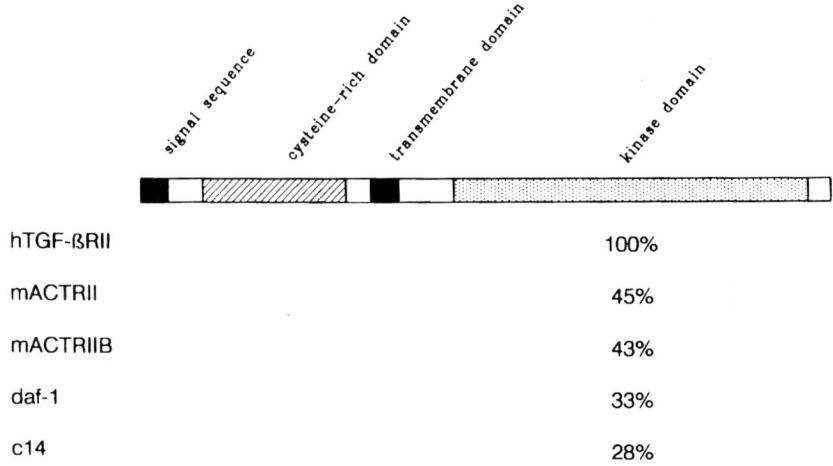

FIG. 4. Similarity of the kinase domain within the TGF-β/activin receptor superfamily. The figure shows the percentage similarity of the amino acid sequences of the serine/threonine kinase domain of the human TGF-β type II receptor, the mouse activin receptors types II and IIB, *Caenorhabditis elegans* daf-1 (1,16,26,28), and the cDNA clone C14 obtained from a rat Sertoli cell cDNA library (3).

POSSIBLE ROLES OF GROWTH FACTORS IN SPERMATOGENESIS

Once the germ cells have entered the stage of differentiating spermatogonia, further development reflects a cascade of genetically programmed events. The differentiating spermatogonia are irreversibly committed to becoming spermatozoa within a restricted time period. The onset of meiosis follows a defined series of spermatogonial divisions, and the duration of germ cell development through meiosis and subsequent spermatid formation is constant for a given species.

In this context, it can be speculated that possible roles of non-steroidal ligand-receptor systems mainly concern cell survival signals (such as SCF/*c-kit*) and effects on spermatogonial proliferation (27), or inductive interactions that do not interfere with the postulated genomic programming of the germ cells.

TGF-βs, possibly secreted by spermatocytes and spermatids (44), might act on Sertoli cells, in view of observations on biochemical effects of TGF-β1 on cultured porcine Sertoli cells (29). In addition, nerve growth factor and other, undefined, germ cell factors may act on Sertoli cells (22,40). This type of interaction may activate Sertoli cells to develop the cyto-architecture that is required for maintenance of spermatogenesis. Most notable in this respect is the cyclic regulation of Sertoli cell activities (22,32), such as the opening and closure of the Sertoli cell barrier during transport of developing germ cells from the basal to the adluminal compartment of the tubules. As discussed above, spermatid elongation involves the intensification of structural Sertoli cell-germ cell contacts. These contacts might be a conditio sine qua non for the complex process of spermatid elongation, and their selective disassembly could take part in the regulation of spermiation. Little is known about cell surface expression of proteins involved in the formation of Sertoli cell-germ cell contacts, such as cadherins and integrins (31). Some stimulatory effect on the assembly or disassembly of these cell-cell and cell-matrix contacts might be one possible outcome of ligand-receptor mediated Sertoli cell-germ cell communication.

Much more information is needed about the occurrence and actions of growth factors and their receptors in the testis. Many aspects remain to be studied, such as the local concentration gradients of growth factors and the threshold levels for receptor activation, binding affinities of the ligands to different receptors and the expression of receptor isoforms, the attachment of growth factors to extracellular matrix components, and so forth. The elucidation of the regulatory mechanisms involved in these and other Sertoli cell-germ cell interactions is an appreciable challenge for the future.

CONCLUDING COMMENT

It was discussed in the introduction to this chapter, that the embryonic and spermatogenic stages of sperm development are part of an integrated series of events. Similarly, there must be a link between the testicular and post-testicular stages of the life-history of spermatozoa. Unless experimental data indicate otherwise, it cannot be excluded that expression of receptor genes in spermatids has no role to play during spermatogenesis but is rather involved in sperm function. Alternatively, the encoded receptors might be active at both stages. Although not belonging to a family of growth factor receptors, the recently described PH-30 protein (6) may illustrate this point. The integral membrane protein PH-30 is a sperm surface protein involved in sperm-egg fusion, and it was postulated that this protein might also play a role in attachment of spermatogenic cells to Sertoli cells (6). A search for functions of receptors expressed by spermatogenic cells therefore should not disregard a possible role in some aspect of sperm function.

REFERENCES

1. Attisano, L., Wrana, J.L., Cheifetz, S. and Massagué, J. (1992) Novel activin receptors: Distinct genes and alternative mRNA splicing generate a repertoire of serine/threonine kinase receptors. Cell, 68:97-108.
2. Baarends, W.M., Themmen, A.P.N., Blok, L.J., Mackenbach, P., Brinkmann, A.O., Meijer, D., Faber, P.W., Trapman, J. and Grootegoed, J.A. (1990) The rat androgen receptor gene promoter. Mol. Cell. Endocrinol., 74:75-84.
3. Baarends, W.M., Helmond, M.J.L. van, Themmen, A.P.N. and Grootegoed J.A. (1992) Cloning of androgen-induced genes expressed in rat Sertoli cells using subtractive hybridization. 7th European Workshop on Molecular and Cellular Endocrinology of the Testis, Miniposter 27.
4. Bardin, C.W., Cheng, C.Y., Musto, N.A. and Gunsalus G.L. (1988) The Sertoli cell. In: The physiology of reproduction, edited by Knobil, E., Neil J.D. et al., pp 933-974. Raven Press, New York.
5. Bartlett, J.M.S., Weinbauer, G.F. and Nieschlag, E. (1989) Differential effects of FSH and testosterone on the maintenance of spermatogenesis in adult hypophysectomised rat. J. Endocrinol., 1:49-58.
6. Blobel, C.P., Wolfsberg, T.G., Turck, C.W., Myles, D.G., Primakoff, P. and White, J.M. (1992) A potential fusion peptide and an integrin ligand domain in a protein active in sperm-egg fusion. Nature, 356:248-252.
7. Blok, L.J., Mackenbach, P., Trapman, J., Themmen, A.P.N., Brinkmann, A.O. and Grootegoed, J.A. (1989) Follicle-stimulating hormone regulates androgen receptor mRNA in Sertoli cells. Mol. Cell. Endocrinol., 63:267-271.
8. Blok, L.J., Bartlett, J.M.S., Bolt-de Vries, J., Themmen, A.P.N., Brinkmann, A.O., Weinbauer, G.F., Nieschlag, E. and Grootegoed, J.A. (1992) Effect of testosterone deprivation on expression of the androgen receptor in rat prostate, epididymis and testis. Int. J. Androl., 15:182-198.
9. Blok, L.J., Hoogerbrugge, J.W., Themmen, A.P.N., Baarends, W.M., Post, M. and Grootegoed J.A. (1992) Transient down-regulation of androgen receptor mRNA expression in Sertoli cells by follicle-stimulating hormone is followed by up-regulation of androgen receptor mRNA and protein. Endocrinology, (in press).
10. Blok, L.J., Themmen, A.P.N., Peters A.H.F.M., Baarends, W.M., Hoogerbrugge, J.W. and Grootegoed, J.A. (1992) Transcriptional regulation of the androgen receptor (I): Effect of FSH on Sertoli cells. 7th European Workshop on Molecular and Cellular Endocrinology of the Testis, Miniposter 18.
11. Boer, P.J. den, Mackenbach, P. and Grootegoed, J.A. (1989) Glutathione metabolism in cultured Sertoli cells and spermatogenic cells from hamsters. J. Reprod. Fert., 87:391-400.
12. Boer, P.J. den, Poot, M., Verkerk, A., Jansen, R., Mackenbach, P. and Grootegoed, J.A. (1990) Glutathione-dependent defence mechanisms in isolated round spermatids from the rat. Int. J. Androl., 13:26-38.
13. Camp, T.A., Rahal, J.O. and Mayo, K.E. (1991) Cellular localization and hormonal regulation of follicle-stimulating hormone and luteinizing hormone receptor messenger RNAs in the rat ovary. Mol. Endocrinol., 5:1405-1417.
14. Cunha, G.R., Chung, L.W.K., Shannon, J.M., Taguchi, O. and Fujii, H. (1983) Hormone-induced morphogenesis and growth: role of mesenchymal-epithelial interactions. Recent Prog. Horm. Res. 39.559-598.
15. Dolci, S., Williams, D.E., Ernst, M.K., Resnick, J.L., Brannan, C.I., Lock, L.F., Lymans, S.D., Boswell, H.S. and Donovan, P.J. (1991) Requirement for mast cell growth factor for primordial germ cell survival in culture. Nature, 352:809-811.
16. Georgi, L.L., Albert, P.S. and Riddle, D.L. (1990) Daf-1, a *C. elegans* gene controlling dauer larva development, encodes a novel receptor protein kinase. Cell, 61:635-645.
17. Godin, I., Deed, R., Cooke, J., Zsebo, K., Dexter, M. and Wylie, C.C. (1991) Effects of the steel gene product on mouse primordial germ cells in culture. Nature, 352:807-808.
18. Grootegoed, J.A., Peters, M.J., Mulder, E., Rommerts, F.F.G. and Molen, H.J. van der (1977) Absence of a nuclear androgen receptor in isolated germinal cells of rat testis. Mol. Cell. Endocrinol., 9:159-167.
19. Grootegoed, J.A., Jansen, R. and Molen, H.J. van der (1985) Intercellular pathway of leucine catabolism in rat spermatogenic epithelium. Biochem. J., 226:889-892.
20. Grootegoed, J.A. and Boer, P.J. den (1989) Energy metabolism of spermatids: a review.

In: Cellular and molecular events in spermiogenesis, edited by Hamilton, D.W., Waites, G.M., pp 193-216. Cambridge University Press, Cambridge.
21. Grootenhuis, A.J., Timmerman, M.A., Hordijk, P.L. and Jong, F.H. de (1990) Inhibin in immature rat Sertoli cell conditioned medium: a 32 kDa $\alpha\beta$-B dimer. Mol. Cell. Endocrinol., 70:109-116.
22. Jégou, B., Syed, V., Sourdaine, P., Byers, S., Gérard, N., Velez de la Calle J., Pineau, Ch., Garnier, D.H., and Bauché, F. (1992) The dialogue between late spermatids and Sertoli cells in vertebrates: A century of research. In: Spermatogenesis-Fertilization-Contraception. Molecular, Cellular and Endocrine Events in Male Reproduction, edited by Nieschlag, E., Habenich, U.-F. pp 57-95. Springer-Verlag, Berlin.
23. Jessell, T.M. and Melton, D.A. (1992) Diffusable factors in vertebrate embryonic induction. Cell, 68:257-270.
24. Kerr, J.B., Maddocks, S. and Sharpe, R.M. (1992) Testosterone and FSH have independent, synergistic and stage-dependent effects upon spermatogenesis in the rat testis. Cell Tissue Res., 268:179-189
25. Klaij, I.A., Toebosch, A.M.W., Themmen, A.P.N., Shimasaki, S., Jong, F.H. de and Grootegoed, J.A. (1990) Regulation of inhibin α- and β_B-subunit mRNA levels in rat Sertoli cells. Mol. Cell. Endocrinol., 68:45-52.
26. Lin, H.Y., Wang, X.-F., Ng-Eaton, E., Weinberg, R.A. and Lodish, H.F. (1992) Expression cloning of the TGF-β type II receptor, a functional transmembrane serine/threonine kinase. Cell, 68:775-785.
27. Mather, J.P. and Krummen, L.A. (1992) Inhibin, activin and growth factors: paracrine regulators of testicular function. In: Spermatogenesis-Fertilization-Contraception. Molecular, Cellular and Endocrine Events in Male Reproduction, edited by Nieschlag, E., Habenicht, U.-F., pp 169-200. Springer-Verlag, Berlin.
28. Mathews, L.S. and Vale, W.W. (1991) Expression cloning of an activin receptor, a predicted transmembrane serine kinase. Cell, 65:973-982.
29. Morera, A.M., Esposito, G., Ghiglieri, C., Chauvin, M.A., Hartmann, D.J., and Benahmed, M. (1992) Transforming growth factor $\beta 1$ inhibits gonadotropin action in cultured porcine Sertoli cells. Endocrinology, 130:831-836.
30. Nemere, I. and Norman, A.W. (1991) Steroid hormone actions at the plasma membrane: induced calcium uptake and exocytotic events. Mol. Cell. Endocrinol., 80:C165-C169.
31. Palombi, F., Salanova, M., Tarone, G., Farini, D. and Stefanini, M. (1992) Distribution of beta-1 integrins in the rat seminiferous epithelium. 7th European Workshop on Molecular and Cellular Endocrinology of the Testis, Miniposter 66.
32. Parvinen, M. (1982) Regulation of the seminiferous epithelium. Endocr. Rev., 3:404-417.
33. Pelt, A.M.M. van, and Rooij, D.G. de (1990) The origin of the synchronization of the seminiferous epithelium in vitamin A-deficient rats after vitamin A replacement. Biol. Reprod., 42:677-682.
34. Piquette, G.N., LaPolt, P.S., Oikawa, M. and Hsueh, A.J.W. (1991) Regulation of luteinizing hormone receptor messenger ribonucleic acid levels by gonadotropins, growth factors, and gonadotropin-releasing hormone in cultured rat granulosa cells. Endocrinology, 128:2449-2456.
35. Quarmby, V.E., Yarbrough, W.G., Lubahn, D.B., French, F.S. and Wilson, E.M. (1990) Autologous down-regulation of androgen receptor mRNA. Mol. Endocrinol., 4:22-28.
36. Raff, M.C. (1992) Social controls on cell survival and cell death. Nature, 356:397-400.
37. Rossi, P, Albanesi, C., Grimaldi, P. and Geremia, R. (1991) Expression of the mRNA for the ligand of c-kit in mouse Sertoli cells. Biochem. Biophys. Res. Commun., 176:910-914.
38. Russell, L.D. (1980) Sertoli-germ cell interactions: a review. Gamete REs., 3:179-202.
39. Schlatt, S., Weinbauer, G.F., Arslan, M.A. and Nieschlag, E. (1992) Testosterone induces the appearance of α-smooth muscle actin in peritubular cells of the immature monkey testis: potentiation by FSH. 7th European Workshop on Molecular and Cellular Endocrinology of the Testis, Miniposter 36.
40. Seidl, K. and Holstein, A.F. (1990) Evidence for the presence of nerve growth factor (NGF) and NGF receptors in human testis. Cell Tissue Res., 261:549-554.
41. Sharpe R.M., Donachie, K. and Cooper, I. (1988) Re-evaluation of the intratesticular level of testosterone required for quantitative maintenance of spermatogenesis in the rat. J. Endocrinol., 117:19-26.
42. Skinner, M.K. (1991) Cell-cell interactions in the testis. Endocr. Rev., 12:45-77.
43. Sorrentino, V., Giorgi, M., Geremia, R., Besmer, P. and Pellegrino, R. (1991) Expression of the c-kit proto-oncogene in the murine male germ cells. Oncogene, 6:149-151.

44. Teerds, K.J. and Dorrington, J.H. (1992) Localization of TGF-β1 and TGF-β2 in the rat testis. 7th European Workshop on Molecular and Cellular Endocrinology of the Testis, Miniposter 80.
45. Themmen, A.P.N., Blok, L.J., Post, M., Baarends, W.M., Hoogerbrugge, J.W., Parmentier, M., Vassart, G. and Grootegoed, J.A. (1991) Follitropin receptor down-regulation involves a cAMP-dependent post-transcriptional decrease of receptor mRNA expression. Mol. Cell. Endocrinol., 78:R7-R13.
46. Toebosch, A.M.W., Robertson, D.M., Klaij, I.A., Jong, F.H. de and Grootegoed, J.A. (1989) Effects of FSH and testosterone on highly purified rat Sertoli cells: inhibin α-subunit mRNA expression and inhibin secretion are enhanced by FSH but not by testosterone. J. Endocrinol., 122:757-762.
47. Trapman, J., Klaassen, P., Kuiper, G.G.J.M., Korput, J.A.G.M. van der, Faber, P.W.F., Rooij, H.C.J. van, Geurts van Kessel, A., Voorhorst, M.M., Mulder, E. and Brinkmann, A.O. (1988) Cloning, structure and expression of a cDNA encoding the human androgen receptor. Biochem. Biophys. Res. Commun., 153:241-248.
48. Verhoeven, G. and Cailleau, J. (1988) Follicle stimulating hormone and androgens increase the concentration of the androgen receptor in Sertoli cells. Endocrinology, 122:1541-1550.
49. Winter, J.P. de, Themmen, A.P.N., Hoogerbrugge, J.W., Klaij, I.A., Grootegoed, J.A. and Jong, F.H. de (1992) Activin receptor mRNA expression in rat testicular cell types. Mol. Cell. Endocrinol., 83:R1-R8.
50. Winter, J.P. de, Kant, H.J.G. van de, Hoogerbrugge, J.W., Rooij, D.G. de, Themmen, A.P.N., Grootegoed, J.A. and Jong, F.H. (1992) Activin receptor mRNA expression in germ cells of the male rat. 7th European Workshop on Molecular and Cellular Endocrinology of the Testis, Miniposter 75.
51. Woodruff, T.K., Borree, J., Attie, K.M., Cox, E.T., Rice, G.C. and Mather J.P. (1992) Stage-specific binding of inhibin and activin to subpopulations of rat germ cells. Endocrinology, 130:871-881.
52. Yoshinaga, K., Nishikawa, S., Ogawa, M., Hayashi, S.-I., Kunisada, T., Fujimoto, T. and Nishikawa, S.-I. (1991) Role of c-kit in mouse spermatogenesis: identification of spermatogonia as a specific site of c-kit expression and function. Development, 113:689-699.
53. Zirkin, B.R., Santulli, R., Awoniyi, A. and Ewing, L.L. (1989) Maintenance of advanced spermatogenic cells in the adult rat testis: quantitative relationship to testosterone concentration within the testis. Endocrinology, 124:3043-3049.

Epididymal Control of Sperm Maturation in Mammals

H.D.M. Moore

Institute of Zoology, Regent's Park, London NW1 4RY, UK

INTRODUCTION

Over sixty years ago, Young (1931) showed that guinea-pigs inseminated with spermatozoa from the proximal region of the epididymis, had a pregnancy rate of less than half that for females inseminated with spermatozoa from the distal epididymis. He concluded from these experiments that spermatozoa undergo a maturation process within the epididymal lumen. However, not until the classical ligation experiments, carried out by Orgebin-Crist (29) and Bedford (1) was it fully appreciated that the development of the fertilizing capacity of mammalian spermatozoa was dependent on an essential contribution from the epididymis under the control of androgens. Since this time, the exact region of the epididymis where spermatozoa acquire their fertilising capacity has been established for most laboratory and domestic species by *in vivo* insemination and/or *in vitro* fertilization (see References 18,19). At the gross morphological level, the precise position along the convoluted epididymal duct where spermatozoa first develop fertility may vary between species but when an examination is made at the ultrastructural level, it is associated normally with a similar epithelial morphology, usually in the corpus epididymidis. In a rodent, such as the hamster, for example, the fertilizing capacity of spermatozoa increases from less than 5% in the distal corpus epididymidis to over 75% in the proximal cauda epididymidis. These segments are only 3-5 mm apart and even when the duct is uncoiled represent a tubule length of only 4-6 cm (Fig. 1). During passage through this region, hamster spermatozoa acquire the ability to bind to and penetrate the zona pellucida and undergo fusion with the oolemma (15,22). The development of sperm fertility in the human epididymis is less well defined than in other species, although these is considerable indirect evidence that in the normal male a sperm maturation process does normally occur (6). Compared with ejaculated or cauda epididymal spermatozoa, those recovered from the proximal epididymis of men undergoing vasectomy (24) or from cancer or comatosed patients (13,9) display poor forward motility and have a very limited capacity to bind or penetrate human oocytes or to fuse with zona-free hamster eggs. Furthermore, after epididymovasostomy to relieve obstructive azoospermia due to blockage of the excurrent ducts, the likelihood of producing competent spermatozoa is generally low when the vas is anastomosed to the proximal first centimetre of duct (32). Occasionally, however, a very small proportion (1-3%) of human spermatozoa from the proximal epididymidis do exhibit progressive forward motility.

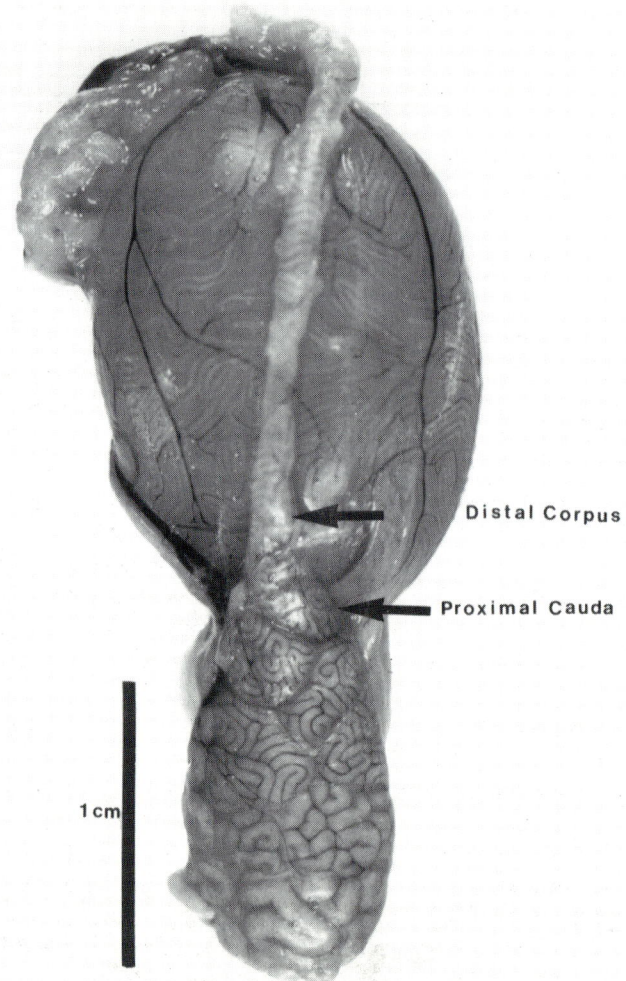

FIG. 1. Hamster testis and epididymis. Spermatozoa acquire their fertilizing capacity when passing from the distal corpus to proximal cauda region

Recently, spermatozoa retrieved by aspiration from the proximal epididymidis or vasa efferentia of men with congenital absence of the vas deferens or with epididymal obstruction have been used to establish pregnancies following *in vitro* fertilization (33,17). While these latter results may suggest that human sperm maturation might be somewhat more pliable than in laboratory species, they should not be taken as indicating that epididymal sperm maturation is insignificant in man. In this chapter, I will review briefly the changes to spermatozoa during maturation and the role the epididymal epithelium plays in promoting and controlling this process.

CHANGES TO EPIDIDYMAL SPERMATOZOA

Motility

The most obvious functional change to spermatozoa during epididymal transit is the development of flagellum movement so that sustained progressive motility is attained in the appropriate medium *in vitro* (16). It should be noted than within the epididymal lumen, spermatozoa remain quiescent, possible due to the ionic composition of the epididymal fluid or the presence of high viscosity proteins which in the rat inhibit tail movement (35,36). The capacity for sperm motility is only partly due to the epididymal milieu. If the distal corpus region of the epididymis is ligated, spermatozoa in the proximal duct obtain motility after 2-3 days although this cannot be sustained as long as for fully mature spermatozoa (1,22). Thus development of sperm motility probably results from intrinsic intracellular changes, i.e. structural stabilization of dense fibres (3) and phosphorylation of signalling proteins in association with epididymal secretory proteins. In the hamster, the development of full sperm motility was associated with a 34 kDa protein secreted by epididymal epithelial cells in the distal caput region (34).

Stabilization of Sperm Chromatin

The chromatin of the eutherian spermatozoon undergoes considerable stabilization during epididymal maturation due to the formation of disulphide bonds within the nuclear protamines (3). The effect of this process on sperm function is unclear, although a rigid sperm head is probably essential for penetration of the zona pellucida (20). For laboratory species, the stabilization of the sperm head occurs uniformly for the entire sperm population, however, human spermatozoa display much variation in nuclear stability as detected by the swelling reaction with detergents (2). This raises the question whether a spermatozoon lacking disulphide bonds is capable of fertilization or maintaining embryonic development. Testicular sperm heads micro-injected into oocytes do form pro-nuclei but embryonic development is curtailed (37).

Sperm Surface Changes

Many investigations have shown that the distribution and density of sperm membrane components alter during epididymal transit (10,19). Some of these changes are due undoubtedly to intrinsic alterations in the composition of the cholesterol/lipid ratio of the plasmalemma thereby affecting the mobility of intramembranous particles, while other changes may be due to specific processing and modifications of endogenous proteins (14). However, the expression of many new surface determinants on epididymal spermatozoa may result from specific antigens secreted by the epididymal epithelium being transferred onto the sperm surface. Over the last decade, studies in my own laboratory with specific antisera or monoclonal antibodies (17,21, 11,25) have shown that the expression of such antigens is often associated with the development of sperm fertilising capacity. Furthermore, these antibodies may block fertilization *in vitro* (21) or *in vivo* (17). Whether this effect is due to a specific masking of a functional epitope or occurs in response to a non-specific steric hindrance is still unclear.

Other Changes to Spermatozoa

In many species, a degree of morphological remodelling occurs during epididymal transit. This involve only the movement of the cytoplasmic droplet, or in the case of Hystricomorphs or marsupials radical changes to the sperm head. In American marsupials, spermatozoa join together to form a pair in the epididymis and remain joined until just before fertilization (18).

THE EPIDIDYMAL EPITHELIUM

The classification of the histology of the epididymis at the light microscope level can be somewhat confusing since in laboratory species, at least, longitudinal sections of duct display numerous segments divided by connective tissue. This led originally to a complex classification system based on epithelial height (31). Currently, however, most investigators divide the epididymis into five main regions represented by the initial segment, proximal and distal caput, corpus and cauda region, since this provides a consistent basis for comparing sperm maturation in various species (19). Compared with laboratory species, the human epididymis exhibits much less morphological differentiation between the various regions although considerable individual differences are observed (23). The pseudostratified epithelium of the epididymis is composed of five cell types. Tall principal cells make up about 85% of the epithelium and are present throughout its length (Fig. 2). These cells have long microvilli on their luminal border and serve but an absorptive and secretory function (see References 5 and 18). Other cell types include the apical and clear cells which have a pinocytotic

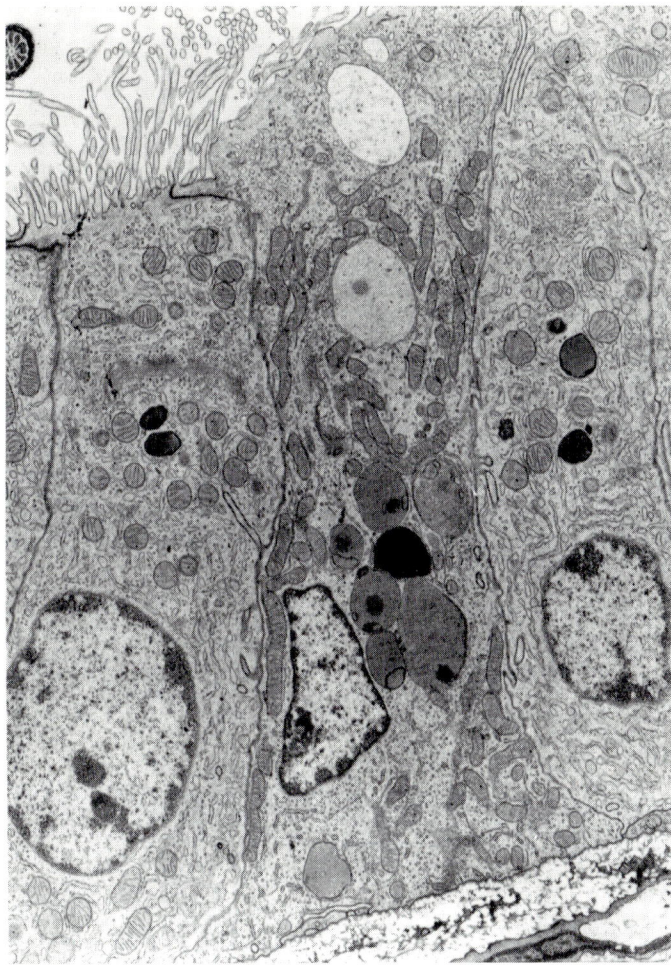

FIG. 2. Electron micrograph of the epididymal epithelium of rat. Principal cells surround a clear cell in the corpus epididymidis.

function and a pronounced carbonic anhydrase activity involved in acidification a basal stem cell, and intraepithelial lymphocytes. Hence, this epithelium serves to provide a continuously altering microenvironment for spermatozoa as they pass along the duct.

The epididymal epithelium is critically dependent on androgens such that castration or hypophysectomy leads to cessation of sperm maturation within 2-3 days (28). Moreover, ligation of the efferent duct in the rat leads to the selective regression of the initial segment and proximal caput epididymidis suggesting that androgens from the peripheral circulation alone are insufficient to maintain epididymal function in these regions and that androgens (bound to androgen biding protein) derived from the rete testis is important in this respect (30). This may not be the case in the human, however, as no consistent gradient of dihydrotestosterone has been observed along the epididymis. One consequence of this may be the poor regional morphological differentiation exhibited by the epididymis in men (22).

CULTURE OF EPIDIDYMAL EPITHELIUM AND *IN VITRO* SPERM MATURATION

Since access to the luminal environment of the epididymis *in situ* is limited, investigators have turned *in vitro* culture techniques to provide a simplified model open to experimental manipulation. Mammalian sperm maturation *in vitro* was first carried out by Orgebin-Crist and Jahad (29) who performed organ culture of rabbit epididymal tubule and with the addition of epididymal cytoplasmic extracts were able to significantly promote sperm fertilizing capacity. Similarly, Blaquier and co-workers increased the fertilizing capacity of immature hamster spermatozoa with crude epididymal cytosolic extracts (8). To provide functional epididymal epithelial cells in culture several techniques have been used including single cell preparations of principal cells, monolayer cultures on permeable supports and inverted epididymal vesicles (22,7). The latter preparation (Fig. 2) has been used in my laboratory to successfully promote the final stages of maturation of hamster spermatozoa (22). The technique consists of recovering immature spermatozoa (5% fertilization rate) from the mid to distal corpus region of the ligated epididymis and incubating them (for 6 hours) with epithelial vesicles from the cauda epididymidis which have been in culture previously for three days. This co-culture leads to a significant improvement in the fertilising capacity of the spermatozoa (30-50% fertilization rate) probably as a result of a pronounced increase in their ability to bind to the zona pellucida (22). Since co-incubation of spermatozoa with epididymal epithelium cultured in the absence of dihydrotestosterone, or with other cell types fail to promote maturation, it can be concluded that specific secretions under the control of androgens are responsible for this *in vitro* sperm maturation.

More recently, a similar procedure has been used also to promote the development of human sperm fertilising capacity *in vitro*. Co-incubation of immature caput epididymal spermatozoa (recovered from men undergoing vasectomy) with 3 day-old epithelial cultures from human cauda epididymidis induced a significant increase in progressive sperm motility and sperm binding to salt-stored human zona pellucidae (Table 1) compared to spermatozoa incubated without epithelium, or with androgen deficient epithelium (25,26). Such an increase in human sperm function was associated with the secretion of specific epididymal proteins of 22, 40 and 66 kDa (26).

Table 1. The effects of co-culture of caput epididymal spermatozoa with cauda epididymal epithelium preparations on sperm motility and sperm binding to salt-stored human zona.

Experiment	Proportion of Motile Sperm (%progressively motile sperm)				Mean Number of Sperm Bound to Zona (5-8 salt-stored zonae/value)			
	0 h	12 h	24 h	48 h	0 h	24 h	48 h	
1	5	15	28	12	12.3	22.5	16.1	
2	2	22	26	18	9.2	54.6**	29.3	
3	7	15	19	8	4.8	12.4	10.5	
4	6	20	31	21[1]	8.9	42.5**	28.2	
	Overall Means (± SD)				Overall means (± SD)			
	4±3	18±4*	26±4*	15±8	8.8±4.6	33.0±24.6*	23.5±16.7	
Ejaculated Sperm (N=4)	82±15	64±12	35±17	16±14	89.0±22.0	41.5±18.5	15.8±11.8	
Caput Sperm + Old Culture (N=2)	5±2	3±4	3±2	0	-	2.4±1.8	0.0	
Caput Sperm Alone (N=4)	4±3	5±5	2±2	0	-	2.9±3.4	0.0	

* significantly different from 0 h value, $P \leq 0.05$.
** significantly different from 0 h value, $P \leq 0.005$.
[1] some motile sperm after 72 h.

CONCLUSION

During epididymal passage, mammalian spermatozoa undergo myriad changes concomitant with their acquisition of fertilising capacity. While some of these changes are intrinsic and are not necessarily due to a direct influence of the epididymis, it is evident that androgen dependent secretions of the epididymal epithelium are required for full sperm fertility. Despite many investigations over the last twenty years, exactly how this maturation occurs still remains to be elucidated. Overall, the observations from both *in vivo* and *in vitro* studies strongly support the view that epididymal-specific determinants transferred onto the surface of spermatozoa are required for sperm-zona recognition and the development of full sperm motility. The recent successes of *in vitro* fertilisation and pregnancy using epididymal spermatozoa from the caput epididymidis and efferent ducts has led to the suggestion that post-testicular human sperm maturation is not an essential requirement. But the very low success rate of this technique achieved by most investigators is indicative of the poor fertilising potential of spermatozoa from the proximal excurrent duct which can only be overcome by using large numbers of oocytes per insemination and very careful pre-selection of a motile sperm population. Long-term epididymal cultures may enable a practical *in vitro* maturation technique to be developed as well as providing an insight in the sperm maturation process.

REFERENCES

1. Bedford, J.M. (1967) Effect of duct ligation on the fertilizing ability of spermatozoa in the epididymis of the rabbit. J. Exp. Zool., 166:271-282.
2. Bedford, J.M., Calvin, H.I. and Cooper, G.W. (1973) The maturation of spermatozoa in the human epididymis. J. Reprod. Fert. Suppl., 18: 99-208.
3. Calvin, H. I. and Bedford, J.M. (1971) Formation of disulphide bonds in the nucleus and accessory structures of mammalian spermatozoa during maturation in the epididymis. J. Reprod. Fert. Suppl., 13:65-75.
4. Chen, J.P., Hoffer, A.P. and Rosen, S. (1976) Carbonic anhydrase localization in the epididymis and testis of the rat: histochemical and biochemical analysis. Biol. Reprod., 14:339-346.
5. Cooper, T.G. (1986) The epididymis, sperm maturation and fertilisation. Springer-Verlag, Heidelberg.
6. Cooper, T.G. (1990) In defense of the human epididymis. Fertil. Steril., 54:965-975.
7. Cooper, T.G., Yeung, C.H., Meyer, R. and Schulze, H. (1990) Maintenance of human epididymal epithelial cell function in monolayer culture. J. Reprod. Fert., 90:81-91.
8. Cuasnicu, P.S., Gonzalez-Echeverria, F., Piazza, A., and Blaquier, J.A. (1984) addition of androgens to cultured hamster epididymis increase zona recognition by immature spermatozoa. J. Reprod. Fert., 70:541-547.
9. Dacheaux, J.L., Chevrier, C. and Lanson, Y. (1987) Motility and surface transformations of human spermatozoa during epididymal transit. Proc. Natl. Acad. Sci., USA., 513:560.
10. Eddy, E.M., Vernon, R.B., Muller, C.H., Hahnel, A.C. and Fenderson, B.A. (1985) Immunodissection of sperm surface modifications during epididymal maturation. Am. J. Anat., 174:225-237.
11. Ellis, D.H., Hartman, T.D. and Moore, H.D.M. (1985) Maturation and function of the hamster spermatozoon probed with monoclonal antibodies. J. Reprod. Immunol., 7:229-314.
12. Jequier, A.M., Cummins, J.M., Gearon, C., Apted, S.L., Yovich, J.M. and Yovich, J.L.

(1990) A pregnancy achieved using sperm from the epididymal caput in idiopathic obstructive azoospermia. Fertil. Steril., 53:1104-1105.
13. Hinrichsen, M.J. and Blaquier, J.A. (1980) Evidence supporting the existence of sperm maturation in the human epididymis. J. Reprod. Fert., 60:291-297.
14. Holt, W.V. (1982) Functional development of the mammalian sperm plasma membrane. Oxford Rev. Reprod. Biol., 4:195-240.
15. Horan, A.H. and Bedford, J.M. (1972) Development of the fertilising ability of spermatozoa in the epididymis of the syrian hamster. J. Reprod. Fert., 30:417-423.
16. Hoskins, D.D. and Casillas, E.R. (1975) Function of cyclic nucleotides in mammalian spermatozoa. In: Handbook of Physiology, Endocrinology V, Section 7, Male Reproductive Tract., edited by Greep, R. and Hamilton, D., pp 453-462. American Physiological Society, Washington.
17. Moore, H.D.M. (1981) Glycoprotein secretion of the epididymis in the rabbit and hamster: Localisation on epididymal spermatozoa and the effect of specific antibodies on fertilization in vivo. J. Exp. Zool., 215:77-85.
18. Moore, H.D.M. (1990) The epididymis. In: Scientific Foundations of Urology, 3rd edition; ed Chisholm, G. and Fair, W., pp 399-410. Heinemann, London.
19. Moore, H.D.M. (1990) Development of sperm-egg recognition processes in mammals. J. Reprod. Fert. Suppl., 42:71-78.
20. Moore, H.D.M. and Bedford, J.M. (1983) The interaction of mammalian gametes in the female. Sperm/egg interactions in vivo. In: Mechanism and Control of Animal Fertilization. Edited by Hartmann, J.F. pp 453-497. Academic Press, New York.
21. Moore, H.D.M. and Hartman, T.D. (1984) Localization by monoclonal antibodies of various surface antigens of hamster spermatozoa and the effect of antibodies on fertilization in vitro. J. Reprod. Fert., 70:175-183.
22. Moore, H.D.M. and Hartman, T.D. (1986) In vitro development of the fertilizing ability of hamster epididymal spermatozoa after co-culture with epithelium from the proximal cauda epididymidis. J. Reprod. Fert., 78:347-352.
23. Moore, H.D.M. and Pryor, J.P. (1980) The comparative ultrastructure of the epididymis in monkeys and man; A search for a suitable animal model for studying primate epididymal physiology. Am. J. Primatol., 2:231-239.
24. Moore, H.D.M., Pryor, J.P. and Hartman, T.D. (1983) Development of the oocyte penetrating capacity of the human epididymis. Int. J. Androl., 6:310-318.
25. Moore, H.D.M., Curry, M. and Pryor, J.P. (1989) In vitro culture of epididymal epithelium for the study of mammalian sperm maturation. In: In vitro approaches to mammalian gamete maturation and embryonic development, edited by Lauria, A. and Gandolfi, F., pp 1-10. Serovet, Rome.
26. Moore, H.D.M., Curry, M.R., Penfold, L.M. and Pryor, J.P. (1992) The culture of human epididymal epithelium and in vitro maturation of epididymal spermatozoa. Fertil. Steril. (in press)
27. Orgebin-Crist, M.-C. (1967) Maturation of spermatozoa in the rabbit epididymis. Fertilizing ability and embryonic mortality in does inseminated with epididymal spermatozoa. Ann. Biol. Animale Biochim. Biophys., 7:373-389.
28. Orgebin-Crist, M.-C., Danzo, B.J. and Davies, J. (1975) Endocrine control of the development and maintenance of sperm fertilizing ability in the epididymis. In: Handbook of Physiology, Endocrinology V, section 7, Male Reproductive Tract., edited by Greep, R. and Hamilton, D., pp 319-337. American Physiological Society, Washington.
29. Orgebin-Crist, M.-C. and Jahad, N. (1979) The maturation of rabbit epididymal spermatozoa in organ culture: stimulation by epididymal cytosolic extracts. Biol. reprod., 21:511-516.
30. Pelliniemi, L.J., Dym, M., and Gunsalus, G.L. (1980) Immunocytochemical localisation of androgen-binding protein in the male reproductive tract. Endocrinology, 108:925-931.
31. Reid, B.L. and Cleland, K.W. (1957) The structure and function of the epididymis. I. The histology of the rat epididymis. Aust. J. Zool., 5:233-246.
32. Schoysman, R.J. and Bedford, J.M. (1986) The role of the human epididymis in sperm maturation and sperm storage as reflected in the consequences of epididymovasostomy. Fertil. Steril., 46:293-299.
33. Silber, S.J., Balmaceda, J., Borrero, C., Ord, T. and Asch, R., (1988) Pregnancy with sperm aspiration from the proximal head of the epididymis: A new treatment for congenital absence of the vas deferens. Fertil. Steril., 50:525-528.
34. Smith, C.A., Hartman, T.D. and Moore, H.D.M. (1986) A determinant of M_r 34000 expressed by hamster epididymal epithelium binds specifically to spermatozoa in co-culture. J. Reprod. Fertil., 78:337-345.

35. Turner, T.T. and Howards, S.S. (1978) Factors involved in the initiation of sperm motility. Biol. Reprod., 18:571-578.
36. Wong, P.Y.D. and Lee W.M. (1983) Potassium movement during sodium induced motility initiated in the rat caudal epididymal spermatozoa. Biol. Reprod., 28:206-212.
37. Yanagida, K., Bedford, J.M. and Yanagimachi, R. (1991) Cleavage of rabbit eggs after microsurgical injection of testicular spermatozoa. Hum. Reprod., 6:277-279.
38. Young, W.C. (1931) A Study of the function of the epididymis. II. Function changes undergone by spermatozoa during their passage through the epididymis and vas deferens in the guinea-pig. J. Exp. Biol., 8:151-163.

Cell Biology of the Oocyte

R.J. Aitken

MRC Reproductive Biology Unit,
University of Edinburgh Centre for Reproductive Biology
37 Chalmers Street, Edinburgh EH3 9EW, UK

The mammalian oocyte is not only the largest cell in the body but also one of the most complex, displaying a carefully regulated sequence of changes that enable this cell to remain for several decades in an arrested state with the ovary, until stimulated to resume meiosis and prepare itself for fertilization and the programming of embryonic development.

The precursor of the oocyte is evidently a highly motile cell that can respond to chemotaxic stimuli and translocate from its site of origin in the embryonic epiblast to the genital ridge. Once located in the primitive ovary the oogonia proliferate and then, after their final mitotic division undergo one further round of DNA replication before entering meiosis and becoming oocytes. The mammalian oocyte passes through the leptotene, zygotene and pachytene stages of meiotic prophase before arresting at diplotene. At this point the oocyte, wrapped in a covering of squamous prefollicular cells is classified as a primordial follicle. It will remain in this state until recruited into the growing follicle population, which in the case of the human oocyte, will be 1-5 decades later.

The biochemical mechanisms resonsible for controlling this complex sequence of events is unknown. The chemotactic factors which guide the germ cells to the genital ridge, the meiosis inducing substances that stimulate the proliferating oogonia to differentiate into oocytes through the initiation of meiosis, the factors responsible for inducing and maintaining meiotic arrest at the diplotene stage and the factors responsible for the recruitment of the primordial follicle into the growing follicle pool all await elucidation.

Once the primordial follicle has initiated its development, the oocyte enters a phase of rapid growth characterized by enhanced gene transcription and qualitative and quantitative changes in the pattern of proteins synthesized. Where the transcription and translation of specific gene products has been followed in detail (*ZP3, Plat* and *Mos*) mRNA can be detected over a prolonged period following the initiation of oocyte growth, but the timing of translation appears to be very carefully controlled. During this phase of oocyte growth the nucleus remains arrested at the dictyate stage of meiotic prophase and does not resume meiosis until oocyte maturation is initiated in response to the LH surge that induces ovulation. Our knowledge of the mechanisms responsible for the initiation of oocyte growth, the continued suppression of meiosis during folliculogenesis and the sudden release of this inhibition immediately prior to ovulation is still fragmentary. The observation, made more than 50 years ago (2), that removal of a growing oocyte from the follicle prior to the LH surge will lead to the spontaneous initiation of oocyte maturation, led to the conclusion that the ovary must elaborate a suppressive factor that maintains meiotic arrest during folliculogenesis. The fact that the spontaneous maturation of *in vitro* cultured oocytes can be suppressed by strategies that elevated cAMP levels, has promoted the concept that the maintenance of meiotic arrest is cAMP/ protein kinase A-dependent. Recent studies suggest that the follicular factor responsible for elevating cAMP in the arrested oocyte is the phosphodiesterase inhibitor, hypoxanthine (1). Further elucidation of the cellular mechanisms responsible for the control of oocyte growth and maturation, as well as the programming of the oocyte so that it is competent to support embryogenesis, is of importance in a wide variety of contexts. In addition to a fundamental scientific interest in discovering how such fundamental processes as meiosis are controlled, a deeper understanding of oocyte cell biology should have an impact on fields as disparate as the treatment of premature ovarian failure, the survival of rare or endangered species and the creation of transgenic animals. The three papers that follow this introduction serve to illustrate the kind of advances that we are now making in our abililty to understand, and thence manipulate, the biology of this extraordinary cell.

REFERENCES

1. Eppig, J. J. and Downs, S. M. (1987) The effect of hypoxanthine on mouse oocyte growth and development in vitro: maintenance of meiotic arrest and gonadotrophin induced maturation. Dev. Biol., 119:313-320.
2. Pincus, G. and Enzmann, E. V. (1935) The comparative behavior of mammalian eggs *in vivo* and *in vitro*. 1. The activation of ovarian eggs. J. Exp. Med., 62:655-660.

Molecular Basis of Sperm-Egg Interaction

R.J. Aitken

*MRC Reproductive Biology Unit,
University of Edinburgh Centre for Reproductive Biology
37 Chalmers Street, Edinburgh EH3 9EW, UK*

INTRODUCTION

The gamete recognition and activation events that comprise the early stages of fertilization are of strategic importance to the design and development of new approaches to contraception, as well as the diagnosis and treatment of infertility. In order to achieve these clinical aims, the molecular basis of sperm-egg interaction needs to be resolved and the aberrant biochemical mechanisms that lead to the inhibition of fertilization in cases of infertility, understood. In the recent past a number of new insights into the cell biology of mammalian gametes and the molecular basis of fertilization have been obtained, many of which are of direct relevance to the clinical situation. In this brief overview, I shall consider some of these recent developments dealing with the various levels of sperm-egg interaction in sequence, beginning with the passage of spermatozoa through the cumulus oophorus, their subsequent recognition of the zona surface, penetration through the zona matrix and, finally, fusion with the vitelline membrane of the oocyte.

CUMULUS OOPHORUS

In most mammalian species the egg is ovulated surrounded by a cumulus mass comprising a population of follicular cells embedded in an extracellular matrix which is rich in hyaluronic acid. Since the acrosomal vesicle contains hyaluronidase, it was originally thought that the acrosome reaction was a prerequisite for sperm penetration through the cumulus mass. However, recent data suggest that the spermatozoa that penetrate the cumulus matrix are structurally intact (3,23); it is acrosome reacted spermatozoa that appear to be excluded from penetration of the cumulus mass (11). Such findings have lead to the suggestion that the cumulus oophorus acts as a physiological filter allowing only acrosome intact, functionally competent spermatozoa access to the surface of the zona pellucida (11). The fact that inhibition of hyaluronidase activity with myocrisin (20) inhibits the ability of mouse spematozoa to fertilize cumulus-enclosed, but not cumulus-free oocytes, strongly suggests that acrosomal hyaluronidase is released by the spermatozoa as they pass through the cumulus matrix and does play an important role at this stage of fertilization. The corollary of this observation is that hyaluronidase release by spermatozoa traversing the cumulus matrix must occur before any major structural changes are observed in the acrosomal region of the cell. Exteriorization of acrosomal enzymes before morphological signs of vesiculation or loss of the acrosomal membranes, has been reported in the case of acrosin (26) and could certainly occur with a highly soluble enzyme such as hyaluronidase.

Since spermatozoa can fertilize cumulus-free ova without any difficulty we must conclude that the changes induced by the presence of the cumulus mass are facilitatory rather than obligatory. Components of the cumulus complex certainly have the capacity to stimulate sperm motility (5) and support both capacitation and the acrosome reaction in mammalian spermatozoa (2). Moreover, the Fab fragments of polyclonal antibodies raised against the human cumulus complex have been shown to block the fertilization of human ova *in vitro.* (27). The weight of evidence therefore suggests that the cumulus oophorus serves a 'priming' role, preparing the spermatozoa for their subsequent interaction with the zona pellucida by inducing an enhancement of sperm motility and inducing an early stage of the acrosome reaction. The components responsible for this priming function and the way in which their production is controlled have not yet been elucidated. There is some evidence to suggest that the secretory functions of the cumulus mass are stimulated by FSH (5) and that the major products are poorly defined, large molecular weight glycoproteins, that readily coat the surface of mammalian spermatozoa (27).

SPERM-ZONA RECOGNITION

The zona pellucida is a translucent acellular shell that is secreted around the oocyte during folliculogenesis and remains intact until the moment of implantation. It is a complex structure that has evolved to fulfill a number of different functions during fertilization and early embryonic development in mammals. In the Metatheria, for example, the zona pellucida functions primarily as a template for the construction of the unilamellar blastocyst. In the Eutheria, it serves a multitude of functions during fertilization acting as a recognition site for the attachment and the subsequent tenacious binding of capacitated spermatozoa and as a stimulus for the acrosome reaction.

Post-fertilization, the zona pellucida may participate in the block to polyspermy and physically protects the developing embryo during its sojourn through the female reproductive tract to the site of fertilization.

Biochemically the structure of the zona pelludida is relatively straightforward comprising 3 or 4 major glycoprotein species in every species that has been examined, including man (29,30,31). The animal model that has been most thoroughly studied with respect to the composition and function of the zona pellucida is the mouse. In this species the zona pellucida comprises 3 major glycoproteins, ZP1, ZP2 and ZP3, which together account for most of this structure's mass. In terms of three-dimensional structure, the zona is composed of very long filaments constructed of ZP2-ZP3 dimers, with each dimer located approximately every 15 nm along the filaments. The filaments are interconnected by bridges composed of the highest molecular weight zona component, ZP1. Although all three zona components play important roles in creating and maintaining the structural integrity of the zona pellucida, they are highly differentiated with respect to their biological roles (29,30,31).

ZP3 has been identified as the primary sperm receptor, mediating the tenacious binding of capacitated spermatozoa to the zona pellucida during the early stages of fertilization. The evidence that ZP3 performs this important role has come largely from competition experiments whereby incubation of spermatozoa with this glycoprotein has been shown to suppress the subsequent ability of these cells to bind to the zona pellucida. The primary target for the spermatozoa is not the polypeptide backbone of ZP3 but a particular class of O-linked oligosaccharides (Mr 3900) which represent a relatively small fraction of the total O-linked oligosaccharide pool characteristic of this glycoprotein (29,30,31). An idea of the biological efficiency of this recognition event can be gained from the fact that nanomolar quantities of the purified O-linked ZP3 oligosaccharides are able to prevent sperm-zona interaction *in vitro*. Whilst the detailed chemistry of the carbohydrate configurations responsible for sperm binding have not been fully worked out, it is known that a galactose residue, located in α-linkage with the non reducing terminus of the oligosaccharide, plays an important role in this interaction. Removal or modification of this sugar residue destroys the sperm binding capacity of the ZP3 glycoprotein (29,30,31).

The importance of sugar residues in mediating sperm-zona recognition has been emphasized in attempts to identify the complementary receptor for ZP3 on the surface of the spermatozoon. These studies, again conducted exclusively in the mouse, have suggested that the plasma membrane overlying the sperm head expresses a galactosyl transferase that targets a terminal glcNAc residue on ZP3. In the absence of substrate UDPgalactose, the enzyme essentially functions as a lectin, forming stable complexes with its glcNAc binding site on the zona pellucida. This hypothesis is supported by data indicating that pregalactosylation of the zona receptor or glycosidase-mediated modification of this site, impairs the ability of spermatozoa to bind to the zona pellucida (10. 21, 22). Superficially, there would appear to be an (as yet, unresolved) discrepancy between the galactosyl transferase model proposed by Shur (21,22), which requires an available glcNAc residue on the zona pellucida and the Wassarman data (3,31), suggesting the involvement of a terminal α-galactose on ZP3 in mediating sperm zona recognition.

The galactosyl transferase model is not the only mechanism which has been put forward for mediating sperm egg recognition. A 56 kDa protein has been identified on the surface of mouse spermatozoa which binds ZP3 but not ZP2 (3). The fact that this protein binds galactose but not N-acetyl glucosamine is in contradiction to the galactosyltransferase hypothesis but in keeping with a notion that terminal α-galactose on ZP3 is instrumental in mediating sperm-zona interaction. Evidence has also been put forward to support the involvement of a sperm tyrosine kinase in the process of sperm-egg recognition (17). In these studies, addition of solubilized mouse zona proteins to suspensions of murine spermatozoa resulted in an enhancement in the level of tyrosine phosphorylation observed in a 95 kDa protein. This same protein was also found to bind labeled ZP3 suggesting that this 95 kDa protein could serve as a receptor for the zona pellucida and also transduce the egg-recognition signal through the phosphorylation of tyrosine residues. Since the ligands for receptor tyrosine kinases are invariably proteinaceous this hypothesis cannot be easily integrated into a sheme in which carbohydrate residues are thought to play a key role in mediating sperm-egg recognition. On the other hand the fact that receptor tyrosine kinases are capable of being activated by oligomerization (aggregation of the receptor) is in keeping with data indicating that the activation of the spermatozoon by ZP3 involves an aggregation dependent mechanism (18).

SPERM ACTIVATION

ZP3 is not merely a recognition site for spermatozoa, it is also the molecule responsible for sperm activation, inducing exocytosis of the acrosomal vesicle and the generation of a fusogenic equatorial segment capable of initiating fusion with the vitelline membrane of the oocyte. Of all the zona glycoproteins tested for their ability to induce the acrosome reaction, only ZP3 was found to be biologically active (29,30,31). In this respect, ZP3 is as effective a stimulant of the acrosome reaction as the divalent cation ionophore A23187, although the concentration of ZP3 required for this activity is significantly higher than the nanomolar quantities needed to block sperm-egg recognition in competition assays. The ability of ZP3 to activate the spermatozoon is dependent on the integrity of both the O-linked carbohydrate side chains and the peptide backbone of the molecule. Whilst the former is necessary for sperm recognition, the importance of the latter resides in its capacity to cross-link zona recognition sites on the surface the spermatozoa thereby achieving the receptor oligomerization needed to activate the cell (18).

The signal transduction mechanisms whereby the aggregation of zona binding sites on the surface of the spermatozoon leads to the generation of those second messengers involved in precipitating the acrosome reaction, are poorly understood. There is some evidence, cited above (17), suggesting that interaction with ZP3 leads to tyrosine phophorylation in a 95 kDa molecule presumably located in the sperm plasma membrane. There is also some evidence to suggest that a GTP-binding regulatory subunit is involved in transducing the zona recognition signal in murine spermatozoa. The support for this hypothesis derives largely from the inhibitory action of pertussis toxin on the zona-induced acrosome reaction. This toxin catalyzes the ADP-ribosylation of certain G-proteins, including those of the G_i class which are known to be components of mammalian spermatozoa (8,9,12). Peptide mapping studies involving mouse and human spermatozoa suggest that the 41 kDa pertussis toxin substrate of these cells is similar to the a_i moiety of mouse S-49 lymphoma cells (16). The specificity of the pertussis toxin treatment was indicated by the ability of GTPγS (which dissociates the abg heterotrimer and thereby inhibits the ability of this reagent to catalyze αβγ-ribosylation) to prevent pertussis toxin from blocking ZP-induced acrosome reactions. Immunofluorescence studies with an antiserum directed against a conserved region of $G_α$ proteins revealed the presence of the corresponding antigen over the acrosomal region of the cell, in an ideal position to participate in the signal transduction mechanisms involved in sperm-egg interaction. (14,15). Spermatozoa do not appear to contain substrates for cholera toxin-catalysed ADP-ribosylation, suggesting that the G_s regulatory subunit is not a feature of this particular cell type.

The body of evidence therefore suggests that mammalian spermatozoa possess at least 2 different pathways for transducing the zona-recognition signal: one involving a receptor type tyrosine kinase and the other involving the mediation of a G protein. The relationship between these two pathways and other elements thought to be involved in sperm-egg recognition including the 56 kDa protein described by Bleil (3) or the galactosyl transferase described by Shur's group (21,22) is currently unknown. There is agreement, however, over the nature of the second messengers generated as a result of this signal transduction process. The two key messengers that appear to generated when the spermatozoon binds to the zona pellucida are calcium and pH.

The involvement of calcium in the induction of the acrosome reaction has been established in every species investigated (1,15). The omission of calcium from the medium inhibits the acrosome reaction, while this event can be readily induced by divalent cation ionophores in the presence of extracellular calcium (1,24,25). However it is not generally appreciated that the addition of ionophore not only induces an influx of extracellular calcium but also stimulates an efflux of protons leading to an increase in intracellular pH. Alkalinization of the sperm cytoplasm is an important stimulus for exocytosis in its own right, such that a low level of acrosome reaction can be induced in human spermatozoa by elevating pH, in the absence of a calcium influx. Nevertheless, maximal rates of acrosomal loss require the concerted action of both pH and calcium signals (15). The biological significance of these second messengers was indicated by Florman *et al.* (12) who observed elevations of intracellular pH and calcium following the induction of the acrosome reaction in bovine spermatozoa with solubilized bovine zonae pellucidae.

Once the acrosome reaction has occurred a phase of secondary binding ensues involving the zona glycoprotein ZP2 (29). The purpose of such secondary binding is to maintain intimate contact between the advancing spermatozoon and the zona matrix thereby facilitating the interaction between proteolytic enzymes on the inner acrosomal membrane and their substrate. There is an impressive body of evidence indicating that the sperm specific protease, acrosin, may possess both the proteolytic activity necessary to cut the zona matrix and a fucose binding domain capable of effecting secondary binding to the zona pellucida (13,28). Although the target for for acrosin binding has not yet been shown to be ZP2, this molecule locates to the outer surface of the spermatozoon during an early stage of the acrosome reaction (26) in an ideal position to orchestrate the alternating cycles of proteolysis and binding that are thought to characterize the passage of spermatozoa through the zona pellucida.

SPERM-OOCYTE FUSION

The acrosome reaction is not merely an exocytotic event involving the release of the acrosomal contents. It also involves changes in the structure and organization of the sperm plasma membrane required for binding to, and fusion with, the vitelline membrane of the oocyte. Concomitant with the acrosome reaction a discrete band of plasma membrane around the equatorial segment of the sperm head suddenly acquires the ability to recognize and fuse with the oolemma. The molecular basis of this interaction is just beginning to be unravelled. Intriguing new evidence suggests that there are similarities in the way that enveloped viruses fuse with their target cell and the fusion of acrosome reacted spermatozoa with the vitelline membrane of the oocyte. Using the guinea pig as an animal model and a monoclonal antibody (PH-30) that that disrupts sperm-oocyte fusion, a sperm surface component involved in mediating this event has been cloned and sequenced. PH-30 precipitates two, tightly coupled, immunologically distinct subunits (α,β) that behave as a single integral membrane protein (19). This complex finds expression on the posterior surface of the mature sperm head in the appropriate location for a molecular entity involved in sperm-oocyte fusion. Sequence analysis has revealed that the α-subunit comprises a 289 amino-acid protein containing a single membrane spanning domain towards the C-terminus. The most interesting feature of this particular molecule is its structural similarity to viral fusion proteins. The features that are shared with such fusion proteins include central proline residues and a stretch of amino acids that can be modelled as a 'sided' α-helix with most of the hydrophobic residues on one face. This hydrophobic motif is positioned in such a way that it should facilitate the integration of this region of α-subunit of PH-30 into the plasma membrane of the oocyte. Since the carboxyl terminus of this protein is anchored in the sperm plasma membrane, the α-subunit should effectively promote the close apposition and, ultimately, the fusion of the male and female gametes (4).

The β subunit of the PH-30 complex is specialized for sperm-egg recognition. This is achieved through the presence of an integrin-binding domain, similar to the disintegrins found in snake venoms. In the context of fertilization, the significance of an integrin-binding site on the surface of the spermatozoon lies in the results of recent studies indicating that the oocyte expresses an integrin-like receptor (6,7). Micromolar amounts of the integrin-binding peptide, RGD, have been shown to suppress the ability of human spermatozoa to fuse with the oocyte, presumably by competing with the disintegrin domains on a PH-30β-like protein for the integrin receptors on the surface of the oocyte. The tasks of recognizing and fusing with the vitelline membrane of the oocyte are therefore contained within different components of the PH-30 complex: PH-30β bearing the resonsibility for binding the spermatozoon to the surface of the oocyte and PH-30α initiating the process of membrane fusion. Whether an equivalent molecule exists on the human sperm plasma membrane and whether defects in the composition or insertion of this molecule are involved in the many cases of male infertility involving a failure of sperm oocyte fusion, are important topics for future research.

SUMMARY

In summary, the molecular mechanisms involved in the complex cascade of interactions between the male and female gametes at fertilization are rapidly being elucidated. The molecular structure and functional significance of the various components of the zona pellucida have been thoroughly investigated and the results should have implications for fields as diverse as the development of contraceptive vaccines, the cryostorage of oocytes and the treatment of male infertility. The complementary receptors on the surface of the spermatozoon are currently receiving the attention of many laboratories and the fact that multiple candidates have been put forward, may simply mean that the details of sperm-zona interaction are complex and involve a multiplicity of components. The cellular events downstream from sperm-zona binding are less clear and although there is good evidence to suggest that elevations of cytoplasmic pH and calcium are important, the way in which the zona-recognition signal is transduced in order to generate these second messengers, is still far from clear. Finally, recent progress towards a molecular definition of sperm-oocyte fusion has produced results that are not only biologically intriguing but should also provide a sound biochemical basis for understanding the nature of the lesions responsible for the loss of fertilizing potential in cases of male infertility - currently, the largest single, defined, cause of childlessness in couples attending infertility clinics in the United Kingdom.

REFERENCES

1. Aitken, R. J., Ross, A., Hargreave, T., Richardson, D. W. and Best F. S. M. (1984) Analysis of human sperm function following exposure to the ionophore A23187. Comparison of normospermic and oligozoospermic men. J Androl., 5:321-329.
2. Bavister, B. D. (1982) Evidence for a role of post-ovulatory cumulus components in supporting fertilizing ability of hamster spermatozoa. J. Androl., 3:365-372.
3. Bleil, J.D. (1991) Sperm receptors on mammalian eggs. In: Elements of mammalian fertilization, edited by Wasserman, P. M., pp 133-151. CRC Press, Boca Raton.
4. Blobel, C. P., Wolfsberg, T. G., Turck, C. W., Myles, D. G. Primakoff, P. and White, J. M. (1992) A potential fusion peptide and an integrin ligand domain in a protein active in sperm oocyte fusion. Nature, 356:248-252.
5. Bradley, M. P. and Garbers, D. L. (1983) The stimulation of bovine caudal epididymal sperm forward motility by bovine cumulus-egg complexes *in vitro*. Biochem. Biophys. Res. Commun., 115:777-787.
6. Bronson, R. A. and Fusi, F. (1990) Sperm-oolemmal interaction : role of the Arg-Gly-Asp (RGD) adhesion peptide. Fertil. Steril., 54:527-529.
7. Bronson, R. A. and Fusi, F. (1990) Evidence that an Arg-Gly-Asp adhesion sequence plays a role in mammalian fertilization. Biol. Reprod., 43:1019-1025.
8. Endo, Y., Lee, M. A. and Kopf, G. S. (1987) Evidence for the role of a guanine nucleotide-binding regulatory protein in the zona-induced mouse sperm acrosome reaction. Dev. Biol., 119:210-216.
9. Endo, Y., Lee M. A. and Kopf, G. S. (1988) Characterization of an islet activating protein-sensitive site in the mouse sperm that is involved in the zona pellucida-induced acrosome reaction. Dev. Biol., 129:12-24.
10. Fayrer-Hosken, R. A., Caudel, A. B. and Shur, B. D. (1991) Galactosyltransferase activity is restricted to the plasma membranes of equine and bovine spermatozoa. Molec. Reprod. Dev., 28:74-78.
11. Florman, H. M. and Babcock, D. F. (1991) Progress toward understanding the molecular basis of capacitation. In: Elements of mammalian fertilization, edited by Wasserman, P. M., pp105-132. CRC Press, Boca Raton.
12. Florman, H. M., Tombes, R.M., First, N. L. and Babcock, D. F. (1989) An adhesion-associated agonist from the zona pellucida activates G protein-promoted elevations of internal Ca^{2+} and pH that mediate mammalian sperm acrosomal exocytosis. Dev. Biol., 135:133-146.
13. Jones, R. (1991) Identification and functions of mammalian sperm-egg recognition molecules during fertilization. J. Reprod. Fertil. Suppl., 42:89-105.
14. Kopf, G. S. (1990) Zona pellucida-mediated signal transduction in mammalian spermatozoa. J. Reprod. Fertil. Suppl., 42:33-49.
15. Kopf, G. S. and Gerton, G. L. (1991) The mammalian sperm acrosome and the acrosome reaction. In: Elements of mammalian fertilization, edited by Wasserman P. M., pp153-203. CRC Press, Boca Raton.
16. Kopf, G. S., Woolkalis, M. J. and Gerton, G. L. (1986) Evidence for a guanine nucleotide-binding regulatory protein in invertebrate and mammalian sperm: identification by islet-activating protein-catalyzed ADP-ribosylation and immunochemical methods. J. Biol Chem., 261:7327-7331.

17. Leyton, L. and Saling, P. (1989) 95kd sperm proteins bind ZP3 and serve as tyrosine kinase substrates in response to zona binding. Cell., 57:1123-1130.
18. Leyton, L. and Saling, P. (1989) Evidence that aggregation of mouse sperm receptors by ZP3 triggers the acrosome reaction. J. Cell Biol., 108:2163-2168.
19. Primakoff, P. Hyatt, H. and Tredick-Kline, J. (1987) Identification and purification of a sperm surface protein with a potential role in sperm-egg membrane fusion. J. Cell Biol. 104:141-149.
20. Reddy, J. K., Joyce, C. and Zaneveld, J. D. (1980) Role of hyaluronidase in fertilization: the antiferility activity of myocrisin, a nontoxic hyauronidase inhibitor. J. Androl., 1:28-32.
21. Shur, B. D. and Hall, N. G. (1982) A role for mouse sperm surface galactosyltransferase in sperm binding to the egg zona pellucida. J. Cell Biol., 95:574-579.
22. Shur, B. D. and Neely, C. A. (1988) Plasma membrane association, purification, and partial characterization of mouse sperm β-1.4-galactosyl-transferase. J. Biol. Chem., 263: 17706-17714.
23 Storey, B. T., Lee, M. A., Muller, C., Ward, C. R. and Wirtshafter, D. G. (1984) Binding of mouse spermatozoa to the zonae pellucidae of mouse eggs in cumulus: evidence that the acrosomes remain substantially intact. Biol. Reprod. 31:1119-1128.
24. Summers, R. G., Talbot, P., Keough, E. M., Hylander, B. L. and Franklin, L.E. (1976) Ionophore A23187 induces acrosome reactions in sea urchin and guinea pig spermatozoa. J. Exp. Zool, 196:381-386.
25. Talbot, P., Summers, R. G., Hylander, B.L., Keough, E. M. and Franklin, L. E. (1976) The role of calcium in the acrosome reaction : an analysis using ionophore A23187. J. Exp. Zool. 198:383-392.
26. Tesarik, J., Drahorad, J., Testart, J. and Mendoza, C. (1990) Acrosin exposure follows its surface exposure and precedes membrane fusion in human sperm acrosome reaction. Development, 110:391-400.
27. Tesarik, J., Pilka, L., Drahorad, J., Cechova, D., and Veselsky, L. (1988) The role of cumulus cell-secreted proteins in the development of human sperm fertilizing ability: implication in IVF. Hum. Reprod., 3:129-132.
28. Topfer-Peterson, E. and Henschen, A. (1988) Zona pellucida-binding and fucose-binding of boar sperm acrosin is not correlated with proteolytic activity. Biol. Chem. Hoppe-Seyler 369:69-76.
29. Wassarman, P. M. (1988) Zona pellucida glycoproteins. Annu. Rev. Biochem. 57:415-442.
30. Wassarman, P. M. (1990) Profile of a mammalian sperm receptor. Development 108:1-17.
31. Wassarman, P. M. (1990) Regulation of mammalian fertilization by zona pellucida glycoproteins. J. Reprod. Fertil. Suppl., 42:79-87.

Cyclin and p34^{cdc2} Kinase Activity in Pig Oocytes During the G2- to M-phase Transition

R. Moor, T. Jung, T. Miyano and P. Barker

*Department of Molecular Embryology,
AFRC Institute of Animal Physiology & Genetics Research,
Babraham, Cambridge CB2 4AT, UK*

INTRODUCTION

A highly productive phase in the study of meiosis was initiated by the discovery of a factor in amphibian oocytes whose activity varied in a cell cycle manner and which on intracellular injection induced the transition from the G2- to M-phase of the meiotic cycle. Not only was this so-called maturation promoting factor (MPF) highly conserved amongst a wide range of species but it was also shown to be central to the progression of both mitosis and meiosis. Despite its biological importance, little progress was made in the chemical analysis of MPF until recently when work on yeast and marine invertebrates lead respectively to the discovery of a cell cycle dependent protein kinase referred to as p34^{cdc2} kinase and a family of cell cycle related molecules called cyclins (see References 16,33). The association of p34^{cdc2} kinase and cyclin B was shown to result in the formation of an inactive or pre-MPF complex whose conversion to an active form depended on selective phosphorylation modifications to its constituent molecules (13,7). Initial optimism that these molecular advances provided the full explanation of cell cycle control has now been replaced by the realisation that the intracellular regulatory machinery extends well beyond that of the synthesis, modification and formation of active MPF. Consequently, interest now focuses on the modulation, compartmentalization and interactions that occur between cell cycle molecules and their intracellular substrates.

In this paper we discuss changes in the key cell cycle molecules during the G2- to M-phase transition in mammalian germline cells during meiosis.

This cell cycle form is unique firstly because of its restriction to a single cell lineage in the body, secondly because of its progression through two M-phases with no intervening S-phase and thirdly because of the consequence of meiosis in halving of the cell's chromosomal complement. In female germline cells (oocytes) a further degree of specialization during meiosis is reflected in two unusual periods of cell cycle arrest in (a) late prophase (germinal vesicle stage; GV) and (b) after the formation of the second metaphase plate. The ideal system for the study of meiotic controls is one in which the cells are not only freely available but where each meiotic cycle stage is extended, clearly defined and can be faithfully reproduced *in vitro*. In mammals, these requirements are most completely met by utilising porcine oocytes obtained from the almost unlimited supply of ovaries from commercially slaughtered pigs. After dissection these oocytes undergo normal meiotic progression *in vitro* as evidenced by their ability to develop into young following fertilization and transfer to the oviduct of an appropriate foster mother (see Reference 18). Moreover, progression from the germinal vesicle to the MII phase of meiosis in pig oocyte takes over 40 h and is one of the most extended meiotic cycles in mammals. This period of so-called oocyte maturation can be further subdivided into an interval from the initiation of maturation (late G2-phase) to the breakdown of the germinal vesicle which takes approximately 24 h and consists of four distinct phases (see Reference 24). Progression through metaphase I takes 6-8 h, the anaphase-telophase transition occurs in under 2 h and leads to a period of meiotic arrest once the second metaphase plate has been established.

Because of its many advantages the porcine oocytes has been selected by us for a detailed analysis of meiosis. Our first priority in this undertaking has been the cloning and expression of key porcine cell cycle genes and the preparation of monoclonal antibodies against regulatory peptide sequences in the corresponding proteins. The resultant molecular reagents are being used in studies on the intracellular concentration, localization and function of these molecules during meiosis.

GENERAL REQUIREMENTS FOR G2- TO M-PHASE TRANSITION IN PORCINE OOCYTES

A variety of studies suggest that exit from the G2- or dictyate phase of the meiotic cycle in porcine cumulus-oocyte complexes requires a gonadotrophic initiation signal followed by transcription, translation, phosphorylation and proteolysis. Inhibition of any one of these metabolic processes is reported to reversibly prevent the G2- to M-phase transition (reviewed in Reference 23).

Transcriptional requirements. Studies initiated in the sheep and later repeated on bovine and porcine oocytes showed that the inhibition of transcription in cumulus-oocyte complexes during the first few hours after response to a gonadotrophic initiator signal invariably blocked exit from the G2-phase (27,9,18). No effect on meiosis was, however, observed when transcription was inhibited at any time after the first 2, 4 or 6 h for sheep, cow and pig oocytes respectively. Using cell manipulation and microinjection approaches we showed that this early transcriptional requirement was restricted solely to the associated cumulus cells and not to the oocyte itself (5). Although not proven, we postulate that this cumulus-specific transcription is required to modify the somatic compartment such that inhibitory signals are suppressed, thus enabling the oocyte to translate or modify proteins required for meiosis.

Protein synthetic requirements. Pig oocytes, in common with those from the sheep and cow, have an absolute dependence on protein synthesis for the G2- to M-phase transition (3,22,9). According to Fulka and colleagues proteins vital for the progression of the cell cycle are synthesised during the period between 8 and 16 h after the gonadotrophic initiator signal. However, more recent studies suggest that pig oocytes, like those of sheep, require protein synthesis continuously until shortly before nuclear membrane breakdown (18). Although these differences require resolution, it is absolutely clear that new protein synthesis is not required for chromatin condensation (Fig. 1) but is indispensable for nuclear membrane breakdown at the G2- to M-phase boundary (12). Differences in the requirements for protein synthesis, coupled with marked differences in the temporal relationship between chromatin condensation, nucleolar disassembly and membrane

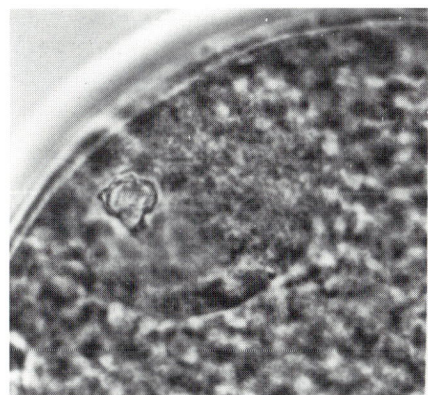
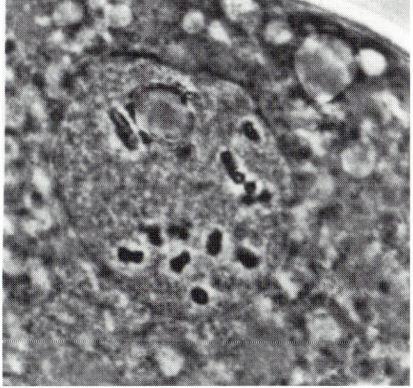

FIG. 1. Chromatin configuration (left panel) in pig oocytes in G2-arrest (or after inhibition of phosphorylation). Inhibition of protein synthesis for 20 h by the addition of cycloheximide (25 µg/ml to the culture medium) blocks nuclear membrane breakdown and nucleolar disassembly but does not inhibit chromatin condensation and bivalent formation in pig oocytes (right panel).

breakdown, indicate that the mechanisms which regulate these three key intranuclear events may differ, thereby imposing a multi-regulatory system on this key meiotic transition phase (see Reference 23).

In addition to the requirement for new protein synthesis, protease and kinase inhibitor studies also indicate an absolute requirement in pig oocytes for proteolysis and phosphoprotein modification before entry into M-phase (12, unpublished observations). The inhibition of proteolysis using 1 mM p-aminobenzamidine arrested oocytes in the germinal vesicle stage with chromatin in a condensed form around the nucleolus. It is noteworthy that while both cycloheximide and p-aminobenzamidine block membrane breakdown, their effect on chromatin condensation differs; blocking proteolysis arrests chromatin condensation at an early stage (Fig. 1: left panel) whilst inhibiting new protein synthesis has no inhibitory effect on condensation or on bivalent formation (Fig. 1: right panel). The inhibition of tyrosine phosphorylation has a similar effect on chromatin and nuclear membrane arrest as that of p-aminobenzamidine (T. Jung & C. Lee, unpublished observations). However, a strong note of caution must be struck about the interpretation of the present proteolysis and tyrosine phosphorylation data; use of p-aminobenzamidine and genistein as inhibitors of proteolysis and phosphorylation also severely inhibit total protein synthesis in porcine oocytes thus raising questions about the specificity of action of these drugs.

In summary, the gonadotrophic initiator signals in porcine oocyte-cumulus complexes act by inducing early and obligatory transcription in the follicle cell compartment followed by protein synthesis in the oocyte. A requirement before entry into M-phase for tyrosine phosphorylation and proteolysis is suggested from inhibitor experiments; however, uncertainty about the interpretation of these results remains because of a lack of specificity of the drugs used. These generalised requirements, in turn, raise questions about the synthesis, degradation, phosphorylation and localization of specific cell cycle proteins during progression through the meiotic cycle. Exploitation of cycloheximide-blocked porcine oocytes (see Reference 12) provides one attractive model for the analysis of mechanisms involved in driving the meiotic cycle through the crucial G2- to M-phase transition. In this model, oocytes are maintained in the G2- phase of cycle (GV) for 20-24 h by culture with cycloheximide. Removal of the inhibitor results in 100% of oocytes undergoing nuclear membrane breakdown within 6 h (see Table 1). Data in this table shows further that the period from cycloheximide release to membrane disassembly can be divided into an early 1.5-2.5 h period of obligatory protein synthesis followed by a further two to four hour interval before membrane breakdown when no further protein synthesis is required. It is with the changes in quantitation and localisation of cell cycle molecules that the remainder of this paper will be concerned.

Table 1. *Time-dependent effects of cycloheximide (10 μg/ml) on nuclear membrane disassembly in porcine oocytes (after Kubelka et al. 1988, Reference 12)*

1st period (20 h) of cycloheximide inhibition	2nd culture without inhibitor (h)	3rd culture period with new cycloheximide inhibition (h)	Percent oocytes undergoing nuclear membrane breakdown
20 h	0	0	0
	2	0	0
	4	0	86
	6	0	100
20 h	1	5	28
	1.5	4.5	53
	2.5	3.5	95

MOLECULAR EVENTS ASSOCIATED WITH NUCLEAR MEMBRANE BREAKDOWN IN PORCINE OOCYTES

A. Porcine cell cycle probes

Two strategies have been adopted for the production of the series of molecular probes required for a detailed analysis of the meiotic cycle. Firstly, the entire range of porcine cell cycle genes are being cloned and expressed to provide sequence data, mRNA and antisense constructs for microinjection plus purified proteins for monoclonal antibody production (C. Hawkins & R. Moor, unpublished observations). In parallel, peptides corresponding to active sites on the cyclin and p34^{cdc2} kinase molecules have been synthesised and appropriate polyclonal and monoclonal antibodies have been produced (A. Hutchings & R. Moor, unpublished observations).

The peptide antibodies specified in Table 2, have been used in results to be outlined in this paper. In addition, analysis of histone H1 kinase activity in single oocytes has been carried out using established procedures (1,13).

Table 2. *Peptide sequences from p34^{cdc2} and cyclin B proteins used for antibody production. Important sites of phosphorylation are indicated by an asterisk adjacent to the appropriate amino acid*

Protein	Antibody	Site of interest	Peptide sequence
p34^{cdc2}	TYG	ATP binding site	EKIGEG**T*Y*G**VVYKGRGKTT
	PSTAIR	Conserved kinase motif	EEGV**PSTAIRE**ISLLKELRH
Cyclin B	METS	Autophosphorylation site	ILVDTAS P**S*PMETS**CAP
	SKYEEM	Conserved sequence	MFIA**SKYEEM**YPPEIGDFAFV
	RASK	cAMP-dependent phosphorylation site	GLGRPLPLHRL**RAS*K**OGEV

B. *Cell cycle molecules in G2-arrested oocytes*

The amount of $p34^{cdc2}$ protein in fully grown porcine oocytes has been examined after polypeptide separation on SDS gels and Western blotting using antibodies specified in Table 2. Our results, like those of others (see Reference 26), show clearly that the level of $p34^{cdc2}$ kinase in porcine oocytes before the gonadotrophin initiator signal is high (T. Jung, R. Moor, A. Hutchings & T. Miyano, unpublished observations). After 20 h of culture in medium containing cycloheximide (25 µg/ml), Western blot analysis showed that the $p34^{cdc2}$ protein levels had not diminished, suggesting that the turnover of this molecular is relatively slow in oocytes.

The levels of putative cyclin B2 as measured by the RASK antibody, are similarly relatively high in oocytes in G2-phase arrest. Caution must be used in this interpretation because of a lack of definitive proof at present that the antibody does not cross-react with cyclin B1.

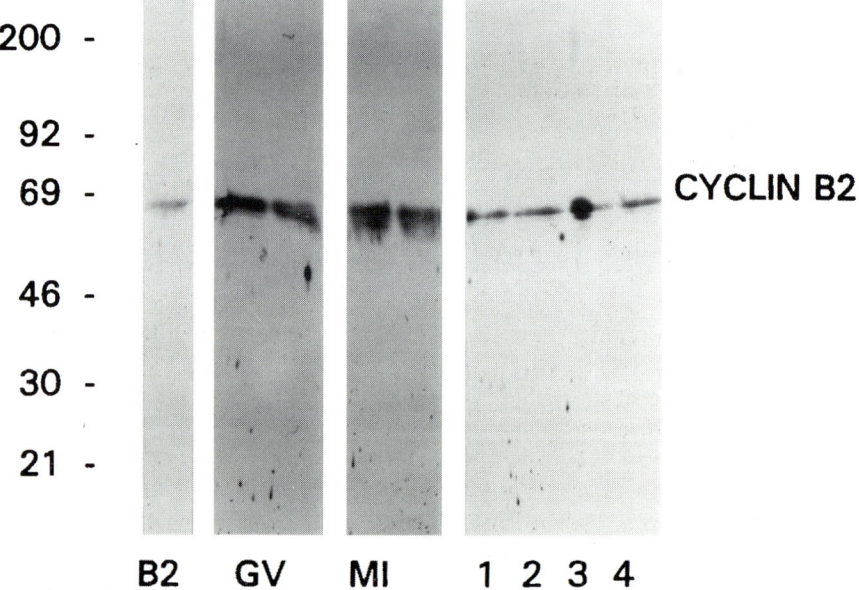

FIG. 2. Level of cyclin B2 antibody in porcine oocytes during G2-arrest (GV), after entry in M-phase (MI) and at hourly intervals after release from 20h of cycloheximide inhibition (lanes marked 1,2,3,4 refer to time (h) after cycloheximide removal). Purified cyclin B2 from *Xenopus laevis* oocytes (gift from T. Hunt) is shown on the extreme left (lane B2). Polypeptides were separated on SDS-PAGE gels, transferred by Western blotting to nitrocellulose and immunoblotted use the polyclonal RASK antibody prepared against the cyclin B2 peptide sequence shown in Table 2.

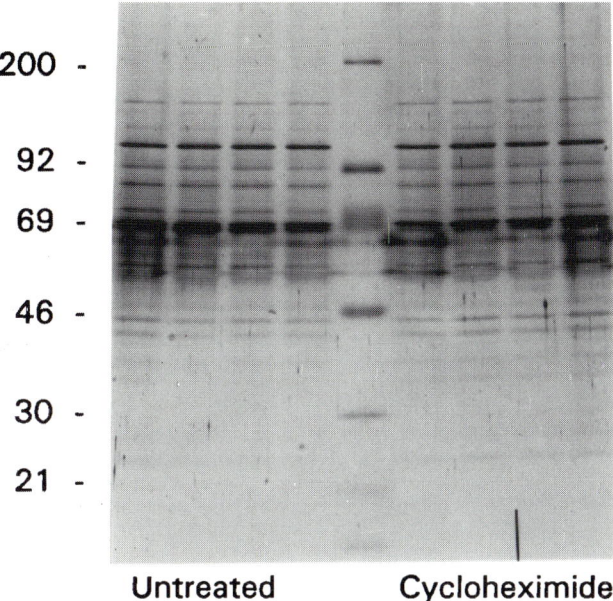

FIG. 3. A comparison of polypeptide profiles, as revealed by silver staining, in porcine in G2-arrest (untreated) and after 20 h of culture with 25 μg/ml of cycloheximide (cycloheximide). Each lane on the gel represents a group of 30 oocytes.

Fig. 2. shows that the levels of B-type cyclins are slightly lower after culture for 20 h in cycloheximide than that in oocytes before inhibition. Nevertheless, it is apparent that substantial amounts of cyclin B remain in the oocyte after culture with protein inhibitors. That cycloheximide treatment does not induce gross changes in the overall levels of major proteins in porcine oocytes is indicated by comparing the silver staining patterns of similar numbers of oocytes taken immediately after dissection from the ovaries (G2-stage arrest) or after 20 h of culture with cycloheximide (Fig. 3).

Despite the presence of both $p34^{cdc2}$ protein and cyclin B2 in oocytes before and during cycloheximide arrest no detectable histone H1 kinase activity was found in either G2-arrested or cycloheximide treated oocytes (see Section C, page 92). It must be reiterated at this point that chromatin condensation and bivalent formation invariably occurred in oocytes cultured in the presence of cycloheximide (see Fig. 1). These results suggest that a separation between condensation and MPF activity may be made, but only to the extent that histone H1 kinase activity can be directly equated to the biological activity of MPF. However, recent findings in mammalian fibroblasts support the contention that chromatin condensation is regulated by a different kinase from the classical $p34^{cdc2}$ type (14).

Two further points about G2-arrested and cycloheximide inhibited porcine oocytes require emphasis. Firstly, our data shows that $p34^{cdc2}$ kinase exists in both a phosphorylated and dephosphorylated form during the G2-phase; cycloheximide inhibition does not appear to alter the ratio of these two forms of p34^{cdc2}. Secondly, immunogold localization studies suggest that the two B-type cyclins, but neither cyclin A nor p34^{cdc2} kinase are strictly compartmentalized in the G2-phase of meiosis (T. Miyano, T. Jung, A. Hutchings, C. Hawkins & R.M. Moor, unpublished observations). This tight compartmentalization represents one crucial mechanism by which cell cycle progression may be regulated.

C. Cell cycle molecules during G2- to M-phase transition

The most precise and reproducible timing of the molecular events that precede entry into M-phase in porcine oocytes occurs after release from cycloheximide inhibition (see Reference 12). In this cellular model, disassembly of both the nucleolus and nuclear membrane occur within 6 to 8 h of cycloheximide removal; for both these processes a period of protein synthesis of 1.5 h immediately after cycloheximide release is obligatory (12).

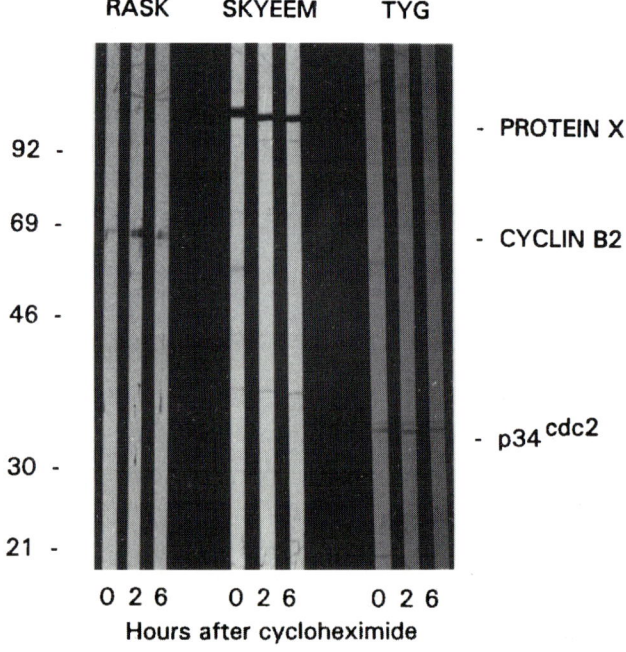

FIG. 4. A comparison of the relative levels of immunoreactive protein in pig oocytes after 20 h of cycloheximide inhibition (befpre cycloheximide release; 0h group) or at 2 h or 6 h after cycloheximide removal. Equal numbers of oocytes were loaded into each well of an 8-15% SDS PAGE gel and, after Western blotting, the nitrocellulose strips were probed (see Table 2) with polyclonal antibodies directed against B-type cyclins (RASK and *SKYEEM*) and p34^{cdc2} protein (TYG). The SKYEEM antibody recognises an unidentified, but oocyte specific protein which probably corresponds with a similar protein in *Xenopus laevis* oocytes described by Kobayashi and colleagues (11).

During this period changes in cyclin and p34^{cdc2} levels have been monitored and are summarised in Fig. 4.

Our results indicate that the total amount of p34^{cdc2} protein in oocytes does not change significantly between cycloheximide release and entry into metaphase. These conclusions are similar to those in other species (26) and show that this cell cycle kinase is continuously present in cells. Indeed, in G2-arrested *Xenopus* oocytes p34^{cdc2} concentrations are roughly 10 times greater than those of the total cyclin content in the cell (11). Our results show that it is probably, but not yet clearly proven, that after cycloheximide release in pig oocytes the level of the phosphorylated form of p34^{cdc2} decreases whilst that of the dephosphorylated form increases slightly.

No measurable differences have been detected in cyclin B1 after cycloheximide release. However, a small but steady increase in the cyclin B2 (recognised by the RASK antibody) is usually observed and [^{32}P] orthophosphate labelling studies during the 6 h post cycloheximide release period suggest that this protein probably becomes increasingly heavily phosphorylated as the oocyte progresses from G2- to M-phase.

Thus, quantitative changes associated with the key cell cycle molecules are surprisingly limited during the 6 h post cycloheximide release period. These apparently small changes are, however, accompanied by very sharp modifications to the levels of histone H1 kinase activity in oocytes during this period (Fig. 5).

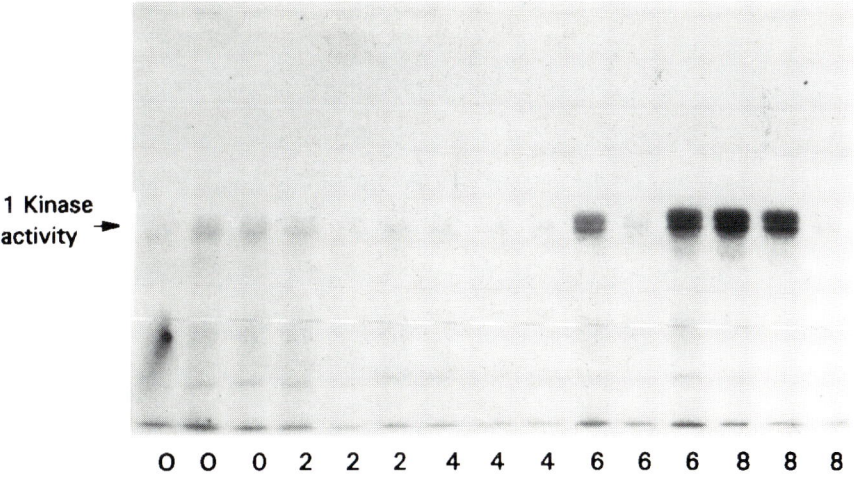

FIG. 5. Histone H1 kinase activity in single pig oocytes after 20 h of culture in medium containing 25 µg/ml cycloheximide (0 h groups) or at two hourly intervals after the removal of the protein synthesis inhibitor. Despite very low levels of H1 kinase activity during the period of protein synthesis inhibition by cycloheximide, chromatin condensation and bivalent formation occurs (see Fig. 1). The sharp increase in H1 kinase activity in oocytes at 6-8 h after release coincides with the time at which nuclear membrane breakdown and nucleolar disassembly occurs.

The results presented in Fig. 5 show the levels of histone H1 kinase activity in individual porcine oocytes at two hourly intervals after release from cycloheximide inhibition. In our culture system nuclear membrane breakdown occurs between 6 and 8 h after cycloheximide release; that nuclear membrane breakdown occurs slightly later than in the earlier studies (12) probably reflects the higher levels of cycloheximide used by us. Nevertheless, the histone H1-kinase levels in oocytes from our experiments are at background levels for the first 4 h and then rise sharply immediately before entry into metaphase.

Our results may therefore be summarised by stressing that porcine oocytes, both during G2-phase arrest and after 20-24 h of cycloheximide inhibition, contain substantial levels of $p34^{cdc2}$ protein and B-type cyclins. In these oocytes, cyclin B is sharply compartmentalised within the cytoplasm. In such cycloheximide-arrested oocytes, chromatin condensation occurs but nucleolar and nuclear membrane disassembly are prevented. After removal of cycloheximide, a short period of protein synthesis (1.5 h) followed by a further synthesis independent interval of 4-6 h, is required for entry into M-phase. During this time cyclin B2-type molecules increase slightly in concentration whilst $p34^{cdc2}$ kinase becomes progressively more dephosphorylated. Entry of B type cyclins into the nuclear compartment is a late event and occurs just before nuclear membrane disassembly. A dramatic and sharp increase in histone-H1 kinase occurs after about 6 h from cycloheximide release and likewise coincides with the breakdown of the nuclear membrane in the oocyte.

CONCLUDING COMMENTS

The results presented in this paper raise three issues of particular importance to the G2- to M-phase transition in mammalian oocytes. These are (i) the differential regulation of individual intranuclear events, (ii) the continuously high levels of the major cell cycle molecules even during periods of G2-arrest and (iii) the tight compartmental localization of B-type cyclins.

The question of whether MPF, when defined as a complex of $p34^{cdc2}$ kinase and cyclin B, is the direct regulator of all intranuclear events or is a central component of a cell cycle cascade is disputed. It is our strong conviction that the condensation of chromatin, nucleolar and nuclear membrane disassembly and spindle formation in oocytes are each controlled in a co-ordinated but differential manner. Of particular interest in this respect is the recent study by Lamb and colleagues (14) on the G2- to M-phase transition in human fibroblasts. These authors show that the inhibition of cAMP-dependent protein kinase (A-kinase) at any stage of the mitotic cycle induces rapid chromatin condensation and a characteristic M-phase-like reorganisation of the microtubular network. However, disassembly of the nuclear membrane does not accompany these intranuclear changes unless the levels of p34^{cdc2} kinase are increased. Although apparently against current dogma, results on isolated nuclei show in turn that active p34^{cdc2} kinase produces little or no chromatin condensation (28). Taken together both the results in meiosis and mitosis suggest that chromatin condensation and spindle formation can be clearly separated at a regulatory level from nuclear membrane disassembly.

The detection of high levels of cyclins and p34^{cdc2} kinase in G2- arrested porcine oocytes corresponds closely with recent findings of a similar accumulation of cell cycle molecules in arrested stage VI *Xenopus laevis* oocytes (11). In that species, concentrations of 4×10^8 and 2×10^9 molecules of cyclin B1 and B2 respectively are present in oocytes before initiation of maturation by progesterone stimulation. The levels of cyclin B1 increase steadily during maturation from about 30 pg to 60-80 pg in metaphase II. However, at the G2- to M-phase transition a sharp but small increase in cyclin B2 synthesis occurs followed by equally rapid degradation at the metaphase I-anaphase transition. The existing high p34^{cdc2} protein levels in stage VI *Xenopus* oocytes are further supplemented during maturation by new p34^{cdc2} synthesis. The significance of these changes in cell cycle components during maturation is, however, far from clear. Thus, microinjection of mRNA coding for cyclin B into stage VI amphibian oocytes results in the rapid breakdown of the nuclear membrane and entry into metaphase (29). These observations together with those showing that cyclin must be synthesised after fertilisation in order to induce mitosis indicate that new cyclin synthesis is necessary for the G2- to M-phase transition (20,25). By contrast, a recent study by Minshull and colleagues (21) reports a contrary observation and suggests that new cyclin synthesis in *Xenopus* oocytes is neither required for the G2- to M-phase transition nor for the entry into second meiotic metaphase. These conclusions were derived from experiments in which antisense oligonucleotides, when injected into G2-arrested *Xenopus* oocytes blocked cyclin synthesis, but did not prevent histone H1 kinase activation. However, oocytes that lacked cyclin mRNAs (as a consequence of antisense oligonucleotide injection) failed to show classical activation responses when injected with calcium. The results with pig oocytes are similar to those in amphibia but our reservations about the specificity of antisense oligonucleotides limit the range of conclusions we are currently willing to draw from our work. Thus, injection of cyclin B1 mRNA into G2-arrested pig oocytes induces rapid histone H1 kinase activation and entry into metaphase (R.M. Moor, A. Hutchings, C. Hawkins & T. Jung, unpublished observations). Conversely, antisense oligonucleotides against B-type cyclins induce hypercondensation (cell damage) in 30-40% of oocytes while the remainder progress through the G2- to M-phase transition (R.M. Moor, & A. Northrop, unpublished observations). It is possible that our results indicate that in physically undamaged oocytes (hypercondensation equates to cell damage) new cyclin B synthesis is not required for progression to M-phase. However, extreme caution is required in interpreting antisense oligonucleotide results (34,15) and until more controls are done we are unwilling to draw firm conclusions from our results.

Evidence has been presented to show that B-type cyclin become phosphorylated and that this phosphorylation is closely associated with the appearance of histone H1 kinase activity (6,29,19). Furthermore, a role for *c-mos* in cyclin B phosphorylation has been demonstrated (32). Notwithstanding all the above evidence, however, a new study by Izumi and Maller (10) using site-directed mutagenesis now casts doubt on the need for cyclin phosphorylation during maturation in *Xenopus* oocytes. Thus, although B-type cyclins are synthesised and phosphorylated in *Xenopus* oocytes before entry into M-phase, neither process is reputedly vital for passage across this crucial meiotic cycle transition phase.

Of considerable current interest is the degree to which B-type cyclin are confined to the cytoplasmic compartment of mitotic cells during interphase and only translocated to the nucleus at the onset of mitosis (30,4). It is further suggested the cyclin B1 interacts with centrosomes and that these interactions may form an important regulatory mechanism in cell-cycle control (2). We find equally tight compartmental localization of B-type cyclins in porcine oocytes and strongly support the view that the stage-specific entry of cyclin into the nuclear compartment is of considerable importance in meiotic cycle regulation. It is our view that it is clearly premature to produce integrated models of cell cycle control at present. However, the data presently available suggests that the control mechanisms will involve firstly a combination of translation, phosphorylation and translocation regulators. Secondly, these controls will probably act not only on cyclins and $p34^{cdc2}$ protein but also crucially on other kinase and phosphatase systems as well.

ACKNOWLEDGEMENTS

The authors thank their colleagues for assistance and access to unpublished data referred to in this paper. We are also indebted to Linda Notton for her expertise in preparing this manuscript for publication. Support from a DFG Fellowship (T.J.) and from a Japanese Government Overseas Research Scholars' fellowship (T.M.) is gratefully acknowledged.

REFERENCES

1. Arion, D., Meijer, L., Brizuela, L. and Beach, D. (1988) cdc2 is a component of the M phase specific histone-H1 kinase: Evidence for identity with MPF. Cell, 55:371-378.
2. Bailly, E., Motlik, J. Fulka, J. and Jilek, F. (1992) Cytoplasmic accumulation of cyclin B1 in human cells: association with detergent-resistant compartment and with the centrosome. J. Cell Sci., 101:529-545.

3. Fulka Jr. J., Motlik, J., Fulka, J. and Jilek, F. (1986) Effect of cycloheximide on nuclear maturation of pig and mouse oocytes. J. Reprod. Fertil., 77:281-285.
4. Gallant, P. and Nigg, E.A. (1992) Cyclin B2 undergoes cell cycle-dependent nuclear translocation and, when expressed as a non-destructible mutant, causes mitotic arrest in HeLa cells. J. Cell Biol., 117:213-224.
5. Galli, C. and Moor, R.M. (1991) Somatic cells and the G2 to M-phase transition in sheep oocytes. Reprod. Nut. Dev., 31:127-134.
6. Gautier, J. and Maller, J.L. (1991) Cyclin B2 and pre-MPF activation in *Xenopus* oocytes. EMBO J., 10:177-182.
7. Gould, K.L. and Nurse, P. (1989) Tyrosine phosphorylation of the fission yeast cdc+ protein kinase regulates entry into mitosis. Nature, 342:39-45.
8. Hunt, T. (1989) Maturation promoting factor, cyclin and the control of M-phase. Curr. Opin. Cell Biol., 1:268-274.
9. Hunter, A.G. and Moor, R.M. (1987) Stage dependent effect of inhibiting RNA and protein synthesis on meiotic maturation of bovine oocytes *in vitro*. J. Dairy Sci., 70:1646-1651.
10. Izumi, T. and Maller, J.L. (1991) Phosphorylation of *Xenopus* cyclins B1 and B2 is not required for cell cycle transitions. Mol. Cell. Biol., 1:3860-3867.
11. Kobayashi, H., Minshall, J., Ford, C., Golsteyn, R., Poon, R. and Hunt, T. (1991) On the synthesis and destruction of A- and B-type cyclins during oogenesis and meiotic maturation in *Xenopus laevis*. J. Cell Biol., 114:755-765.
12. Kubelka, M., Motlik, J., Fulka Jr. J., Prochazka, R., Rimkevicova, Z. and Fulka, J. (1988) Time sequence of germinal vesicle breakdown in pig oocytes after cycloheximide and P-amino-benzamidine block. Gamete Res., 19:423-431.
13. Labbé, J-C., Capony, J-P., Caput, D., Cavadore, J-C., Derancourt, J., Kaghdad, M., Lelias, J-M., Picard, A. and Dorée, M. (1989) MPF from starfish oocytes at first meiotic metaphase is a heterodimer containing one molecules of cdc2 and one molecule of cyclin B. EMBO J., 8:3052-3058.
14. Lamb, N.J.C., Cavadore J-C., Labbé J-C., Maurer, R.A. and Fernandez, A. (1991) Inhibition of cAMP-dependent protein kinase plays a key role in the induction of mitosis and nuclear envelope breakdown in mammalian cells. EMBO J., 10:1523-1533.
15. Leonetti, J.P., Mechti, N., Degols, G., Gagnor, C. and Lebi, B. (1991) Intracellular distribution of microinjected antisense oligonucleotides. Proc. Natl. Acad. Sci. USA, 88:2702-2706.
16. Masui, F.C. and Markert, C.L. (1971) Cytoplasmic control of nuclear behaviour during meiotic maturation of frog oocytes. J. Exp. Zool., 177:129-146.
17. Mattioli, M., Bacci, M.L., Galeati, G. and Seren, E. (1989) Developmental competence of pig oocytes matured and fertilized *in vitro*. Theriogenology, 31:1201-1207.
18. Mattioli, M., Galeati, G., Bacci, M.L. and Barboni, B. (1991) Changes in maturation-promoting activity in the cytoplasm of pig oocytes throughout maturation. Mol. Reprod. Dev., 30:119-125.
19. Meijer, L., Azzi, L. and Wang, J.Y.J. (1991) Cyclin B targets p34^{cdc2} for tyrosine phosphorylation. EMBO J., 10:1545-1554.
20. Minshull, J., Blow, J. and Hunt, T. (1989) Translation of cyclin mRNAs is necessary for extracts of activated *Xenopus* eggs to enter mitosis. Cell, 56:947-956.
21. Minshull, J., Murray, A., Colman, A. and Hunt, T. (1991) *Xenopus* oocyte maturation does not require new cyclin synthesis. J. Cell Biol., 114:767-772.
22. Moor, R.M., and Crosby, I.M. (1986) Protein requirements for germinal vesicle breakdown in ovine oocytes. J. Embryol. Exp. Morph., 94:207-220.
23. Moor, R.M., Mattioli, M., Ding, J. and Nagai, T. (1990) Maturation of pig oocytes *in vivo* and *in vitro*. J. Reprod. Fert. Suppl., 40:197-210.
24. Motlik, J. and Fulka, J. (1976) Breakdown of the germinal vesicle in pig oocytes *in vivo* and *in vitro*. J. Exp. Zool., 198:155-162.
25. Murray, A.W. and Kirschner, M.W. (1989) Cyclin synthesis drives the early embryonic cell cycle. Nature, 339:275-279.
26. Nurse, P. (1990) Universal control of mechanism regulating onset of M-phase. Nature, 344:503-508.
27. Osborn, J.C. and Moor, R.M. (1983) Time-dependent effects of α-amanitin on nuclear maturation and protein synthesis in mammalian oocytes. J. Embryol. Exp. Morph., 73:317-338.
28. Peter, M., Nakagawa, P.M., Dorée M., Labbé, J-C. and Nigg, E.A. (1990) *In vitro* disassembly of the nuclear lamina and M-phase specific phosphorylation of lamins by cdc2 kinase. Cell, 61:591-602.

29. Pines, J. and Hunt, T., (1987) Molecular cloning and characterization of the mRNA for cyclin from sea urchin eggs. EMBO J., 6:2987-2995.
30. Pines, J. and Hunter, T., (1989) Isolation of a human cyclin cDNA: evidence for cyclin mRNA and protein regulation in the cell cycle and for interaction with $p34^{cdc2}$. Cell, 58:833-846.
31. Pines, J. and Hunter, T., (1991) Human cyclins A and B1 are differentially located in the cell and undergo cell cycle-dependent nuclear transport. J. Cell Biol., 115:1-17.
32. Roy, L.M., Sing., B., Gautier, J., Arlinghaus, R.B., Nordeen, S.K. and Maller, J.L. (1990) The cyclin B2 component of MPF is a substrate for the c-*mos* proto-oncogene product. Cell, 61:825-831.
33. Smith, L.D. and Ecker, R.E. (1971) The interaction of steroids with *Rana pipiens* oocytes in the induction of maturation. Dev. Biol., 25:233-247.
34. Smith, R.C., Bement, W.M., Dersch, M.A., Dworkin-Rastl, E., Dworkin, M.B. and Capco, D.G. (1990) Nonspecific effects of oligodeoxynucleotide injection in *Xenopus* oocytes: a re-evaluation of previous D7 mRNA ablation experiments. Development, 110:769-779.

Protein Tyrosine Phosphorylation/Dephosphorylation and Control of Meiosis in Rat Oocytes

N. Dekel and S. Goren

*Department of Hormone Research, The Weizmann Institute of Science
Rehovot 76100, Israel*

INTRODUCTION

The two major events that represent an actively dividing eukaryotic cell are replication of the genetic material in the S phase of the cell cycle and segregation of the replicated DNA to daughter cells during the M-phase. In most types of cells a G1 phase separates the completion of M-phase from the beginning of S-phase, whereas a G2 phase separates S-phase from M-phase. Both G1 and G2 have been identified as control points in the cell cycle.

Germ cells undergo a special type of cell division known as meiosis. Meiosis in oocytes, unlike that in sperm cells, is a protracted process with the fully grown oocyte arrested at a G2-like phase. In response to hormones, these oocytes enter M-phase and mature into metaphase-arrested unfertilized eggs. Thus, at maturation, oocytes undergo a cell cycle comprising a G2 to M transition Very little was known until quite recently about the biochemical control of cell division in general, and that of meiosis in particular. However, during the last four years, the importance of the maturation promoting factor (MPF) at the onset of M-phase in both meiotic and mitotic cells has been established, particularly with respect to critical protein phosphorylation/dephosphorylation events that drive cells to the metaphase state (15).

The mechanism of activation of MPF involves interaction between the two components of this factor. One of which, a 34 kDa protein that is homologous to the product of the cdc2 gene of the fission yeast (7,8), is termed $p34^{cdc2}$. This protein, which is highly conserved among eukaryotes, is a serine/threonine kinase. The level of $p34^{cdc2}$ is not altered during the cell cycle. The other component of MPF is a 45 kDa protein known as cyclin. The cytoplasmic levels of cyclin fluctuate during the cell cycle; concentrations rise just before cell division, turning on the MPF kinase activity. The cyclin concentrations then drop sharply and the kinase activity also declines allowing the cells to complete the division cycle. Resynthesis of the cyclin can then trigger another round of division (13, 16). Binding to cyclin induces both tyrosine and threonine phosphorylation of the previously unphosphorylated $p34^{cdc2}$, rendering it inactivated. The transition into M-phase involves both a reduction in the rate of $p34^{cdc2}$ phosphorylation on tyrosine and an increase in the rate of dephosphorylation (18). Dephosphorylation of tyrosine and threonine residues of the $p34^{cdc2}$ is accompanied by reciprocal phosphorylation of the cyclin (12).

Changes in the pattern of cell phosphoproteins that involve protein phosphorylation/dephosphorylation on tyrosine residues are clearly associated with the transition from G2 to M-phase. Furthermore, it is very well established that protein tyrosine phosphorylation, associated with the binding of mitogenic ligands, plays an important role in the control of cell growth (21). This information combined with our earlier findings that epidermal growth factor (EGF) successfully promotes resumption of meiosis in rat oocytes (4), led us to investigate the involvement of protein tyrosine kinases and phosphatases in regulation of oocyte maturation in this animal model.

As already stated, fully grown oocytes are naturally arrested at a G2-like phase. These oocytes, therefore, serve as a perfect model system for investigation of the control of cell cycle. Meiotically arrested mammalian oocytes resume meiosis *in vivo* in response to the preovulatory surge of the pituitary gonadotropin luteinizing hormone (LH; 10). These oocytes can also resume meiosis *in vitro*, spontaneously upon their release from the surrounding ovarian follicles (17). It has been demonstrated in several mammalian species that cAMP plays a dominant role in keeping the oocyte at the G2-arrested stage and that a drop in intraoocyte concentrations of this cyclic nucleotide is associated with the transition from G2 to M-phase (5). The biochemical events occurring downstream to this drop in cAMP are still unknown. Due to the availability of large amounts of synchronized samples, *Xenopus* oocytes have been widely used to study regulation of the cell cycle during meiosis (11). However, since the amounts of mammalian oocytes that can be easily obtained are very limited, there is hardly any information concerning the regulation of the meiotic cell cycle in mammals.

The experiments described in this chapter were designed to explore the following issues:
1. Involvement of protein tyrosine kinases in maturation of rat oocytes.
2. Involvement of protein tyrosine phosphatases in maturation of rat oocytes.
3. Identification of the target protein(s) for tyrosine kinases and tyrosine phosphatases in maturing rat oocytes.
4. Correlation between intraoocyte cAMP levels and the phosphorylation/dephosphorylation events.

INVOLVEMENT OF PROTEIN TYROSINE KINASES IN MATURATION OF RAT OOCYTES.

The possibility that protein tyrosine phosphorylation is essential for resumption of meiosis was studied by using tyrphostins, a class of novel protein tyrosine kinase (PTK) inhibitors (20). Tyrphostins are low molecular weight compounds derived from the benzylidene malononitrile nucleus. These compounds can traverse the cell membrane and their inhibitory effect is fully reversible. They are competitive with the substrate of the EGF receptor kinase and not with adenosine triphosphate (ATP). They are much more selective to the tyrosine kinase domain of the EGF receptor as compared to that of the insulin receptor. The compounds of this class are diverse in their inhibitory potency which is correlated with their affinity to the substrate binding site of the receptor kinase domain.

The effect of tyrphostins on spontaneous maturation of rat oocytes
The effect of tyrphostins was tested *in vitro* using two types of cultured oocytes:

I. *Cumulus-enclosed oocytes.*

When released from the ovarian follicles, oocytes resume meiosis spontaneously (17). Using tyrphostins that are inhibitors of PTK, we tried to clarify whether this enzyme participates in the process of oocyte maturation. Specifically, the potential of different tyrphostins to inhibit spontaneous maturation of isolated cumulus-enclosed rat oocytes has been examined. Confirming our earlier results (3), we found that after 4 h of incubation in tyrphostin-free medium 85% of the cumulus-enclosed oocytes resumed meiosis. Resumption of meiosis in this experiment, as well as in the other experiments described later in this chapter, was diagnosed by the disappearance of the nuclear structure known as germinal vesicle breakdown (GVB). In cumulus-enclosed oocytes that were incubated in the presence of tyrphostins for a similar period of time the fraction of GVB oocytes was significantly reduced. The effect of the several compounds of this series that have been tested was dose dependent, but they differed in their inhibitory potency. For example, the half maximal effective dose (ED_{50}) for AG-12, which is one of the tyrphostins tested, was 100 µM while that of another tyrphostin, AG-18, was 20 µM. A third tyrphostin of this series, AG-9, which is a less selective inhibitor for the EGF-dependent tyrosine kinase, failed in inhibiting oocyte maturation.

To eliminate the possibility that tyrphostin-inhibited oocyte maturation is a result of a toxic effect of these compounds, reversibility of their influence was examined. Cumulus-enclosed oocytes were incubated for 2 h in the presence of 50 µM of AG-18 and then washed and transferred to tyrphostin-free medium for further incubation. Maturation was monitored in these oocytes after a total culture period of 5 h. Almost 70% of the oocytes recovered from the inhibitory effect showing GVB while the oocytes that were continuously incubated in the presence of AG-18 remained meiotically arrested.

II. *Cumulus-free oocytes.*

The cumulus cells are the immediate cellular neighbours of the oocyte in the ovarian follicle. These cells are known to mediate some of the oocyte responses to external stimuli (6). Demonstration of the tyrphostins effect on the cumulus-enclosed oocyte system may represent a cumulus-mediated action of these PTK inhibitors. To test whether tyrphostin action is exerted directly on the oocyte, cumulus-free oocytes were isolated into culture medium containing either AG-18 (100 µM) or AG-34 (50 µM). Both these tyrphostins were fully effective in inhibiting maturation of cumulus-free oocytes. After 4 h of incubation in the presence of AG-18, only 13.5% of these oocytes resumed meiosis while AG-34 totally blocked meiosis resumption. Being incubated in tyrphostin-free medium 89% of the cumulus-free oocytes resumed meiosis. These results suggest that PTK activity, essential for maturation of rat oocytes, apparently takes place in the oocyte itself. This conclusion remains in accordance with an earlier demonstration of an enhanced rate of tyrosine phosphorylation in mouse oocytes committed to resume meiosis (1).

Timing of the protein tyrosine phosphorylation during oocyte maturation

Maturation of the oocyte consists of a programmed cascade of biochemical events, one of which is apparently represented by tyrosine phosphorylation. In order to pinpoint the time during the maturation process at which the tyrosine phosphorylation event takes place, the following experimental protocol was designed. Cumulus-enclosed rat oocytes were isolated into tyrphostin-free medium. Tyrphostins were added to the medium at 0,15, 30, 45 and 60 min after initiation of incubation. The time at which the addition of the tyrphostin to the incubation medium will no longer inhibit oocyte maturation was determined. We found that when 50 µM of AG-34 were present from the very beginning of incubation, maturation of the oocytes was totally blocked. However, exposure of the oocytes to tyrphostin-free medium for 30 min, followed by addition of AG-34 at this time point resulted in 50% inhibition of maturation while the addition of AG-34 at 45 min after initiation of incubation allowed all the oocytes to resume meiosis. These last results combined with those described earlier in this chapter suggest that protein tyrosine phosphorylation is an obligatory step for reinitiation of meiosis which takes place within 30 min after the initiation of this process.

INVOLVEMENT OF PROTEIN TYROSINE PHOSPHATASES IN MATURATION OF RAT OOCYTES

The effect of vanadate on spontaneous maturation of rat oocytes

Mouse 3T3 fibroblasts cdc2 was shown to be tyrosine-phosphorylated and dephosphorylated in a cell-cycle-dependent manner; its phosphotyrosine content was maximal in late G2, and became abruptly dephosphorylated at the entry to M-phase (14). To test the possibility that tyrosine dephosphorylation is essential for meiosis reinitiation in rat oocytes, cumulus-enclosed G2-arrested oocytes were isolated in vanadate-containing medium. Vanadate is a reported inhibitor of protein tyrosine phosphatases (9,19). We found that vanadate effectively inhibited the spontaneous maturation of rat cumulus-enclosed oocytes. Vanadate action was dose-dependent with an apparent ED_{50} at 0.17 mM. The inhibitory effect of vanadate was reversible, with 75% of the oocytes resuming meiosis upon its removal from the culture medium. Exposure of the oocytes to vanadate-free medium that was followed by its addition to the incubation medium at 45-60 min after their isolation from the ovarian follicles has allowed them to complete the maturation process. These results suggest that protein tyrosine dephosphorylation is another obligatory step for the resumption of meiosis in rat oocytes and that this biochemical event takes place at about 45-60 min after reinitiation of this process.

DETECTION OF PROTEIN TYROSINE PHOSPHORYLATION/DEPHOSPHORYLATION DURING OOCYTE MATURATION

To detect the target protein(s) for tyrosine kinases and phosphatases that participate in meiosis resumption, immunoblot analysis using specific anti-phosphotyrosine antibodies was performed. Using this technique, we studied the state of protein tyrosine phosphorylation in isolated rat oocytes undergoing meiotic maturation spontaneously as compared to that in oocytes maintained in meiotic arrest by either tyrphostins or vanadate. We found in spontaneously maturating oocytes an intensive tyrosine phosphorylation on a 105 kDa protein while a 34 kDa protein showed only partial phosphorylation on its tyrosine residues. In oocytes that are kept meiotically arrested by the presence of vanadate (50 µM), these two proteins and an additional protein of 42 kDa were found to be highly phosphorylated on their tyrosine residues. Tyrosine phosphorylation of these three proteins, but to a lesser extent, was detected in oocytes exposed to AG-34 (50 µM). These results demonstrate that at least three proteins are phosphorylated on their tyrosine residues in the G2-arrested oocytes. Two of these proteins undergo immediate dephosphorylation upon their release from the ovarian follicle. This later biochemical event, that is inhibited by vanadate, is apparently essential for resumption of meiosis. Attempts, to identify the 34 kDa protein as the $p34^{cdc2}$ component of the MPF, are presently being made in our laboratory by employing anti-$p34^{cdc2}$ antibodies. Maturation-associated $p34^{cdc2}$ dephosphorylation has also been suggested in mouse oocytes (2).

CORRELATION BETWEEN INTRAOOCYTE cAMP LEVELS AND THE PHOSPHORYLATION/DEPHOSPHORYLATION EVENTS

As stated in the Introduction, maturation of rat oocytes is negatively regulated by intracellular concentrations of cAMP. Phosphodiesterase inhibitors that prevent the degradation of this cyclic nucleotide are therefore effective inhibitors of spontaneous maturation of rat oocytes (3). We investigated the possible interrelationships between intraoocyte cAMP, and protein tyrosine phosphorylation/dephosphorylation events. We found that in the presence of a phosphodiesterase inhibitor (isobutylmethylxanthine, IBMX, 0.2 mM) in the culture medium, the concentrations of cAMP within the oocyte were 1.42 fmoles. Intracellular concentrations of cAMP in the oocyte at 2 h after isolation from the ovarian follicles into IBMX-free medium dropped to 0.84 fmoles. Tyrphostins seem to prevent at least partially the maturation-associated drop in intraoocyte concentrations of cAMP (1.1 fmoles/oocyte). On the other hand, in the presence of vanadate (50 µM), cAMP concentrations in the oocyte did drop in spite of the inhibitory effect of this agent on oocyte maturation. These findings suggest that the vanadate-inhibited protein tyrosine dephosphorylation event occurs downstream to the maturation-associated drop in intraoocyte cAMP levels.

CONCLUDING REMARKS

Protein phosphorylation involves the transfer of phosphate from a nucleotide to a substrate protein, catalyzed by a protein kinase. The protein kinases that catalyze such reactions act upon one or more specific substrate proteins by transfer of phosphate to the hydroxyl group of serine, threonine or tyrosine residues. The vast majority of phosphorylations occur in serine. While tyrosine phosphorylation is a rare event in a cell, it provides a mechanism for the regulation of numerous crucial processes, one of which is progression through the cell cycle. Our experiments demonstrate that protein tyrosine phosphorylation/dephosphorylation events are included among a number of obligatory steps leading to spontaneous maturation of rat oocytes. One of the most pressing questions to be addressed concerns the nature of the substrate proteins which are phosphorylated on tyrosine and the roles they play in regulation of meiosis in rat oocytes. Detection of the state of tyrosine phosphorylation in these target proteins has been accomplished by the use of antiphosphotyrosine antibodies. These antibodies are specific for phosphotyrosine and do not recognize other phosphorylated amino acids or unphosphorylated tyrosine. Because of their sensitivity they can easily be used for immunoblot analysis of the limited-sized samples of mammalian oocytes. Analysis of the state of tyrosine phosphorylation of proteins in rat oocytes at different stages of meiosis allowed the detection of the target proteins for the cell-cycle dependent phosphorylation/dephosphorylation events. Their identification is presently being attempted in our laboratory by employing specific antibodies against proteins that seem to be good candidates to participate in regulation of the meiotic process.

REFERENCES

1. Bornslaeger, E.A., Mattei, P.M. and Schultz, R.M. (1988) Protein phosphorylation in meiotically competent and incompetent mouse oocytes. Mol. Reprod. Dev., 1:19-25.
2. Choi, T., Aoki, F., Mori, M., Yamashita, M., Nagahama, Y. and Kohmoto, K. (1991) Activation of p34^{cdc2} protein kinase activity in meiotic mitotic cell cycles in mouse oocytes and embryos. Development, 113:789-795.
3. Dekel, N. and Beers, W.H. (1978) Rat oocyte maturation *in vitro*: Relief of cyclic AMP inhibition by gonadotropins. Proc. Natl. Acad. Sci. USA, 75:4369-4373.
4. Dekel, N. and Sherizly, I. (1985) Epidermal growth factor induces maturation of rat follicle-enclosed oocytes. Endocrinology, 116:406-409.
5. Dekel, N. (1988a) Regulation of oocyte maturation: The role of cAMP. Ann. N.Y. Acad. Sci., 541:211-216.
6. Dekel, N. (1988b) Regulation of oocyte maturation by cell-to-cell communication. Cell-to-cell Communication in Endocrinology, edited by Piva, F., Burdin, C.W., Forti, G. and Motta, M., pp 131-194. Raven Press.
7. Dunphy, W.G., Brizuela, L., Bach, D. and Newport, S. (1988) The Xenopus cdc2 protein is a component of MPF, a cytoplasmic regulator of mitosis. Cell, 54:423-431.
8. Gautier, J., Norbury, C., Lohka, M., Nurse, P. and Maller, J. (1988) Purified maturation promoting factor contains the product of a Xenopus homolog of the fission yeast cell cycle control gene cdc^2. Cell, 54:433-439.
9. Klarlund, J.K. (1985) Transformation of cells by an inhibitor of phosphatases acting on phosphotyrosine in proteins. Cell, 41:707-717.
10. Lindner, H.R., Tsafriri, A., Lieberman, M.E., Zor, U., Koch, Y., Bauminger, S. and Barnea, A. (1974) Gonadotrophin action on cultured Graafian follicles: Induction of maturation division of the mammalian oocyte and differentiation of the luteal cell. Recent Prog. Horm. Res., 30:79-138.
11. Maller, J.L. (1990) Xenopus oocytes and biochemistry of cell division. Biochemistry, 29:3157-3166.
12. Meijer, L., Azzi, L. and Wang, J.Y.J. (1991) Cyclin B targets p34^{cdc2} for tyrosine phosphorylation. EMBO J., 10:1545-1554.
13. Minshull, J., Blow, J.J. and Hunt, T. (1989) Translation of cyclin mRNA is necessary for extracts of activated Xenopus eggs to enter mitosis. Cell, 56:947-956.
14. Morla, A.O., Draetta, G., Beach, D. and Wang, J.Y.J. (1989) Reversible tyrosine phosphorylation of cdc2: Dephosphorylation accompanies activation during entry into mitosis. Cell, 58:193-203.
15. Murray, A.W. and Kirschner, M.W. (1989a) Dominoes and clocks: The union of two views of two views of the cell cycle. Science, 246:614-621.
16. Murray, A.W. and Kirschner, M.W. (1989b) Cyclin synthesis drives the early embryonic cell cycle. Nature, 339:275-280.
17. Pincus, G. and Enzmann, E.V. (1935) The comparative behaviour of mammalian eggs *in vivo* and *in vitro*. I. The activation of ovarian eggs. J. Exp. Med., 62:665-675.
18. Solomon, M.J., Glotzer, M., Lee, T.H., Phillippe, M. and Kirschner, M.W. (1990) Cyclin activation of p34^{cdc2}. Cell, 63:1013-1024.
19. Tonks, N.K., Diltz, C.D. and Fischer, E.H. (1988) Characterization of the major protein-tyrosine-phosphatases of human placenta. J. Biol. Chem., 263:6731-6737.
20. Yaish, P., Gazit, A., Gilon, C. and Levitzki, A. (1988) Blocking of EGF-dependent cell proliferation by EGF receptor kinase inhibitors. Science, 242:933-935.
21. Yardan, Y. and Ullrich, A. (1988) Growth factor receptor tyrosine kinases. Annu. Rev. Biochem., 57:443-478.

Development-Related Gene Expression in Oocytes

J.J. Eppig

The Jackson Laboratory, Bar Harbor, Maine, USA

INTRODUCTION

Progression of the earliest stages of embryo development depend upon resources produced during oocyte development. Obviously, the structural components of the embryo are derived from the structural elements of the oocyte and the metabolism of the early embryo resembles the metabolism of the oocyte in several ways. This presentation, however, focuses on regulatory factors produced during oocyte development that profoundly affect early embryogenesis. Understanding of the existence and function of these factors has been obtained through a variety of experimental approaches, but I will emphasize our studies on the developmental capacity of mouse embryos derived from oocytes that underwent maturation and fertilization *in vitro*.

Shortly after the initiation of meiosis in oocytes during fetal life, this process becomes arrested at the diplotene stage. This arrest is sustained by the presence of meiosis-arresting substances within the oocyte (6) and by the absence of factors essential for the progression of meiosis (1). As the oocytes near completion of their growth phase, about the time of follicular antrum formation, they become competent to resume meiosis but remain arrested within the follicle because of the meiosis-arresting action of the somatic cells comprising the follicle wall (11,16,28). Meiosis normally resumes in response to the preovulatory surge of luteinizing hormone (LH) (12), but also resumes spontaneously, in the absence of gonadotropins, when the oocyte is removed from the follicle and cultured in a supportive medium (2,14). Some oocytes in early antral follicles are competent to resume meiosis but are unable to progress to metaphase II (23). Therefore, germinal vesicle breakdown (GVB) and subsequent completion of meiosis I are distinctly separable in oocytes and are sequentially acquired. Furthermore, oocytes must become capable of producing additional factors to progress beyond the initial stages of oocyte maturation.

The final goal of oocyte development is to produce a gamete competent to become fertilized and initiate embryogenesis. Maternal regulatory factors persist in preimplantation embryos and are critical for successful development. Messenger RNA coding for Oct-3, a transcription factor, is detectable in growing and mature oocytes, but not in primordial (resting) oocytes (18,19). Zygotes failed to cleave to the 2-cell stage after fertilized eggs were injected with oligonucleotides antisense to Oct-3 mRNA, suggesting that Oct-3 is a maternal factor essential for first cleavage (17). These results show that regulatory molecules essential for early embryogenesis are synthesized in oocytes and support the hypothesis that translation products of maternal messages are required for first cleavage (8).

Oocyte culture systems are extremely valuable experimental tools for studying the mechanisms regulating oogenesis and subsequent embryogenesis. For example, in the classic experiments of Pincus and his colleagues (14, 15), oocytes were isolated from Graafian follicles and placed in culture where they subsequently underwent spontaneous GVB. This led to the hypothesis that somatic follicular components function to maintain the oocytes in meiotic arrest, a hypothesis supported by research in several laboratories. Observations on spontaneous maturation *in vitro* also led to the conclusion that oocytes sequentially acquire competence to initiate, and and subsequently complete, the first meiotic division (23). In early studies, oocytes matured in culture could not be fertilized and this led to the opinion that oocyte maturation *in vitro* did not lead to the production of a normal gamete. It seemed that oocytes matured outside the follicle were deficient in some way; although 'nuclear maturation' was apparently normal, 'cytoplasmic maturation' was not. The cytoplasmic deficiency appeared to involve a failure to produce a male pronuclear growth factor (26). Since those early studies, however, it has been shown that oocytes of mice (20), rats (21,29), sheep (24), cattle (22,27), and cats (9) can be successfully fertilized after maturation *in vitro*. These results demonstrated that spontaneous maturation may produce a gamete competent to undergo fertilization and embryogenesis if maturation is carried out using appropriate culture conditions. This does not imply, however, that the mechanisms initiating spontaneous maturation *in vitro* and *in vivo* are the same.

EMBRYONIC DEVELOPMENTAL COMPETENCE OF MOUSE OOCYTES MATURED *IN VITRO*: CORRELATION WITH FOLLICULAR DEVELOPMENT

Since a large group of follicles develops almost synchronously in neonatal and juvenile mice, oocytes and follicles at increasing stages of development can be isolated from mice of increasing ages until the animals are about 1 month old (3,13) (Fig. 1). *In vitro* studies with such oocytes recovered from immature mice have shown that the percentage of *in vitro* matured ova that cleave to the 2-cell stage after insemination increases with advancing follicular development (Fig. 2) (3). Likewise, the competence of 2-cell stage embryos to develop to the blastocyst stage also increases with follicular development (Fig. 2) (3). The highest percentage of ova that cleave to the 2-cell stage is achieved by oocytes isolated from 20-day-old mice but the highest percentage of development of 2-cells to the blastocyst stage is not achieved until the oocyte donors are 24 days old. Accordingly, the ratio of ova that cleave to the 2-cell stage to embryos that develop from the 2-cell stage to blastocyst is high when the oocyte donors are 18 days old; more than three times as many ova reach the 2-cell stage as complete the 2-cell stage to blastocyst transition (Fig. 2). In contrast, the 2-cell:blastocyst ratio reach a minimum when the donors are 24 days old: only 1.3 times as many ova reach the 2-cell stage as complete the 2-cell stage to blastocyst transition (Fig. 2). These results suggest that developing oocytes acquire competence to complete the 2-cell stage to blastocyst transition after becoming competent to cleave to the 2-cell stage.

The differing developmental capacities in oocytes isolated from donors of increasing age probably reflect differences in content of regulatory molecules essential for successful embryogenesis. What are the factors that determine whether oocytes contain or can produce these regulatory molecules? This question was investigated with regard to the effect of stimulation with gonadotropin *in vivo* and *in vitro*.

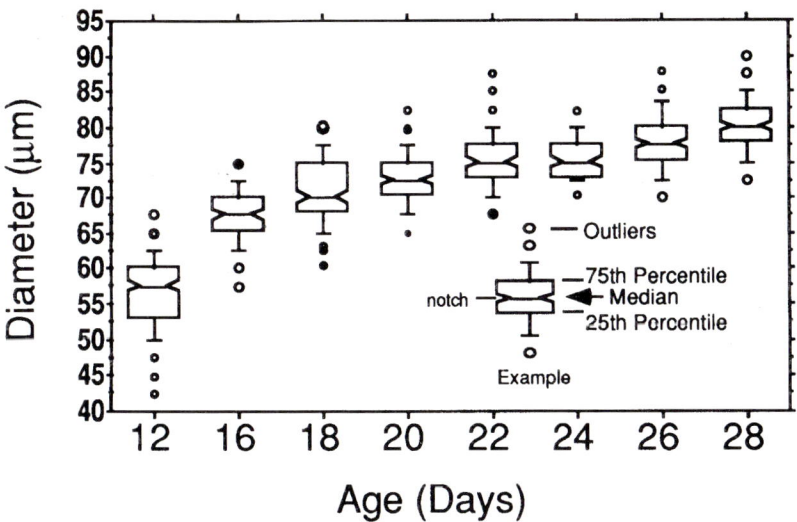

FIG. 1. Diameter of oocytes 12 to 28 days old. Diameters are presented using notched box-and-whisker plots as the percentile distribution of oocytes (see example). Non-overlapping notches between groups indicates a significant difference ($P < 0.05$) in the populations (10). Data adapted from Reference 3.

To assess the effect of gonadotropins on the developmental competence of oocytes, pregnant mares' serum gonadotropin (PMSG), which stimulates follicular development *in vivo*, was injected into 20- and 24-day-old mice and the germinal vesicle (GV)-stage oocytes were isolated 48 h later when the mice were either 22- or 26-days old. The rationale for comparing the developmental capacity of oocytes from 22- and 26-day-old mice is that overall follicular development is slightly more advanced in the older group thereby enabling comparison of the influence of follicles at slightly different stages of development. Oocytes were matured and fertilized *in vitro*. The frequency of cleavage to the 2-cell stage was the same in all groups, 80-90% (Fig. 3a). The percentage that completed the 2-cell stage to blastocyst (2C to B) transition was also determined. There was no difference between the untreated and gonadotropin-treated 22-day-old groups, but gonadotropin injection resulted in an increase in the percentage of oocytes from the 26-day-old group that completed the 2C to B transition.

In the next experiment, the effect of FSH-treatment of oocyte-cumulus cell complexes maturing *in vitro* on competence to complete the 2C to B transition was determined. In experiments using mice not treated with PMSG, FSH had no effect on this competency in oocytes isolated from 22-day-old mice, but increased this capacity when the complexes were isolated from 26-day-old mice (Fig. 3b). In contrast, FSH did not increase the developmental competence of oocytes isolated from PMSG-primed 26-day-old mice above that already increased by PMSG in vivo (Fig. 3c). However, FSH-treatment of complexes from 26-day-old mice not treated with PMSG increased the developmental capacity to approximately the same level as that resulting from PMSG treatment (Fig. 3b and c).

Taken together, therefore, the above results indicate that gonadotropins can have profound effects on the preimplantation developmental competence of oocytes, and that these effects are dependent upon the age of the donor mice. Although the age-dependent effect is probably related to differing stages of follicular development, PMSG-treatment dramatically accelerates follicular development in mice of both ages. In fact, the distribution of follicles of various sizes is about the same in PMSG-treated mice of both ages (4). Therefore, although the development of the somatic components of the follicles is accelerated by PMSG, the developmental capacity of the oocytes contained therein does not appear to be coordinately accelerated. Nevertheless, 2 to 3 times more oocytes are recovered from the ovaries of both ages after PMSG-treatment, so gonadotropins accelerate oocyte development coordinately with follicular development at some stage(s) of follicular development, probably the later stages.

FSH-treatment of *in vitro* maturing oocytes promoted the acquisition of increased developmental competence only when the oocytes were isolated from 26-day-old mice not previously treated with PMSG *in vivo*. In this way, FSH-treatment *in vitro* mimicked PMSG-treatment *in vivo*, but, although the result of both gonadotropin treatments had the same end result (increased

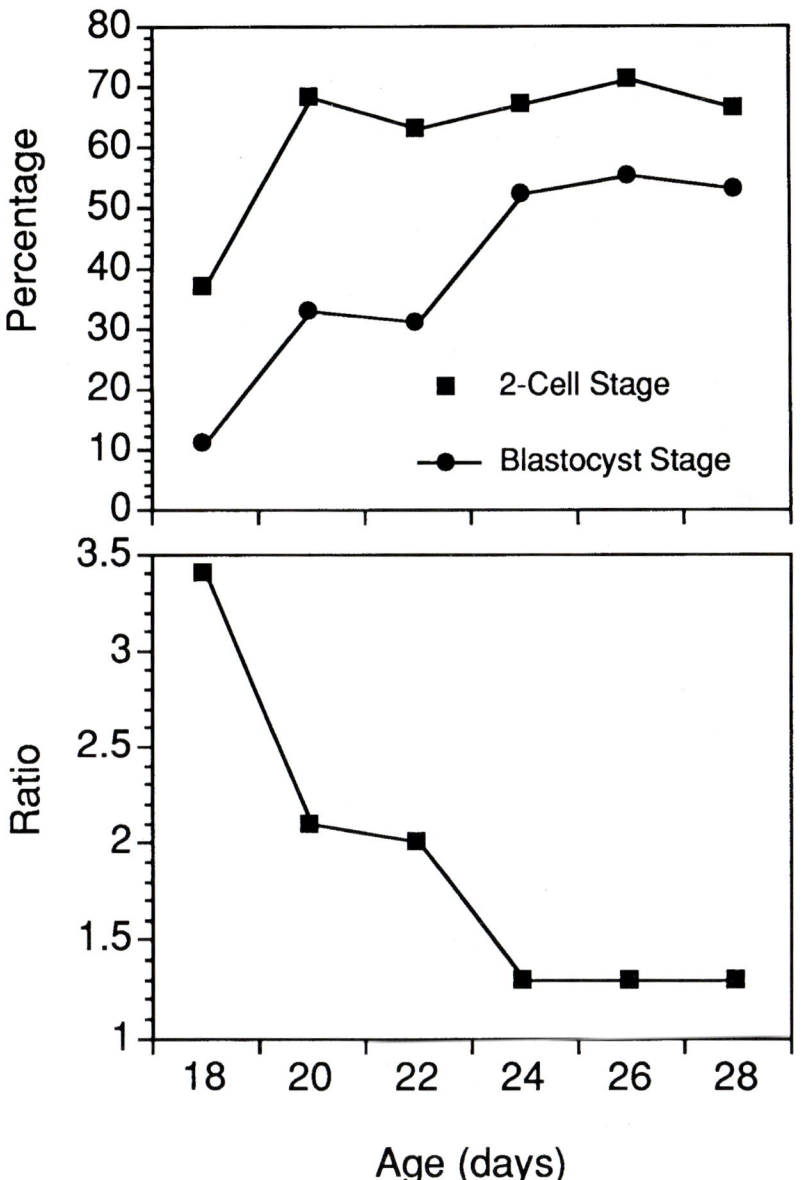

FIG. 2. Development of embryos derived from in-vitro matured oocytes isolated from mice 18 to 28 days old. The top panel shows the percentage of oocytes that cleaved to the 2-cell stage after insemination and the percentage of 2-cell stage oocytes that developed to blastocysts. These percentages were used to calculate the ratio of embryos that cleaved to the 2-cell stage to the embryos that completed the 2C- to B transition shown in the bottom panel. Data adapted from Reference 3.

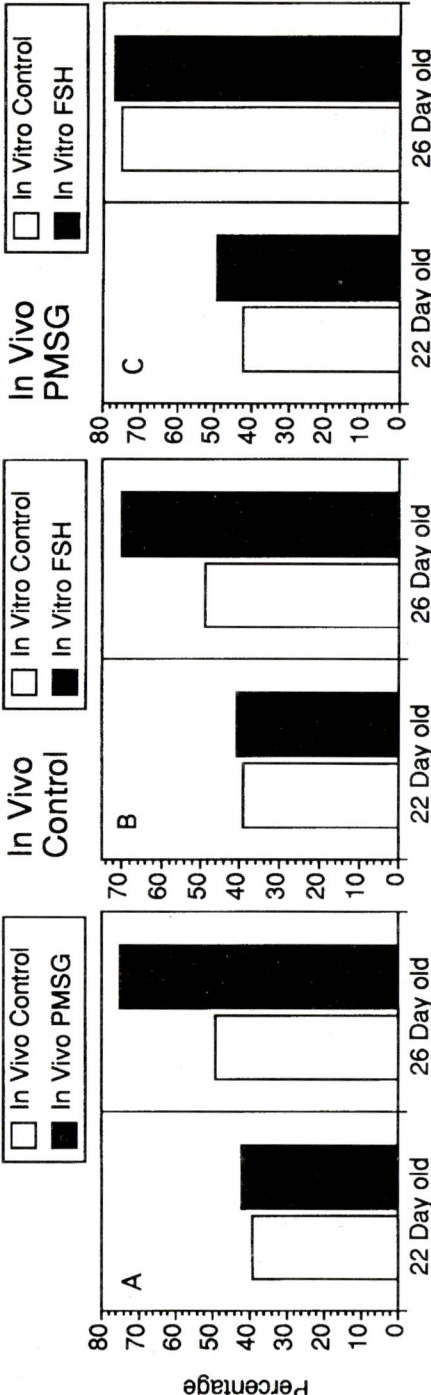

FIG. 3. Percentage of 2-cell stage embryos that developed to blastocysts after maturation of oocytes *in vitro*. Data adapted from Reference 4.
A. Oocytes were isolated at the GV-stage from mice 48 h after injection with PMSG or from uninjected control mice.
B. Oocytes were isolated at the GV-stage from mice not treated with PMSG and matured in the presence or absence of FSH (1 μg/ml).
C. Percentage of 2-cell stage embryos that developed to blastocysts after maturation *in vitro*. Oocytes were isolated at the GV-stage from mice injected 48 h previously with PMSG and matured in the presence or absence of FSH.

frequency of completion of the 2C to B transition), it is not known whether the processes leading to that end are the same. Oocytes affected by PMSG treatment *in vivo* are in the GV-stage and are situated in the complex system of cell-to-cell communications existing in the intact follicle. In contrast, oocytes affected by FSH treatments *in vitro* are undergoing maturation and are isolated from these complex cellular interactions of the intact follicle. It is possible that PMSG treatment *in vivo* initiates some events of maturation before GVB in some oocytes; they may in fact be 'more mature' in some ways than many, but not all, of the oocytes present in the follicles of the untreated mice. This more advanced level of maturation must be related in some way to the oocytes' capacity to carry out processes associated with the 2C to B transition. This leads to the question whether the oocytes contain the critical molecules for this transition before undergoing GVB or whether the molecules are produced during GVB. The observation that FSH-treatment of maturing oocytes can also increase the frequency of 2C to B transition seems to argue that the critical molecules for this transition are synthesized during maturation. Oocytes in less developed follicles, as are many of those in 22-day-old mice, are probably incompetent to produce the critical molecules that promote the acquisition of the capacity to complete the 2C to B transition. Thus it appears that there are at least two critical steps in oocyte development that relate to competence to complete the 2C to B transition: (A) production of molecules that regulate the synthesis of transition factor(s) and (B) the synthesis of the transition factor(s).

Because the cumulus cells of complexes isolated from the 22-day-old mice did not promote the synthesis of transition factor(s) in response to FSH during maturation *in vitro*, it was important to establish whether the cumulus cells of these complexes are capable of responding to FSH. That they can respond to FSH is evident from the observation that virtually all of the cumuli oophori from both 22- and 26-day-old mice underwent expansion in response to FSH whether they were isolated from PMSG-treated or untreated mice. In addition, FSH stimulated elevated cyclic adenosine monophosphate (cAMP) levels in complexes from all groups (Fig. 4). Cyclic AMP levels attained after treatment of complexes from PMSG-treated mice with FSH were about ten-fold greater than those from untreated mice, but there was no difference in the cAMP levels attained in complexes treated with FSH whether the complexes were obtained from 22- or 26-day-old mice. The level of cAMP attained by complexes in response to FSH, therefore, seems to be unrelated to the ability of the complexes to produce transition factor(s); the factor was produced in response to FSH in complexes isolated from 26-day-old mice, not treated with PMSG, but not in those isolated from 22-day-old mice, yet there was no difference in the levels of cAMP produced in response to FSH.

Based on these observations, I hypothesize that many of the follicles in 22-day-old mice are restricted in their ability to complete the 2C to B transition because they are incompetent to produce the transition factor(s) and/or because the somatic components of the follicles are incompetent to

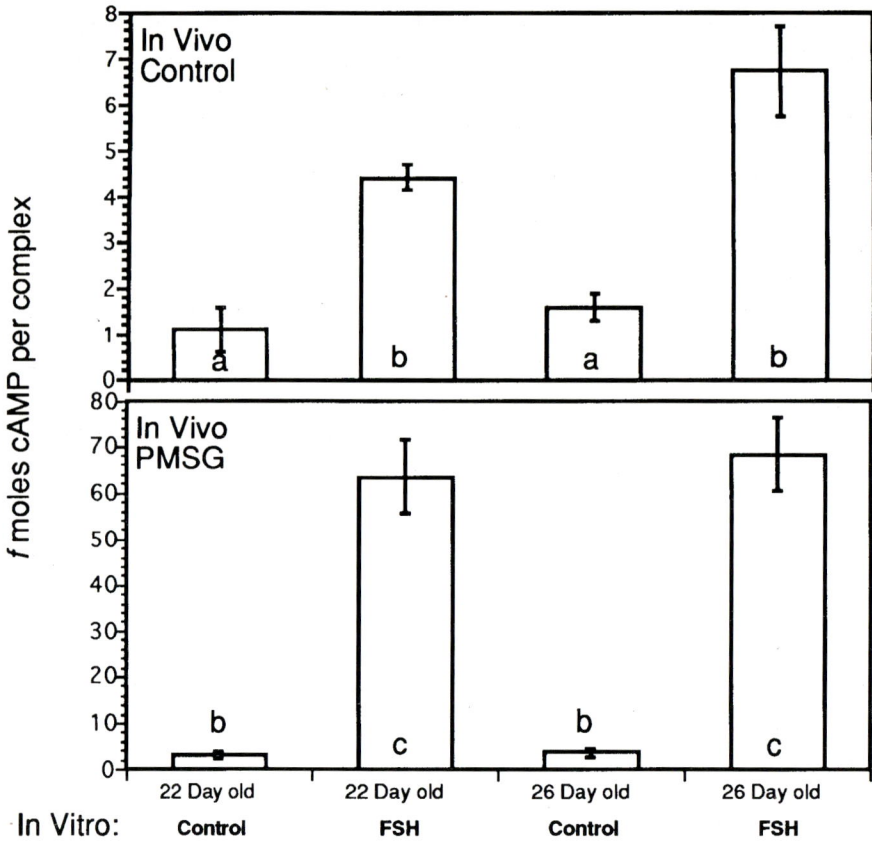

FIG. 4. Cyclic AMP content of oocyte-cumulus cell complexes. Cyclic AMP was determined using radioimmunoassay of complexes cultured for 2 h. in medium with or without FSH (1 µg/ml), both in the presence of the cAMP-phosphodiesterase inhibitor isobutyl methylxanthine (50 µM). Error bars indicate the standard error of the mean. The significance of differences between means were evaluated using the Student-Newman-Keuls Multiple Range Test of log transformed data; different letters on the bars indicate $P < 0.05$ (N=4).

signal the oocyte appropriately to become competent. I also hypothesize that somatic cells of more advanced follicles, such as those more commonly found in the older mice, signal the oocyte in response to gonadotropin to produce the critical transition factor(s). Obviously, the molecules that regulate the acquisition of the capacity to complete the 2C to B transition, as well as those that actually promote the transition, must be identified, and the mechanisms by which the follicular somatic cells participate in this aspect of oocyte development are critical questions of developmental and reproductive biology.

I propose that oocytes restricted in their ability to complete the 2C to B transition exist in a distinct stage of oocyte development. A classification of GV-stage mouse oocytes based on characteristics of competence to complete meiosis and preimplantation development is presented in Table 1. According to this system, embryogenesis restricted oocytes are classified as Stage IV oocytes. Although Stage IV oocytes are able to complete the nuclear events of meiosis and progress to metaphase II, producing the first polar body, and although they are able to cleave to the 2-cell stage after fertilization, they are unable to support development from the 2-cell stage to the blastocyst stage. Many of the embryos from Stage IV oocytes that fail to complete the 2-cell stage to blastocyst transition block at or near the 2-cell stage, although some reach morula stage. Failure to activate zygotic transcription results in rapid termination of embryo development. In mice, zygotic transcription is initiated in the 2-cell stage (5,25) and inhibition of this transcription results in developmental arrest at this stage (7). I propose that Stage IV oocytes are deficient in a factor(s) necessary for the normal sequence of activation of the zygotic genome and, therefore, embryos derived from Stage IV oocytes are unable to develop significantly beyond the 2-cell stage. Accordingly, it is hypothesized that 2C to B transition factors participate in activation of the zygotic genome.

Table 1. *Classification of GV-Stage Oocytes Based on Competence to Complete Meiosis and Undergo Preimplantaton Development*

	STAGE				
	I	II	III	IV	V
Competence					
GVB	No	No	Yes	Yes	Yes
Metaphase II	No	No	No	Yes	Yes
2-Cell Stage	No	No	No	Yes	Yes
Blastocyst	No	No	No	No	Yes
Other Characteristics					
Growth	'Resting'	Growing	Growing	Nearly Grown	Fully Grown
Follicular Origin	Primordial	Preantral	Early Antral	Antral	Antral

ACKNOWLEDGMENTS

This paper is essentially a reproduction of an early paper presented at the Serono Symposium in Newton, MA, entitled "Preimplantation Development" in 1991. It was organized and vigorously edited by Dr. Barry Bavister of the University of Wisconsin. Most of this paper, including the figures, is from this presentation with the permission of Dr. Bavister and Springer Verlag New York, who published the Newton Symposium. The author is grateful to them for allowing the use of this material. This paper is dedicated to Al Schroeder who died in September 1990. Al was a good friend and a valuable colleague who was an important participant in the studies reviewed here. This research was supported by the National Cooperative Program on Non-Human In Vitro Fertilization and Preimplantation Development, NIH, through cooperative agreement HD 21970. I thank Marilyn O'Brien for her highly skilled and dedicated technical assistance in these studies.

REFERENCES

1. Balakier, H. (1978) Induction of maturation in small oocytes from sexually immature mice by fusion with meiotic or mitotic cells. Exp. Cell Res., 112:137-141.
2. Edwards, R. G. (1965) Maturation in vitro of mouse, sheep, cow, pig, rhesus monkey and human ovarian oocytes. Nature, 208:349-351.
3. Eppig, J. J. and Schroeder, A. C. (1989) Capacity of mouse oocytes from preantral follicles to undergo embryogenesis and development to live young after growth, maturation and fertilization in vitro. Biol. Reprod., 41:268-276.
4. Eppig, J. J., Schroeder, A. C. and O'Brien, M. J. (1992) Developmental capacity of mouse oocytes matured in vitro: effects of gonadotropic stimulation, follicular origin, and oocyte size. J. Reprod. Fertil. (in press).
5. Flach, G., Johnson, M. H., Braude, P. R., Taylor, R. A. S. and Bolton, V. N. (1982) The transition from maternal to embryonic control in the 2-cell mouse embryo. EMBO J., 1:681-686.
6. Fulka, J. (1985) Maturation-inhibiting activity of growing mouse oocytes. Cell Diff., 17:45-48.
7. Golbus, M. S., Calarco, P. G. and Epstein, C. J. (1973) The effects of inhibitors of RNA synthesis (a-amanitin and actinomycin D) on preimplantation mouse embryogenesis. J. Exp. Zool., 186:207-216.
8. Johnson, M. H. (1981) The molecular and cellular basis of preimplantation development. Biol. Rev., 56:463-498.
9. Johnston, L. A., O'Brien, S. J. and Wildt, D. E. (1989) In vitro maturation and fertilization of domestic cat follicular oocytes. Gamete Res., 24:343-356.
10. Kafadar, K. (1985) Notched box-and-whisker plot. Encyclopedia of Statistical Sciences, 6:367-370.
11. Leibfried, L. and First, N. (1980) Effect of bovine and porcine follicular fluid and granulosa cells on maturation of oocytes in vitro. Biol. Reprod., 23:699-704.
12. Lindner, H. R., Tsafriri, A., Lieberman, M. E., Zor, U., Koch, Y., Bauminger, S. and Barnea, A. (1974) Gonadotropin action on cultured Graafian follicles: induction of maturation division of the mammalian oocyte and differentiation of the luteal cell. Recent Prog. Horm. Res., 30:79-138.
13. Mangia, F. and Epstein, C. J. (1975) Biochemical studies of growing mouse oocytes: preparation of oocytes and analysis of glucose-6-phosphate dehydrogenase and lactate dehydrogenase activities. Dev. Biol., 45:211-220.
14. Pincus, G. and Enzmann, E. V. (1935) The comparative behavior of mammalian eggs in vivo and in vitro. I. The activation of ovarian eggs. J. Exp. Med., 62:655-675.
15. Pincus, G. and Saunders, B. (1939) The comparative behavior of mammalian eggs in vivo and in vitro. IV. The maturation of human ovarian ova. Anat. Rec., 75:537-545.
16. Racowsky, C. and Baldwin, K. V. (1989) In vitro and in vivo studies reveal that hamster oocyte meiotic arrest is maintained only transiently by follicular fluid, but persistently by membrana/cumulus granulosa cell contact. Dev. Biol., 134:297-306.
17. Rosner, M. H., De Santo, R. J., Arnheiter, H. and Staudt, L. M. (1991) Oct-3 is a maternal factor required for the first mouse embryonic division. Cell, 64:1103-1110.
18. Rosner, M. H., Vigano, M. A., Ozato, K., Timmons, P. M., Poirier, F., Rigby, P. W. J. and Staudt, L. M. (1990) A POU-domain transcription factor in early stem cells and germ cells of the mammalian embryo. Nature, 345:686-692.
19. Schöler, H. R., Hatzopoulos, A. K., Balling, R., Suzuki, N. and Gruss, P. (1989) A family of octamer-specific proteins present during mouse embryogenesis: evidence for germline-specific expression of an Oct factor. EMBO J., 8:2543-2550.
20. Schroeder, A. C. and Eppig, J. J. (1984) The developmental capacity of mouse oocytes that matured spontaneously in vitro is normal. Dev. Biol., 102:493-497.

21. Shalgi, R., Dekel, N. and Kraicer, P. F. (1979) The effect of LH on the fertilizability and developmental capacity of rat oocytes matured in vitro. J. Reprod. Fertil., 55:429-435.
22. Sirard, M. A., Parrish, J. J., Ware, C. B., Leibfried-Rutledge, M. L. and First, N. L. (1988) The culture of bovine oocytes to obtain developmentally competent embryos. Biol. Reprod., 39:546-552.
23. Sorensen, R. A. and Wassarman, P. M. (1976) Relationship between growth and meiotic maturation of the mouse oocyte. Dev. Biol., 50:531-536.
24. Staigmiller, R. B. and Moor, R. M. (1984) Effect of follicle cells on the maturation and developmental competence of ovine oocytes matured outside the follicle. Gamete Res., 9:221-229.
25. Taylor, K. D., and Piko, L. (1987) Patterns of mRNA prevalence and expression of B1 and B2 transcripts in early mouse embryos. Development, 101:877-892.
26. Thibault, C. (1977) Are follicular maturation and oocyte maturation independent processes? J. Reprod. Fertil., 51:1-15.
27. Trounson, A. O., Willadsen, S. M. and Rowson, L. E. A. (1977) Fertilization and developmental capacity of bovine follicular oocytes matured in vitro and in vivo and transferred to the oviducts of rabbits and cows. J. Reprod. Fertil., 51:321-327.
28. Tsafriri, A. and Channing, C. P. (1975) An inhibitory influence of granulosa cells and follicular fluid upon oocyte meiosis *in vitro*. Endocrinology, 96:922-927.
29. Vanderhyden, B. C. and Armstrong, D. T. (1989) Role of cumulus cells and serum on the in vitro maturation, fertilization, and subsequent development of rat oocytes. Biol. Reprod., 40:720-728.

Vascular Control of Testicular Function

A.R.J. Bergh

Department of Pathology, University of Umeå, S-901 87 Umeå, Sweden

INTRODUCTION

The perfusion of the testis by blood is usually regarded as a steady-state process, where changes only come about as a consequence of varying metabolic demands. However, during recent years several studies suggest that the testicular vasculature, which show several unique features, could be more actively involved in modulating testicular functions. The cells in testicular blood vessels are apparently integrated in the paracrine network of cell-cell interactions that control testicular function. Interactions between different testicular cells and the vasculature could also be of importance for the understanding of testicular pathophysiology.

BLOOD FLOW AND THE ROLE OF THE PAMPINIFORM PLEXUS

The testicular vasculature shows several peculiarities. The testicular artery originates from the abdominal aorta. In its lower part it is coiled and enveloped by the venous return channels, the pampiniform plexus. One function of the pampiniform plexus is to enable countercurrent exchange of heat and thus to be a part of testicular temperature control (13,27). A slight reduction in flow markedly reduced the capacity of this system to prevent increased intratesticular temperature during heat exposure (26). Vasoactive substances like prostaglandins and serotonin secreted in the testis may by countercurrent transfer in the plexus reduce flow in the testicular artery (13). It has also been suggested that there are arterio-venous anastomoses in the plexus. The physiological role of this shunting, whether it is constant or modulated by different physiological demands is, however, unknown.

BLOOD FLOW AND ITS EFFECTS ON ENDOCRINE FUNCTION

Testicular blood flow is the main pathway for the transport of nutrients and secretory products to and from the testis. There is a strong positive correlation between testicular blood flow and the secretion of testosterone into the testicular vein in the normal rat testes (8). Retarded flow limits testosterone secretion. Most factors that influence the testicular vasculature reduce flow (13,27,28). Vasoconstrictors with rapid effects like catecholamines, prostaglandins, serotonin, arginine-vasopressin (AVP) (13,39), and stimulation of sympathetic nerves (13) may consequently reduce testosterone secretion immediately. In testes with cryptorchidism- or irradiation-induced damage to the seminiferous tubules testosterone secretion is limited principally as a result of impaired blood flow (9,28). Why blood flow is reduced is, however, unexplored.

The only known substances that may increase testicular blood flow are those stimulating Leydig cell function (1). LH/hCG and LHRH treatment in high doses is associated with a delayed (after 12 h for LH and after 2 h for LHRH) increase in testicular blood flow (1,38,39). This increase in flow obviously promote testosterone secretion, but since it occurs after the peak in Leydig cell testosterone synthesis its role in enhancing testosterone secretion is obscure. Moreover, flow is not increased after stimulation with moderate doses of LH (38).

These factors stimulating Leydig cell function also increase vascular permeability (see below) and consequently lymph flow (1,29). Lower doses of LH are apparently needed to increase permeability than to increase blood flow (2). The transport mechanisms and pathways by which secretory products leave the testis are not fully understood. Testosterone is supposed to diffuse rapidly into testicular veins, but active transport can not be excluded (20). Testosterone in interstitial fluid (IF) is bound to proteins and large proteins and sulphated steroids leave the testis preferably by the lymph drainage (20). A substantial part of the inhibin synthesized in the testis is secreted via the lymph (19). Interestingly, the lymph drainage from one testis is directed to the ipsilateral epididymis and prostate (20). Factors regulating lymph formation and composition (flow and permeability) may thus influence activities in other organs.

Secretory products from Sertoli cells and germ cells are bidirectionally secreted into the lumen of the seminiferous tubules and into the interstitial space. Inhibin, and therefore possibly also other substances, secreted into the seminiferous tubules, may however in rats be reabsorbed by the venous plexus surrounding the rete testis (22). If factors modulate flow and permeability in this plexus locally they could be of large importance for the route and magnitude of testicular secretions.

TESTICULAR MICROCIRCULATION

The testicular microcirculation shows several unique features in both structure and function. The pressure in testicular capillaries is the lowest among all organs studied, and is only slightly higher than in the venules (36). The main reason for the high precapillary resistance is probably the long and coiled artery. In spite of the low pressure gradient, fluid is filtered from the microvasculature and the rate of lymph flow is fairly high (28). How is this possible? The capillary endothelium is unfenestrated and with few vesicles (27,28). Endothelia of this type generally only allow a slow passage of macromolecules (25) and testicular blood vessels are impermeable to dyes that normally penetrate into the interstitium in other organs. Therefore, the blood-testis barrier was originally presumed to be located in the blood vessel walls (27,28). In spite of this, the permeability to albumin is higher than in most organs and the protein concentration in testicular lymph is similar to serum and immunoglobulins are present (28). The mechanism behind this high permeability of macromolecules is not fully established. We have shown that LH stimulation, by mechanisms still largely unknown but to some extent involving polymorphonuclear leukocytes (PMNs), is able to induce endothelial cell contraction and opening of the interendothelial cell junctions in postcapillary venules (2). Opening of these interendothelial cell clefts results in a major inflammation-like increase in vascular permeability. The underlying reason why the size of the interendothelial cell junctions are hormonally modulated, and why permeability is so high also in the unstimulate testis is unknown. The high permeability and the resulting small osmotic pressure gradient between plasma and interstitium may be necessary to secure filtration in an organ where capillary pressure, due to the peculiar anatomy, is so low. If this is the underlying reason, it can be postulated that factors decreasing permeability could be deleterious for the testis. Hypothetically, a high permeability may also be necessary to secure the uptake of macromolecules (for example lipoproteins), to increase lymph flow (see above), to facilitate secretion from the testis, and the PMNs may mediate paracrine signals to testicular cells.

Since there is no osmotic pressure gradient opposing capillary pressure transvascular fluid exchange may to a large extent be influenced by changes in pressure (28,36). The factors regulating testicular capillary pressure are however unknown, but it is apparently constant over a wide variation in systemic systolic pressure (36). Interestingly there are rhythmical variations in capillary blood flow in the rat testis, periods with rapid flow alternate with periods with no flow, so called vasomotion (10). Vasomotion, which is induced by myogenic activity in precapillary arterioles, influences transvascular exchange (fluid is forced into the interstitium during flow and it returns to the vasculature during stops) and precapillary resistance in other organs (18). The physiological role of vasomotion and its regulation in the testis are largely unknown, but vasomotion could be postulated to play a significant role in a microcirculation so dependent on pressure changes. Testicular vasomotion is apparently hormonally and developmentally regulated, but the factors regulating contractility in testicular blood vessels are unknown. Vasomotion is established during puberty and it is inhibited by LH/hCG stimulation in high doses. LH/hCG induced inhibition of vasomotion is associated with an increase in the volume of interstitial fluid in the testis (10,11), suggesting increased filtration. In the absence of a colloid osmotic pressure gradient it is unclear why fluid is resorbed in the venules. The periods of flow stops may be important for this. Hypothetically, local increases in interstitial pressure, caused by contractions in the peritubular myoid cells or in the capsule, could also be of significance.

LOCAL CONTROL OF TESTICULAR MICROCIRCULATION

The precapillary (total flow and vasomotion) and postcapillary (permeability) parts of the testicular microcirculation can be modulated by changes in Leydig cell activity. The mediators are unexplored and it appears that different factors influence the pre- and post-capillary part of the vasculature (1). Changes in testosterone secretion are probably one of the key elements in the control of testicular blood flow (1). The mechanism by which testosterone has this effect is unknown. The effect could be mediated by testosterone-dependent effects in the seminiferous tubules since blood flow, vasomotion and interstitial fluid volume are normalized by testosterone treatment in Leydig cell-depleted rats (12,21). Moreover, there is in some conditions a close correlation between the mass of tubules seminiferous and testis blood flow (28,30). The volume of interstitial fluid is increase by selective removal of late spermatids (33). Collectively these data suggest that the tubules influence testicular blood vessels, but the mechanisms are unknown. Specific vasoactive factors or more general effects induced by altered tubule metabolism? FSH stimulation apparently does not influence the testicular vasculature (5). Recent studies do however suggest that the effects of testosterone on testicular blood flow may not necessarily be mediated via the tubules since immunoreactive androgen receptors are present in the muscular layer of testicular arterioles (4) and considerably lower levels of testosterone are needed to normalize blood flow than spermatogenesis in Leydig cell-depleted animals (own unpublished observations). The role of testicular vascular androgen receptors is totally unknown, but interestingly androgens may have regulatory effects on other parts of the cardiovascular system (35). The locally produced factors regulating vascular permeability are discussed below.

Is the hormonal regulation of the testicular microcirculation of physiological importance? Leydig cells in most species secrete their products into the testicular lymph in the interstitial space. The seminiferous tubules, which constitute up to 90% of the testicular volume, are avascular and therefore dependent on transport of nutrients and hormones from the interstitium for their function. Thus, the composition of the interstitial fluid is important for testicular function since it serves as a medium for communication between tubules, Leydig cells and blood vessels (31,32,34). It is obvious that by modulating testicular blood flow, microcirculation and vascular permeability it is possible to influence both the secretion of hormones from the testis and the local milieu within the testis, and in this manner, achieve paracrine control of testicular cells (31,32,34). A large number of substances which have been suggested to be involved in hormonal, paracrine and autocrine control of testicular cells. For example, Corticotrophin-releasing factor, β-endorphin, ACTH, α-melanocyte stimulating hormone, AVP, oxytocin, IL-1, atrial naturetic factor, TGFβ, nerve growth factor, substance P, histamine, serotonin, β-adrenergic agents, renin-angiotensin II, prostaglandins, and leukotrienes are known to have direct effects on blood vessels and/or blood cells in other organs. Thus, it can not be excluded that some of the effects induced by such factors could involve the testicular vasculature.

TESTICULAR MICROCIRCULATION AND INFLAMMATORY/IMMUNE REACTIONS

Testicular germ cells, including spermatogonia, are antigens and immune responses are therefore continonusly suppressed in order to avoid autoimmune orchitis (24). How this is accomplished is not established, but immunosupressive substances are locally produced (24). Indirect evidence suggest that testicular blood vessels could also be important in maintaining this local milieu. Endothelial cells, by expressing different adhesion molecules regulate the traffic of immunocompetent cells into organs, and by contraction regulate vascular permeability and immunoglobulin passage into the interstitial space (23). The observation that vascular permeability is not increased by common inflammation-mediators like histamine, bradykinin, serotonin, leukotriene B4 (3) suggest local adaptions of endothelial cell function in the testis. Interestingly, the vascular sensitivity to the proinflammatory effect of IL-1 (but not of other mediators) is markedly enhanced by hCG treatment (own unpublished observations).

LH/hCG treatment induces, in a dose-dependent way, accumulation of PMNs in testicular venules and an inflammation-like increase in venular permeability. Apparently both leukocyte-dependent and nonleukocyte-dependent mediators are involved (1) but their nature remains unknown. The physiological role of this LH-induced response is also unknown (see above) but it occurs after physiological LH doses, and a very similar reaction is seen in the ovary after the preovulatory LH-peak (2,14).

Considering the importance of protection of the testis from autoimmune reactions it would not be surprising if the LH-induced inflammatory response was found to be tightly controlled by an inhibitory system. We have recently developed a method to deplete testicular macrophages (6). In such testes blood flow and vasomotion are apparently unaffected, but the inflammatory response to hCG increased (6,7). An inflammation inhibitor may be produced by testicular macrophages. Hypothetically, the postulated inflammation-inhibiting system may be down regulated by hCG treatment. Further studies are needed to explain how the local immunological milieu in the testis is protected to avoid autoimmune reactions in an organ where one of the principal hormonal regulators is able to induce an inflammation-like response!

THE VASCULATURE AND TESTICULAR PATHOPHYSIOLOGY

Several studies suggest that overstimulation of the testis with LHRH and hCG in a single dose or after prolonged treatment may induce vascular changes that eventually result in focal seminiferous tubule damage in intact testes (15,37). Treatment of adult unilaterally cryptorchid rats induces a tremendous increase of testicular vascular permeability (9), leading to a glaucoma-like increase in intratesticular pressure in the abdominal testis (16). Similar changes are also noted in hCG-treated cryptorchid boys (17). These data suggest that the ability of hCG/LH to influence the testicular vasculature may be of importance also for testicular pathophysiology.

Another area of testicular pathology, in which vascular factors are of obvious importance, is varicocele. Varicocele is a common vascular abnormality in man consisting of dilatation of the testicular vein and pampiniform plexus and associated with subfertility. The reason why varicocele impaires testicular function is unknown but possibly related to the increase in venous pressure which must have dramatic effects on microcirculation and transvascular fluid exchange in the testis (36). Blood flow is probably decreased and retarded flow markedly impairs the ability of the pampiniform plexus to protect the testis during heat exposure (26).

GENERAL CONCLUSION

In this overview, several examples are given which illustrate the importance of the vasculature in the control of major testicular functions. It is, however, also evident that this area of testicular function must be explored further before we can fully understand the role of the vasculature in testicular physiology.

ACKNOWLEDGEMENTS

Our own studies have been supported by the Swedish Medical Research Council (Project 5935) and The Maud and Birger Gustavsson Foundation

REFERENCES

1. Bergh, A., Damber, J.E. and Widmark, A. (1988) Hormonal control of testicular blood flow, microcirculation and vascular permeability. In: Molecular and Cellular Endocrinology of the Testis, edited by Cooke B.A., Sharpe, R.M., Serono Symposia Series no 50. pp 123-133. Raven Press, New York,.
2. Bergh, A., Damber, J.-E. and Widmark, A. (1990) A physiological increase in LH may influence vascular permeability in the rat testis. J. Reprod. Fert., 89:23-31
3. Bergh, A. and Söder, O. (1990) Interleukin-1β, but not interleukin-1α induces acute inflammation-like changes in the testicular microcirculation of adult rats. J Reprod Immunol 17:155-165.
4. Bergh, A. and Damber, J.-E. (1992) Immunohistochemical localization of androgen receptors on testicular blood vessels. Int. J. Androl., in press.
5. Bergh, A., Damber, J.-E., Lieu, L. and Widmark, A. (1992) Does follicle stimulating hormone or pregnant mare serum gonadotrophin influence testicular blood flow in rats? Int. J. Androl., in press
6. Bergh, A., Damber, J.-E. and van Rooijen, N. (1992) Liposome mediated depletion of macrophages - an experimental approach to study the role of testicular macrophages. J. Endocrinol., in press.
7. Bergh, A., Damber, J.-E. and van Rooijen, N. (1992) The hCG induced inflammatory response is enhanced in macrophage-depleted testes. J. Endocrinol., in press.
8. Damber, J.-E. and Janson, P.O. (1978) Testicular blood flow and testosterone concentrations in testicular venous blood of anaesthetized rats. J. Reprod. Fertil., 52:265-269.
9. Damber, J.-E., Bergh, A. and Daehlin, L. (1985) Testicular blood flow, vascular permeability and testosterone production after stimulation of unilaterally cryptorchid child rats with human chorionic gonadotrophin. Endocrinology 117:1906-1913.
10. Damber, J.-E., Bergh, A., Fagrell, B., Lindahl, O. and Rooth, P. (1986) Testicular microcirculation in the rat studied by videophotometric capillaroscopy, fluorescence microscopy and laser Doppler flowmetry. Acta Physiol. Scand., 126:371-376
11. Damber, J.-E., Bergh, A., and Widmark, A. (1989) Effects of hormones on testicular microvasculature. In: Perspectives in Andrology, Ed: Serio, M., Serono Symposia Rev., vol 23 pp 97-109. Raven Press.
12. Damber, J.-E., Maddocks, S., Widmark, A. and Bergh, A. (1992) Testicular blood flow and vasomotion can be maintained by testosterone in Leydig cell-depleted rats. Int. J. Androl., in press.
13. Free, M.J. (1977) Blood supply to the testis and its role in local exchange and transport of hormones. In: The Testis, edited by Johnson, A.D., Gomes, W.R., pp 4:39-90. Academic Press, New York.
14. Gerdes, U., Gåfvels, M., Bergh, A. and Cajander, S. (1992) Localized increases in ovarian vascular permeability and leukocyte accumulation after induced ovulation in the rabbit. J. Reprod. Fertil., in press.
15. Habenicht, U.-F. and Mueller, B. (1988) Disturbance of peripheral microcirculation by LHRH-agonists. II. Andrologia 20:23-32.
16. Hjertqvist, M., Bergh, A. and Damber, J.-E. (1988) HCG treatment increases intratesticular pressure in abdominal but not in scrotal testes in unilaterally cryptorchid rats. J. Androl., 9:116-120.
17. Hjertkvist, M., Läckgren, G., Plöen, L., and Bergh, A. (1992) Does hCG treatment induce inflammation-like changes in undescended testes in cryptorchid boys? J. Pediatric. Surg., in press
18. Intaglietta, M. (1988) Arteriolar vasomotion: normal physiological activity or defence mechanism, Diabetes Metab. 14: 489-494.
19. Ishida, H., Tashiro, H., Wanatabe, M., Fujii, N., Yoshida, H., Imamura, K., Minowada, S., Shinohara, M., Fukutani, K., Aso, Y. and deKretser, D.M. (1991) Measurement of inhibin concentrations in men: study of changes after castration and comparison with androgen levels in testicular tissue, testicular venous blood, and peripheral venous blood. J. Clin. Endocrinol. Metab., 70:1019-1022.
20. Maddocks, S. and Setchell, B.P. (1988) The physiology of the endocrine testis. In: Oxford Reviews of Reproductive Biology, edited by Clark, J., vol 10. pp 53-123. Oxford University Press, Oxford
21. Maddocks, S. and Sharpe, R.M. (1989a) Interstitial fluid volume in the rat testis: androgen-dependent regulation by the seminiferous tubules. J. Endocrinol., 120:215-222.

22. Maddocks, S. and Sharpe, R.M. (l989b) The route of secretion of inhibin from the rat testis. J. Endocrinol., 120:R5-R8
23. Pober, J.S. and Cotran, R.S. (1990) The role of endothelial cells in inflammation. Transplantation, 50:537-544.
24. Pöllänen, P., von Euler, M. and Söder, O. (1990). Testicular immunoregulatory factors. J. Reprod. Immunol. 18:51-76.
25. Schnitzer, J.E. (1992) gp60 is an albumin-binding glycoprotein expressed by continous endothelium involved in albumin transcytosis. Am. J. Physiol., 262:H246-H254.
26. Sealfon, A.I. and Zorgniotti, A.W. (1991) A theoretical model for testis thermoregulation. In: Temperature and environmental effects on the testis, edited by Zorgniotti, A.W., pp 123-135. Plenum Press, New York.
27. Setchell, B.P. (1970) Testicular blood supply, lymphatic drainage and secretion of fluid. In: The Testis, edited by Johnson, A.D., Gomes, W.G., Van Demark, N.L., pp 101-239. Academic Press, New York.
28. Setchell, B.P. (1990) Local control of testicular fluids. Reprod. Fertil. Dev., 2:291-309.
29. Setchell, B.P. and Sharpe, R.M. (1981) Effect of injected human chorionic gonadotrophin on capillary permeability, extra cellular fluid volume and the flow of lymph and blood in the testes of rats. J. Endocrinol., 91:245-254.
30. Setchell, B.P., Locatelli, A., Perreau, C., Pisselet, C., Fontaine, I., Kuntz, C., Saumande, J., Fontaine, J. and Hochereau-de Reviers, M.-T. (1991) The form and function of the Leydig cells in hypophysectomized rams treated with pituitary extract when spermatogenesis is disrupted by heating the testes. J. Endocrinol., 131:101-112.
31. Sharpe R.M. (1984) Intratesticular factors controlling testicular function. Biol. Reprod., 30:29-49.
32. Sharpe R.M., Maddocks, S. and Kerr, J.B. (l990) Cell-cell interactions in the control of spermatogenesis as studied using Leydig cell destruction and testosterone replacement. Am. J. Anat., 188:3-20.
33. Sharpe R.M., Bartlett, J.M.S. and Allenby, G. (1991) Evidence for the control of testicular interstitial fluid volume in the rat by specific germ cell types. J. Endocrinol., 128:359-367.
34. Sharpe R.M., (l990) Intratesticular control of steroidogenesis. Clin. Endocrinol., 33:787-807.
35. Stumpf, W.E. (1990) Steroid hormones and the cardiovascular system: direct actions of estradiol, progesterone, testosterone, gluco- and mineral corticoids and soltriol (vitamin D) on central nervous regulatory and peripheral tissues. Experentia, 46:13-25.
36. Sweeney, T., Rozum, J.S., Desjardins, C. and Gore, R.W. (1991) Microvascular pressure distribution in the hamster testis. Am. J. Physiol., 260:H1581-1589.
37. van Vliet, J., Rommerts, F.F.G., de Rooij, D.G., Buwalda, G. and Wensing, C.J.G. (1988) Reduction of testicular blood flow and focal degeneration of tissue in the rat after administration of human chorionic gonadotrophin. J. Endocrinol., 117:51-57.
38. Widmark, A., Damber, J.-E. and Bergh, A. (1989) High and low doses of luteinizing hormone induce different changes in testicular microcirculation. Acta Endocrinol., 121:621-627.
39. Widmark, A., Damber, J.-E. and Bergh, A. (1991) Arginine-Vasopressin induced changes in testicular microcirculation. Int. J. Androl., 14:58-65.

Intratesticular Androgen Action

R.M. Sharpe[1], C. McKinnell[1], M. Millar[1], S. Maddocks[2]
J.B. Kerr[3], T.B. Hargreave[4] and P.T.K. Saunders[1]

[1] MRC Reproductive Biology Unit, University of Edinburgh Centre for Reproductive Biology, 37 Chalmers Street Edinburgh EH3 9EW, U.K.
[2] Department of Animal Science, Waite Agricultural Research Institute, Glen Osmond South Australia 5064, Australia
[3] Department of Anatomy, Monash University Clayton, Victoria 3168, Australia
[4] Department of Urological Surgery, Western General Hospital, Crewe Road, Edinburgh EH4 2XU, U.K.

INTRODUCTION

In the adult male androgens (primarily testosterone) play a central role in the control of spermatogenesis and fertility, though little is known about how they exert their effect on spermatogenesis. Over the past 4-5 years we have addressed this problem by developing and exploiting a 'physiological' model system of androgen withdrawal and replacement in the adult rat in order to identify, at the biochemical and molecular level, how androgens control spermatogenesis. In the longer-term, such information should have value in addressing other key unresolved issues in male reproduction such as the causes of infertility and the development of new contraceptive strategies.

TESTOSTERONE LEVELS WITHIN THE TESTIS

To maintain normal spermatogenesis and fertility it is essential that testosterone levels within the testis are kept at a level much higher than that in peripheral blood. There has been debate in the literature as to just how high intratesticular levels of testosterone need to be to maintain quantitatively normal spermatogenesis (10,16,18), and one of the misleading factors in this respect has been the **artificially** high levels of testosterone which are measured in testicular interstitial fluid collected overnight from the rat testis (7,18). Subsequent studies (8) have shown that the level of testosterone measured in testicular venous (TV) blood (i.e. blood from major veins on the surface of the testis **before** their entry into the mediastinal venous plexus or the pampiniform plexus) provides the most accurate indication of the testosterone levels within the testis. In normal, anaesthetized rats the level of testosterone in TV blood is about 40-fold higher than that in peripheral blood (Fig. 1). In vasectomized men undergoing vasectomy reversal (most of whom subsequently regained their fertility) the TV level of testosterone is more than 200-fold higher than the level in peripheral blood (Fig. 1) In

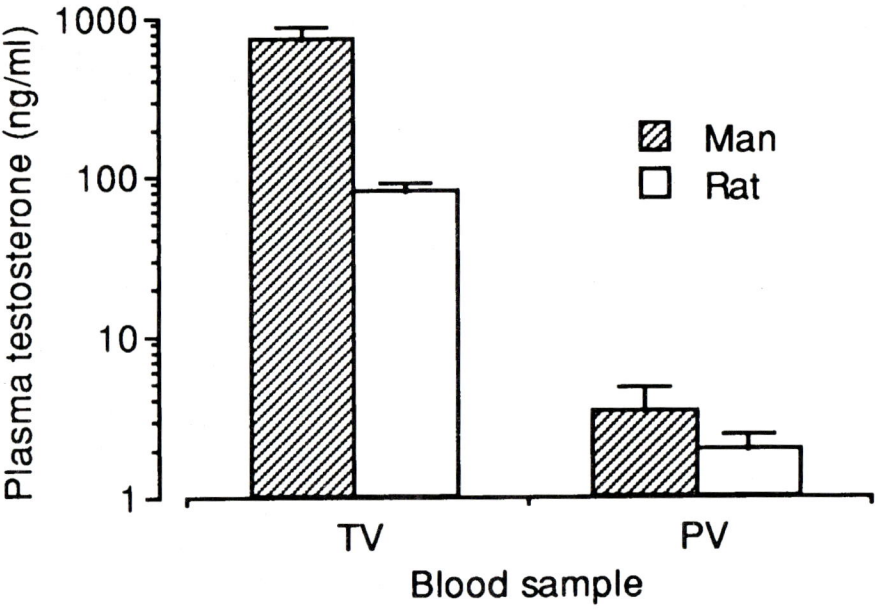

FIG 1. Comparative levels of testosterone in testicular venous (TV) and peripheral venous (PV) plasma in man and the rat. Values are the mean ± SD for either 6 (rat) or 8 (man) individuals. Note that testosterone levels are plotted on a logarimthic scale.

both the rat (18) and man (9) it is established that peripheral administration of androgens which suppress LH secretion and thus lower the intratesticular level of testosterone, results in impairment of spermatogenesis and fertility. So high intratesticular levels of testosterone are essential for normal spermatogenesis, but how and where does testosterone act?

WHERE DOES TESTOSTERONE ACT IN THE TESTIS?

At present, it is presumed that androgens act within the testis via androgen receptors which have been localized immunohistochemically to Sertoli, peritubular and Leydig cells (13) and more recently to arterioles (4). There are apparently no androgen receptors in the germ cells. In the context of spermatogenesis it is therefore presumed that androgens act via the Sertoli and peritubular cells to regulate the process of spermatogenesis (i.e. germ cell development). However, it has been reasonably clear for more than a decade that androgens do not exert an **overall** effect on spermatogenesis, but instead act at a specific stage of the spermatogenic cycle-stage VII in the rat. This evidence derives from studies in which testosterone withdrawal induced by various methods (hypophysectomy, anti-androgens etc.) was shown to result in selective degeneration of some of the germ cells at stage VII as early as 3-4 days after testosterone withdrawal (11,12); no adverse changes were noted at other stages. More recent studies have confirmed these findings by destroying the Leydig cells with ethane dimethane sulphonate (EDS) which rapidly (within 36-48 h) removes **all** Leydig cells and thus depletes **all** testosterone from the testis (3).

In all of these studies, administration of testosterone at appropriately high doses (i.e. to restore normal intratesticular testosterone levels) was able to prevent this germ cell degeneration completely (20). More recent, detailed analysis of the number of degenerating germ cells at stage VII after EDS-induced testosterone withdrawal has, however, revealed that even after 8 days of withdrawal only a small proportion (5% at most) of the germ cells at stage VII are degenerative and this does not seem to get worse (Fig. 2 and Reference 6). So why does spermatogenesis fail after testosterone withdrawal? The answer lies in the stages following stage VII, i.e. stages VIII-XIII. As the period of testosterone withdrawal increases, and especially beyond 5 days, so degenerating germ cells begin to appear at stage VIII, then stages IX, X, XI etc., in ever increasing numbers, such that by day 9 most of the step 11-12 spermatids at stages XI-XII are either degenerating or absent (Fig. 2) (see Reference 6). Throughout this period of time, germ cells at stages I-VI remain completely normal (Fig. 2 and Reference 6).

The best interpretation of these findings is as follows. As germ cells pass through stage VII, they undergo a series of specific changes which are androgen-regulated (via the Sertoli cells) and these changes are essential prerequisites for other subsequent modifications that will occur in stages IX-XII. If the androgen-regulated changes at stage VII do not occur (because of androgen withdrawal) then when these germ cells reach stages IX-XII they are unable to undergo the normal changes at these stages and therefore degenerate and are phagocytosed by the Sertoli cells. In particular, it appears that the elongating spermatids are especially affected as most of these cells subsequently degenerate. This is of interest as these are the cells which undergo nuclear condensation during stages VIII-XIV, raising the possibility that deficiencies in the onset of this change (perhaps during stage VII) may be the causal factor. If so, then it must be presumed that testosterone controls the onset of nuclear condensation in spermatids (see also below).

The above findings are all consistent with testosterone acting at around stages VI-VIII (probably stage VII) of the spermatogenic cycle in the rat and our interest was therefore focused on these stages in order to identify

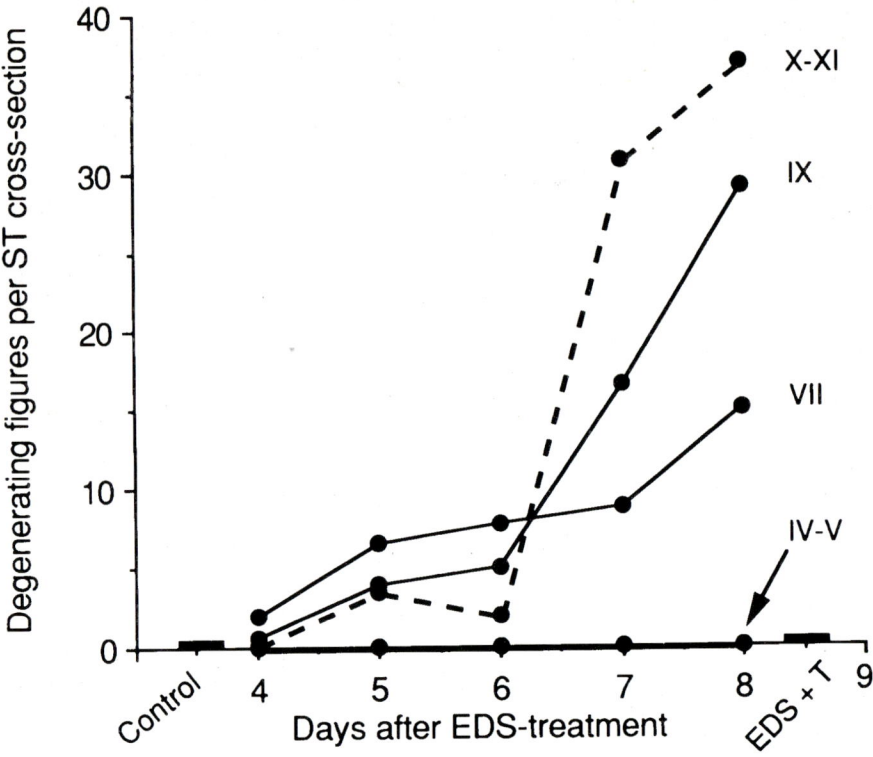

FIG. 2 Incidence of degenerating germ cells at stages IV-V, VII, IX and X-XI at various times after EDS-induced testosterone withdrawal. Degenerating germ cells in control and EDS-treated rats supplemented with testosterone esters (T) were virtually non-detectable at all of the stages assessed. Error bars have been omitted for clarity. For further details see Kerr et al. 1992. (Reference 6).

the biochemical and molecular mechanisms of testosterone action. We chose to restrict our studies to the initial 4-6 days after EDS-induced testosterone withdrawal, for the following reasons. First, germ cell degeneration at stage VII was virtually maximal by day 6 (Fig. 2). Second, seminiferous tubules at later stages of the spermatogenic cycle were still unaffected (day 4) or were only affected slightly (day 6). Third, the germ cell complement at stage VII was still virtually normal, as the number of degenerating germ cells comprised only 0.5-1.5% of all the germ cells present (Fig. 3); the latter was considered particularly important because there is ever-increasing evidence that major reduction in the number of germ cells associated with the Sertoli cell can lead to marked changes in Sertoli cell function (17) and such changes might obscure any selective effects of testosterone withdrawal.

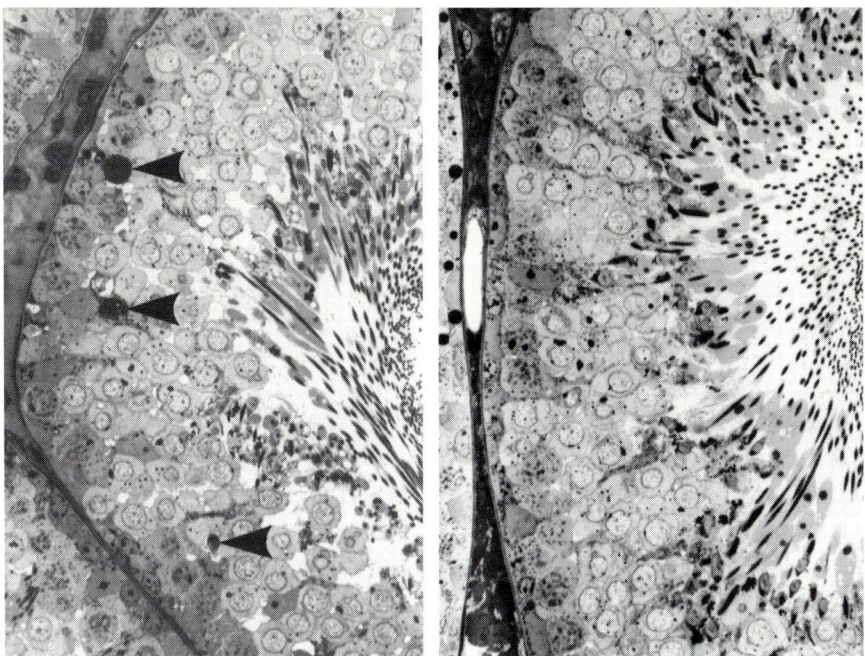

FIG. 3. Representative morphology of stage VII seminiferous tubules from a control (right) and from a rat treated 4 days earlier with EDS (left); note the degenerating germ cells (arrowheads) in the latter.

EFFECTS OF TESTOSTERONE WITHDRAWAL ON PROTEIN SECRETION BY ISOLATED SEMINIFEROUS TUBULES

Based on the principles described above, ST at stages II-V (i.e. preceding the androgen-dependent stages), VI-VIII (androgen-dependent) or IX-XII (following the androgen-dependent stages) were isolated from control rats and from rats treated 2-6 days earlier with EDS, some of which had been supplemented with injection of long-acting testosterone esters (TE). It should be noted that the dose of TE administered (25 mg every 3 days, commencing on day 0) has been shown to maintain virtually normal spermatogenesis and fertility in EDS-treated rats for at least 10 weeks (19). The isolated seminiferous tubules were cultured in the presence of 60 µCi ^{35}S-labelled methionine for 22-24 h at 34°C as detailed elsewhere (21); the culture conditions were selected on the basis of previous studies showing that changes in Sertoli cell function *in vivo* could be accurately reproduced *in vitro* (1,2).

Somewhat surprisingly, the first major finding was that EDS-induced testosterone withdrawal led within 3 days to a significant decrease in overall protein secretion by seminiferous tubules at stages VI-VIII, as judged by the incorporation of ^{35}S-methionine into secreted proteins (Fig. 4). This decrease was maximal by day 4, by which time protein secretion had fallen by over half, and remained at this low level up to day 6. There were no comparable changes at stages II-V or IX-XII and administration of TE to EDS-treated rats prevented completely the EDS-induced decrease in protein secretion by seminiferous tubules at stages VI-VIII, at least up to day 5 (Fig. 4). However, re-examination of this data and that from controls revealed that EDS-induced testosterone withdrawal had **prevented** the

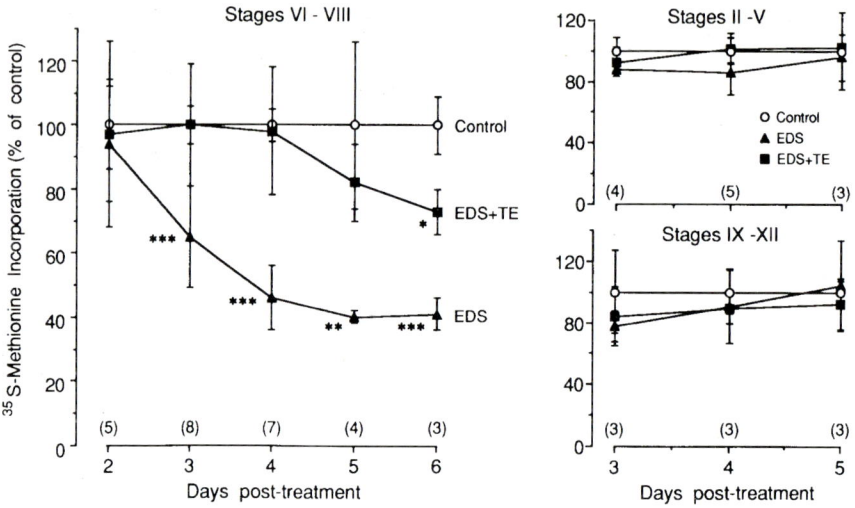

FIG. 4. Effect of treatment with EDS ± supplementation with testosterone esters (TE) on the incorporation of ^{35}S-methionine into proteins secreted by isolated seminiferous tubules (10cm) at stages VI-VIII or stages II-V and IX-XII. Results have been expressed as a percentage of the respective mean control value at each time-point. Mean ± SD for the number of animals shown in parentheses. *$P<0.05$, **$P<0.01$, ***$P<0.001$, in comparison with respective control group. Reproduced with permission from Sharpe et al. (1992) (Reference 21).

normal **increase** in protein secretion that occurs as seminiferous tubules transform from stages II-V to VI-VIII (Fig. 5) rather than causing an actual **decrease** in protein secretion by the tubules. This shows clearly that one of the ways in which testosterone controls spermatogenesis appears to involve an overall effect on protein secretion by the seminiferous tubules. This change may well be a consequence of the increased volume of mitochondria and rough endoplasmic reticulum described in Sertoli cells at stages VII-VIII (5,23).

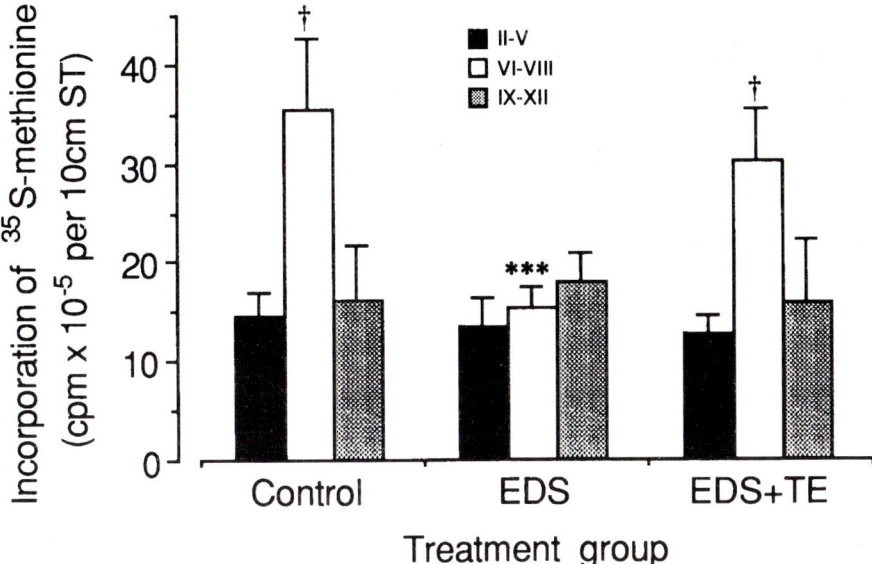

FIG.5. Androgen-dependence of the normal increase in total protein secretion by isolated seminiferous tubules at stages VI-VIII of the spermatogenic cycle when compared with stages II-V and IX-XII. Values are the mean ± SD for 4 rats in each group. EDS was administered 4 days prior to tubule isolation. ***$P<0.001$, in comparison with stages VI-VIII in control. † $P<0.001$, in comparison with stages II-V and IX-XII in control. Reproduced with permission from Sharpe et al. (1992) (Reference 21).

IDENTIFICATION OF ANDROGEN-REGULATED PROTEINS (ARPS) SECRETED BY SEMINIFEROUS TUBULES AT STAGES VI-VIII

Analysis by 2-dimensional SDS-PAGE of the proteins secreted by seminiferous tubules from the various treatment groups, revealed that the secretion of nearly 40 proteins by seminiferous tubules at stages VI-VIII was reduced following EDS-induced testosterone withdrawal and was prevented by TE-supplementation (21). Of these proteins, seven were classified subsequently as being androgen-regulated proteins (ARPs) on the basis that, in the normal spermatogenic cycle in controls, these proteins were secreted primarily at stages VI-VII rather than at other stages and that this secretion was testosterone-dependent (21) (see Fig. 6). The identity of the ARPs is not known though some share certain similarities with known proteins. For example, ARP-6 and ARP-7 are of comparable molecular weight and pI to the A- and B-forms of P-Mod-S, a protein secreted *in vitro* under androgen control by isolated peritubular cells from immature

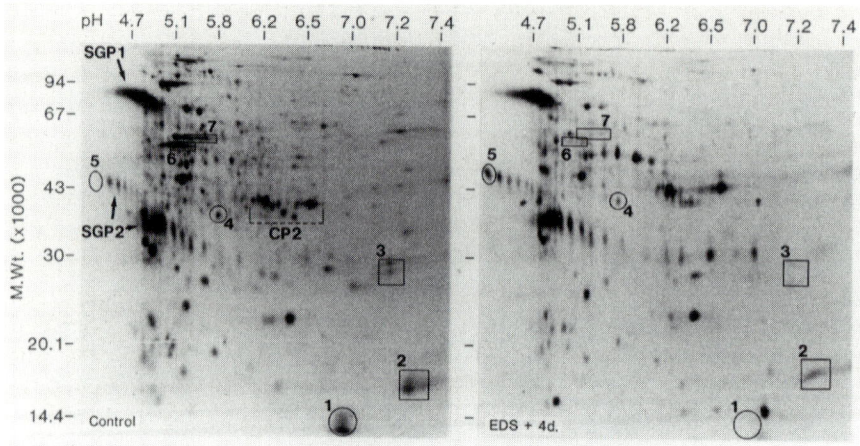

FIG. 6. Representative two-dimensional SDS-PAGE of ^{35}S-labelled proteins secreted by stage VI-VIII seminiferous tubules from a control rat (left) and a rat treated 4 days earlier with EDS (right). Seven putative androgen-regulated proteins (see text) are numbered and circled and the Sertoli cell-secreted proteins SGP-1, SGP-2 and cyclic protein-2 (CP-2) are indicated for reference in the control.

rats (22). ARP-5, which is regulated negatively by testosterone, is a charge isomer of sulphated glycoprotein-2 (SGP-2) and may have a different degree of sulphation and/or glycosylation compared with higher pH forms of SGP-2 (Fig. 6). ARP-1 and ARP-2 are the most abundant of the ARPs and are in the molecular weight range for growth factors. Studies are currently in progress to isolate and identify the ARPs and to characterize their role in spermatogenesis.

USE OF SUBTRACTION HYBRIDIZATION TO IDENTIFY ANDROGEN-REGULATED GENES IN THE SEMINIFEROUS TUBULE

The basis for this approach is outlined in Fig.7 (see Reference 15). Essentially, it seeks to isolate androgen-regulated genes by taking a 10-fold excess of mRNA isolated from seminiferous tubules at stages VI-VIII from rats treated 6 days earlier with EDS (and which are presumed to be **depleted** of androgen-regulated mRNAs) and hybridizing this to single-stranded radiolabelled cDNA generated from mRNA isolated from seminiferous tubules at stages VI-VIII from control rats or from EDS-treated rats supplemented with TE (both of which should contain androgen-regulated mRNAs). After removal of double-stranded cDNA-mRNA duplexes (representing mRNA's common to both control and EDS-treated groups and therefore not androgen-regulated) and single-stranded mRNA (the excess mRNA from EDS-treated rats), the remaining single-stranded cDNAs (presumed to be androgen-regulated) were made double-stranded and then amplified by 'lone-linker' PCR (15).

To date, more than 30 genes have been cloned using this subtraction approach and they are currently being sequenced and their androgen-dependence assessed using Northern and in-situ hybridizations. One clone (AA-8) for which the sequence has been determined and compared to Genbank, has proved to be transition protein-2 (TP-2). This is one of the DNA-binding proteins that fulfills an intermediary role during the replacement of histones by protamines in condensation of the nuclear DNA during spermatogenesis. Analysis in-situ of stage-dependent expression of the mRNA for TP-2, using a digoxygenin-labelled riboprobe, shows that this gene is first transcribed at stage VII of the spermatogenic cycle when its

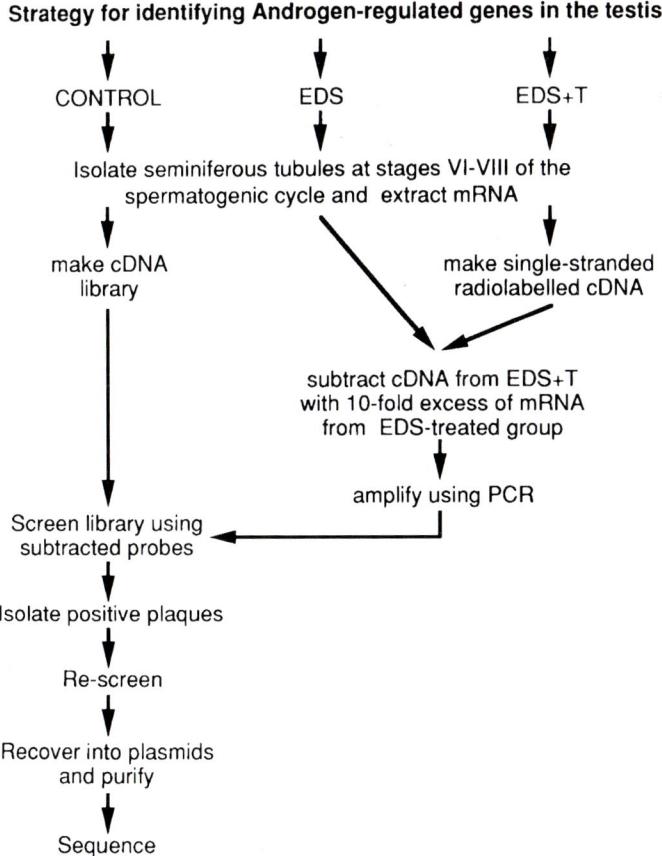

FIG.7. Flow diagram illustrating the principles underlying the isolation of androgen-regulated genes using subtraction hybridization.

expression is restricted to step 7 spermatids (Fig. 8). The level of expression of the mRNA for TP-2 is then at its highest in step 8-12 spermatids at stages VIII-XII of the spermatogenic cycle before disappearing by stage XIV when nuclear condensation is virtually complete. Although the mRNA for TP-2 was first detectable at stage VII (the androgen-dependent stage), further in-situ and Northern analyses using RNA from control, EDS-treated and EDS+ TE-treated rats failed to reveal any detectable evidence for the androgen-dependent expression of TP-2 (14). Isolation and cloning of the TP-2 gene using the subtraction hybridization procedure described above, probably occurred because it is a highly abundant mRNA at stages VII-VIII. However,

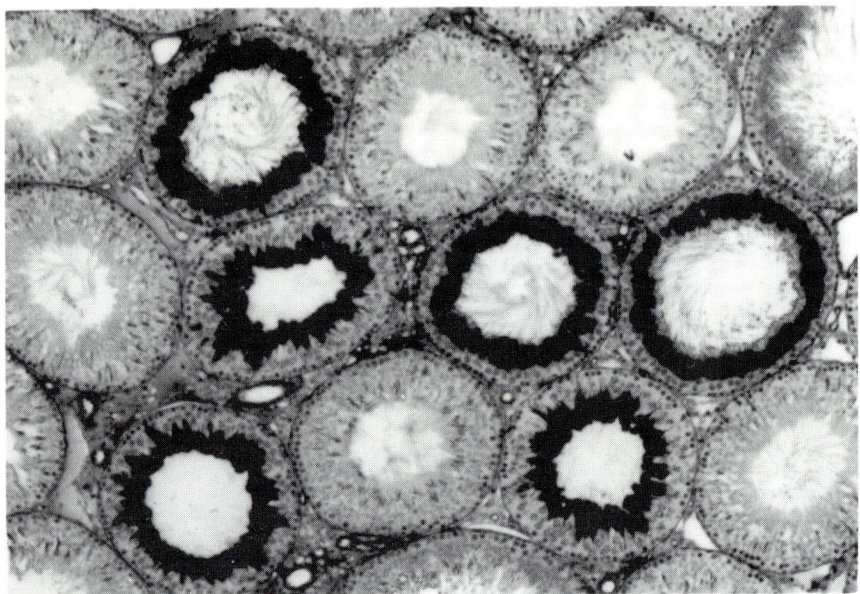

FIG. 8. Stage-dependent expression of the mRNA for transition protein-2 using a digoxygenin-labelled riboprobe.

it is of particular interest that our studies had shown clearly that it is the spermatids expressing TP-2 which are the most vulnerable to the effects of testosterone withdrawal (Fig. 3), and that it is primarily via the degeneration of these cells that spermatogenesis fails after testosterone withdrawal (6). It may yet prove that some aspect of the process of nuclear condensation of spermatids is androgen-regulated.

CONCLUSIONS

Our studies have used the ultimate biological endpoint of testosterone action in the testis (i.e. the maintenance of normal germ cell numbers) to identify a time-frame within which the molecular and biochemical mechanisms of testosterone action on the seminiferous tubule can be identified. Using this time-frame we have identified novel effects of testosterone on overall protein secretion as well as the secretion of specific proteins by seminiferous tubules at stages VI-VIII. These findings, or identification of androgen-regulated genes by subtraction hybridization, should enable future characterization of the mechanisms via which testosterone drives spermatogenesis. In turn, these results should lead to improved ability to manipulate reproductive potential in man.

REFERENCES

1. Allenby, G., Foster, P.M.D. and Sharpe, R.M. (1991). Evaluation of changes in the secretion of immunoactive inhibin by adult rat seminiferous tubules in-vitro as an indicator of early toxicant action on spermatogenesis. Fundamental and Applied Toxicology, 16:710-724.
2. Allenby, G., Foster, P.M.D. and Sharpe, R.M. (1991). Evidence that secretion of immunoactive inhibin by seminiferous tubules from the adult rat testis is regulated by specific germ cell types: correlation between in-vivo and in-vitro studies. Endocrinology, 128: 467-476.
3. Bartlett, J.M.S., Kerr, J.B. and Sharpe, R.M. (1988). The selective removal of pachytene spermatocytes using methoxyaceticacid as an approach to the study in-vivo of paracrine interactions in the testis. J. Androl., 9:31-40.
4. Bergh, A. and Damber, J.E. (1992). Immunohistochemical demonstration of androgen receptors on testicular blood vessels. International J. Androl. (in Press).
5. Kerr, J.B. (1988). A light microscopic and morphometric analysis of the Sertoli cell during the spermatogenic cycle of the rat. Anat. Embryol., 179:191-203.
6. Kerr, J.B., Millar, M., Maddocks, S. and Sharpe, R.M. (1992). Stage-dependent changes in spermatogenesis and Sertoli cells following withdrawal and restoration of testosterone. Anat. Rec. (in Press).
7. Maddocks, S. and Setchell, B.P. (1989). Testosterone concentrations in testicular interstitial fluid collected with a push-pull cannula or by drip-collection from adult rats given testosterone or aminoglutethimide. J. Endocrinol., 121:303-309.
8. Maddocks, S. and Sharpe, R.M. (1989). Dynamics of testosterone secretion by the rat testis: implications for measurement of the intratesticular levels of testosterone. J. Endocrinol., 122:323-329.
9. Morse, H.C., Horike, N., Rowley, M.J. and Heller, C.G. (1973). Testosterone concentrations in testes of normal men: effects of testosterone propionate administration. J. Clin. Endocrinol. Metab., 37: 882-886.
10. Rommerts, F.F.G. (1988). How much androgen is required for maintenance of spermatogenesis? J. Endocrinol., 116:7-9.
11. Russell, L.D. and Clermont, Y. (1977). Degeneration of germ cells in normal, hypophysectomized and hormone treated hypophysectomized rats. Anat. Rec., 187:347-366.
12. Russell, L.D., Malone, J.P. and Karpas, S.L. (1981). Morphological pattern elicited by agents affecting spermatogenesis by disruption of its hormonal stimulation. Tissue Cell, 13:369-380.
13. Sar, M., Lubahn, D.B., French, F.S. and Wilson, E.M. (1990). Immunohistochemical localization of the androgen receptor in rat and human tissues. Endocrinology, 127: 3180-3186.
14. Saunders, P.T.K., Millar, M.R., Maguire, S.M. and Sharpe, R.M. (1992). Stage-specific expression of rat transition protein 2 mRNA and possible localization to the chromatoid body of step 7 spermatids by in-situ hybridization using a non-radioactive riboprobe. Mol. Reprod. Dev. (in Press).
15. Saunders, P.T.K., Millar M.R. and Sharpe, R.M. (1992). Mitochondrial cytochrome C

oxidase II mRNA is expressed at high levels in a stage-dependent manner in pachytene spermatocytes during spermatogenesis in the rat. Biol. Reprod. (submitted).
16. Sharpe, R.M. (1987). Testosterone and spermatogenesis. J. Endocrinol., 113:1-2.
17. Sharpe, R.M. (1992). Experimental evidence for Sertoli-germ cell and Sertoli-Leydig cell interactions. In: The Sertoli Cell, edited by L.D. Russell & M.D. Griswold. Cache River Press (in Press).
18. Sharpe, R.M., Donachie, K. and Cooper, I. (1988). Re-evaluation of the intratesticular level of testosterone required for quantitative maintenance of spermatogenesis in the rat. J. Endocrinol., 117:19-26.
19. Sharpe, R.M., Fraser, H.M. and Ratnasooriya, W.D. (1988). Assessment of the role of Leydig cell products other than testosterone in spermatogenesis and fertility in adult rats. Int. J. Androl., 11:507-523.
20. Sharpe, R.M., Maddocks, S. and Kerr, J.B. (1990). Cell-cell interactions in the control of spermatogenesis as studied using Leydig cell destruction and testosterone replacement. Am. J. Anat., 188:3-20.
21. Sharpe, R.M., Maddocks, S., Millar, M., Saunders, P.T.K., Kerr, J.B. and McKinnell, C. (1992). Testosterone and spermatogenesis: identification of stage-dependent, androgen-regulated proteins secreted by adult rat seminiferous tubules. J. Androl., 13:172-184.
22. Skinner, M.K., Fetterolf, P.M. and Anthony, C.T. (1988). Purification of a paracrine factor, P-Mod-S, produced by testicular peritubular cells that modulates Sertoli cell function. J. Biol. Chem., 263:2884-2890.
23. Ueno, H. and Mori. H. (1990). Morphometrical analysis of Sertoli cell ultrastructure during the seminiferous epithelial cycle in rats. Biol. Reprod., 43: 769-776.

Nonsteroidal Regulation of Testicular Function

M.K. Skinner

Reproductive Endocrinology Center, University of California, San Francisco, CA 94143-0556, USA

INTRODUCTION

The physiology of an organ such as the testis is significantly more complex than the functions associated with an individual cell type. This intricate physiology reflects the ability of different cell types within the organ to interact and communicate. Therefore, an understanding of the regulation of testis function requires a consideration of the interactions between different cell types. Several cell types make up the testis and the seminiferous tubules where the process of spermatogenesis occurs. The epithelial-like Sertoli cells form the tubule and provide the physical support and microenvironment required for germinal cell development. The mesenchymally derived peritubular cells surround and provide structural integrity to the tubule. Within the interstitium between tubules are the Leydig cells responsible for the production of androgen. The androgens act on the seminiferous tubules to maintain the process of spermatogenesis.

The endocrine regulation of testis function primarily involves the actions of the pituitary gonadotropins, follicle stimulating hormone (FSH) and luteinizing hormone (LH). These are two essential nonsteroidal agents required in the regulation of testis function. LH acts specifically on Leydig cells to induce the production of androgen that subsequently acts on the seminiferous tubule at either peritubular cells or Sertoli cells. This action of LH is also required to maintain normal circulating levels of androgens. FSH acts specifically on Sertoli cells to provide cellular differentiation during pubertal development and maintain optimal function in the adult testis. The remaining nonsteroidal agents involved in the regulation of testis function mediate local cell-cell interactions. In general, these cellular interactions are induced or influenced by gonadotropins and/or androgen.

The two primary and essential functional parameters of the testis are the production of sperm and androgen. The complex network of cell-cell interactions mediated, by both steroidal and nonsteroidal agents, have evolved to maintain and control the spermatogenic and steroidogenic processes. The two aspects of cellular physiology that require regulation are growth and differentiation. Growth and differentiation are interrelated, but controlled by distinct regulatory agents. During pubertal development cell growth is required and at the onset of puberty individual cell types have specific growth requirements. A class of nonsteroidal regulatory factors involved in this growth regulation are growth factors. The influence that hormones have on cell proliferation often are indirectly mediated through the local production of these growth factors. Throughout testis development and particularly at the onset of puberty, cellular differentiation is induced and maintained for various cell types to acquire specific functions. Therefore, another class of nonsteroidal regulatory factors are involved in the control of cell differentiation. In considering the regulation of testicular function the factors involved include 1) the ability of gonadotropins to act on the testis, 2) cell-cell interactions mediated by both steroidal and nonsteroidal factors, 3) the control of cellular growth and differentiation, and 4) the maintenance of the spermatogenic and steroidogenic processes. Examples of nonsteroidal factors involved in this process will be discussed.

GROWTH REGULATION

All the cell types in the testis proliferate during fetal development and prepubertally. At the onset of puberty Sertoli cell growth is arrested and cell differentiation is induced. Germinal cell growth is increased and the spermatogenic process initiated. Leydig cell and peritubular cell growth is decreased but continues at a reduced rate in the adult (1). Therefore a number of changes in cell growth are required at the onset of puberty. A number of different growth factors have been shown to be produced in the testis (2) and have been postulated to mediate numerous cell-cell interactions in that gland (Table 1) (3).

The ability of FSH to influence Sertoli cell growth factor production will be used as an example of nonsteroidal growth regulation. Sertoli cells have been shown to produce the growth stimulators transforming growth factor-alpha (TGFα) (4) and fibroblast growth factor (FGF) (5), as well as the growth inhibitor transforming growth factor-beta (TGFβ) (6). Observations have been obtained on the developmental and hormonal regulation of TGFα, TGFβ and FGF expression and action. TGFα expression declines gradually during pubertal development to constant level and is not responsive to hormones. TGFα acts at the epidermal growth factor receptor (EGFR) that was found to be expressed by Leydig, peritubular, Sertoli and germinal cells. Peritubular cells and Leydig cells were responsive to TGFα *in vitro*. FGF

Table 1. *Growth Factors in the Testis*

Growth Factor	Proposed Site Production	Proposed Site of Action	Proposed Function*
IGF-1	Leydig Peritubular Sertoli	Leydig Peritubular Sertoli Germinal	+Steroidogenesis +Growth +Growth/Differentiation ?
TGF-α	Peritubular Sertoli Leydig	Leydig Peritubular Sertoli Germinal	−Steroidogenesis +Growth ±Differentiation ?
TGF-β	Peritubular Sertoli	Leydig Peritubular Sertoli Germinal	−Steroidogenesis −Growth/+Differentiation +Differentiation ?
IL-1	Sertoli	Leydig Germinal	−Steroidogenesis ?
FGF	Sertoli	Leydig Sertoli	±Steroidogenesis +Growth
NGF	Germinal	Sertoli	?

* (+) denotes an increase, (−) indicates a decrease and (?) represents an unknown function.

expression by Sertoli cells remained relatively constant during development and was found to be induced by FSH. FGF has been shown to act on Sertoli cells to promote cell proliferation (5,7) and localize in germinal cells (8). FSH induced Sertoli cell FGF expression may provided an indirect mechanism to control Sertoli and/or germinal cell growth. The three isoforms of TGFβ (TGFβ1, TGFβ2 and TGFβ3) have distinct patterns of expression during development. TGFβ1 remains relatively constant during development and is not hormone responsive. Interestingly, TGFβ3 expression by Sertoli cells has a dramatic transient increase in expression at the onset of puberty that declines after the induction of the spermatogenic process. Therefore, TGFβ3 may be involved in the induction of the pubertal process and germinal cell development. This transient increase in TGFβ3 is not responsive to hormones such as FSH or androgen. TGFβ2 expression by Sertoli cells was only present prepubertally and declined to negligible levels at the onset of puberty. TGFβ2 production was dramatically suppressed by the actions of FSH. Therefore, at the onset of puberty FSH actions on Sertoli cells cause a suppression of TGFβ2 expression and increase in FGF expression. The absence of a growth inhibitor such as TGFβ2 may allow growth stimulators such as TGFα and FGF to promote germinal cell proliferation that is inhibited prepubertally by the growth inhibitor.

This observation of the actions of FSH on Sertoli cells demonstrates that hormones can act on the testis to influence the local production of growth factors. These growth factors subsequently mediate cell-cell interactions and influence testis growth. Hormones can indirectly through the actions of these nonsteroidal agents, influence cell proliferation and tissue growth.

DIFFERENTIATION REGULATION

During development all testis cell types undergo alterations in cellular differentiation to acquire unique and essential cellular functions. Leydig cells are derived from the precursor mesenchymal cell population in the interstitium during fetal and pubertal development to maintain a high basal androgen production in the adult. Peritubular cells differentiate in response to androgens prior to puberty. Sertoli cells differentiate throughout pubertal development. Germinal cell differentiation and development is initiated at the onset of puberty. Gonadotropins and androgens have an important role in the differentiation process of these cell types. Equally important, however, is the local production of nonsteroidal agents that act as differentiation-type factors and regulate this process Table 2.

Table 2. *Regulation of Cellular Differentiation/Function*

	Source	Agent	Action
Sertoli	Endocrine	FSH	Increase
	Peritubular	PMODS	Increase
	Leydig	Androgen	(?)Increase
		POMC	Modulate FSH
	Germinal	(?) Factors	Increase
Leydig	Endocrine	LH	Increase
	Sertoli	(?)Factors	Increase/Decrease
Peritubular	Leydig	Androgen	Increase
	Sertoli	(?)Factors	Increase
Germinal	Sertoli	(?)Factors	Increase

(?) Represents uncharacterized factors.

The agents that influence Sertoli cell differentiation will be used as an example of nonsteroidal differentiation regulation. The induction of Sertoli cell differentiation results in the expression of a large number of unique secretory products postulated to be essential for germinal cell development. An example of such a Sertoli cell product is transferrin that can bind and transport iron to developing germinal cells. FSH can promote Sertoli cell differentiation and the production of most of these secretory products. Although androgen actions on the seminiferous tubule are essential for the maintenance of Sertoli cell differentiation *in vivo*, the *in vitro* actions of androgens on Sertoli cells are negligible. Androgens, however, also act on peritubular cells that can produce a paracrine factor termed PModS that induces Sertoli cell differentiation (9). PModS appears to be a differentiation-type factor and has a more dramatic effect on Sertoli cell functions *in vitro* than any individual agent previously identified, including FSH (9,10). A cascade of cell-cell interactions is proposed in that LH acts on Leydig cells to promote androgen production that acts on peritubular cells to promote PModS production which subsequently induces Sertoli cell differentiation and functions required for germinal cell development.

This observation of the regulation of Sertoli cell differentiation demonstrates that hormones can act on the testis to influence the local production of differentiation factors. These differentiation-type factors subsequently mediate cell-cell interactions and influence testis physiology. Through the actions of these nonsteroidal agents, hormones can indirectly influence testis development and cellular differentiation.

SUMMARY

The examples given of the regulation of Sertoli cell growth and differentiation demonstrates that a complex network of cell-cell interactions are mediated by nonsteroidal agents. These nonsteroidal agents play an integral role in the regulation of testis function. The ability of gonadotropins and androgen to influence testis physiology is critical, however, this underlying network of cellular interactions and nonsteroidal growth and differentiation agents provide the actual mechanism by which testis function is regulated. The elucidation of how testis function is regulated will require an understanding of these cellular interactions and the nonsteroidal agents involved.

As previously noted, all of these cellular interactions and this complex regulation of testis function is required to control the steroidogenic and spermatogenic processes. In understanding the regulation of testis function, several aspects of testis physiology must be considered. In the adult testis, spermatogenesis is optimal with minimal regulation and androgen levels within the testis are an order of magnitude greater than that required to stimulate testis function. Therefore, adult testis function is an optimal steady state condition that requires maintenance, but not an active regulation to alter cellular functions. The endocrine regulation and the local network of cell-cell interactions in the adult testis is required to maintain optimal testis function. Factors such as androgens, gonadotropins and paracrine growth and differentiation factors keep testis function maintained. Although an active regulation of testis function is required during fetal and pubertal development, in the adult testis maintenance of optimal function is required. In considering the function of nonsteroidal factors in the testis, this aspect of testis physiology needs to be considered.

REFERENCES

1. Teerds, K.J., DeRooij, D.G., Rommerts, F.F.G., Van Der Tweel, I. and Wensing C.J.G. (1989) Turnover time of Leydig cells and other interstitial cells in the testis of the adult rat. Arch. Androl., 23:105-111.
2. Bellve, A.R. and Feig, L.A., (1984) Cell proliferation in the mammalian testis: biology of the seminiferous growth factor. Recent Prog. Horm. Res., 40:531-561.
3. Skinner, M.K., (1991) Cell-cell interactions in the testis. Endocr. Rev., 12:45-77.
4. Skinner, M.K., Takacs, K. and Coffey, R.J. (1989) Transforming growth factor-alpha gene expression action in the seminiferous tubule: peritubular cell-Sertoli cell interactions. Endocrinology, 124:845-854.
5. Smith, E.P., Hall, S.H., Monaco, L., French, F.S., Wilson, M.W. and Conti, M. (1989) A rat Sertoli cell factor similar to basic fibroblast growth factor increases c-fos messenger ribonucleic acid in cultured Sertoli cells. Mol. Endocrinol., 3:954-961.
6. Skinner, M.K. and Moses, H.L. (1989) Transforming growth factor beta gene expression and action in the seminiferous tubule: peritubular-Sertoli cell interactions. Mol. Endocrinol., 3:625-634.
7. Jaillard, C., Chatelain, P.G. and Saez, J.M. (1987) In vitro regulation of pig Sertoli cell growth and function: effects of fibroblast growth factors and somatomedin-C. Biol. Reprod. 37:665-674.
8. Mayerhofer, A. Russell, L.D., Grothe, C., Rudolf M. and Gratzl, M. (1991) Presence and localization of a 30-kDa basic fibroblast growth factor-like protein in rodent testes. Endocrinology, 129:921-924.
9. Skinner, M.K., Fetterolf P.M., Anthony C.T. (1988) Purification of the paracrine factor, P-Mod-S, produced by testicular peritubular cells that modulates Sertoli cell function. J. Biol. Chem., 263:2884-2890.
10. Anthony, C.T., Rosselli M. and Skinner M.K. (1991) Actions of the testicular paracrine factor (P-Mod-S) on Sertoli cell transferrin secretion throughout pubertal development. Endocrinology, 129:353-360.

Paracrine Control of Ovarian Endocrine Function

C.D. Smyth, P.F. Whitelaw, I.M. Turner, F. Miró,
C.M. Howles* and S.G. Hillier

*Reproductive Endocrinology Laboratory, Department of Obstetrics & Gynaecology,
University of Edinburgh Centre for Reproductive Biology, 37 Chalmers Street,
Edinburgh EH3 9EW, UK
* Serono Laboratories (UK) Ltd, 99 Bridge Road East,
Welwyn Garden City, Herts. AL7 1BG, UK*

INTRODUCTION

During the follicular phase of the human menstrual cycle, the follicle destined to ovulate grows to a diameter of over 20 mm and becomes the major ovarian source of secreted oestrogen. The oestrogen-secretory stage in its development encompasses a programmed sequence of cell growth and differentiation in the follicle wall which terminates in ovulation and transformation of the follicle into a corpus luteum (3). This entire sequence of events depends upon primary endocrine stimulation of the ovaries by the gonadotrophins FSH and LH. It is also assumed to involve secondary paracrine control emanating within the follicle itself (4,5,7). In this article, we assess the basis for that assumption, and report new evidence that paracrine signalling between granulosa and thecal cells actually occurs.

THE FOLLICULAR PARACRINE CONCEPT

Paracrine regulation is a generalised form of bioregulation whereby one cell-type in a tissue selectively influences the activity of an adjacent cell-type through the biosynthesis and release of chemical messengers which diffuse into the parenchyma and act specifically on neighbouring target cells (2). The term 'paracrine' was initially coined to explain cell-cell interactions in the digestive tract mediated by locally produced gut peptides (8). The particular relevance of paracrine control to the coordination of thecal and granulosa cell function in the ovarian follicle has become increasingly apparent hand-in-hand with the application of modern cell and molecular biology techniques to study the growth and differentiation of follicular cells *in vitro* (4,5,7).

The 'two-cell, two-gonadotrophin' model of oestrogen synthesis in the preovulatory follicle not only explains gonadotrophic requirements for oestrogen synthesis (1) but also provides a conceptual framework for paracrine signalling within the follicle wall. Gonadotrophic regulation of oestrogen synthesis hinges on the fact that granulosa cells exclusively express FSH receptors whereas thecal cells express LH receptors (4). Granulosa cells only express LH receptors during advanced preovulatory development stimulated by FSH. FSH receptors in granulosa cells are coupled via cyclic AMP mediated intracellular signalling to genes encoding proteins upon which differentiated function depends, including LH receptors and the steroidogenic enzyme crucial to oestrogen synthesis, cytochrome P450arom (aromatase). LH receptors on thecal cells are also coupled to steroidogenesis via cyclic AMP, the major steroidogenic enzyme under LH control being cytochrome P450c17 (17-hydroxylase/C17-20 lyase). This enzyme is crucial for follicular androgen synthesis, and hence the provision of aromatase substrates for FSH-stimulated granulosa cells. Granulosa cells do not measurably express 17-hydroxylase/C17-20 lyase, whereas thecal cells do not express aromatase. That both androgens and oestrogens accumulate in ovarian follicular fluid constitutes *prima facie* evidence for steroid mediated cell-cell communication in the preovulatory follicle, and it follows that steroidal and nonsteroidal factors could also function as paracrine signals at this site.

EVIDENCE FOR INTRAFOLLICULAR PARACRINE SIGNALLING

Most evidence for paracrine communication between granulosa cells and theca cells is indirect, mainly being based on the demonstrated ability of a particular factor(s) that is known to be produced within one or other cell-type to exert a potential physiologically important action on the other cell-type *in vitro* (4-7). Previous attempts to demonstrate paracrine signalling in the ovarian follicle *in vivo* have generally been hampered by the unavailability of suitably pure forms of exogenous FSH with which to experiment. Almost all pituitary or urinary preparations available to-date contain finite amounts of LH. Injection of such LH-contaminated FSH preparations into experimental animals therefore activates thecal cell function via direct stimulation of the LH receptors that are constitutively present on thecal cells, possibly obscuring any FSH-activated paracrine control by granulosa cells. The recent availability of recombinant human FSH (rh-FSH) expressed in Chinese Hamster Ovary cell lines offers a unique opportunity to test the follicular paracrine concept, since this form of FSH is completely devoid of LH.

A series of pilot studies was recently completed, demonstrating that injection of rh-FSH into immature female rats dose-dependently stimulates the level of the ovarian mRNA transcript that encodes cytochrome P450c17 (Smyth, C.D. et al., in preparation). The response to daily treatment with 36 IU rh-FSH for two days is shown in Fig. 1. Although rh-FSH is completely devoid of LH it stimulates a similar degree of P450c17 nRNA expression to that elicited by a single injection of 15 IU pregnant mares' serum gonadotrophin, which contains both FSH and LH bioactivity.

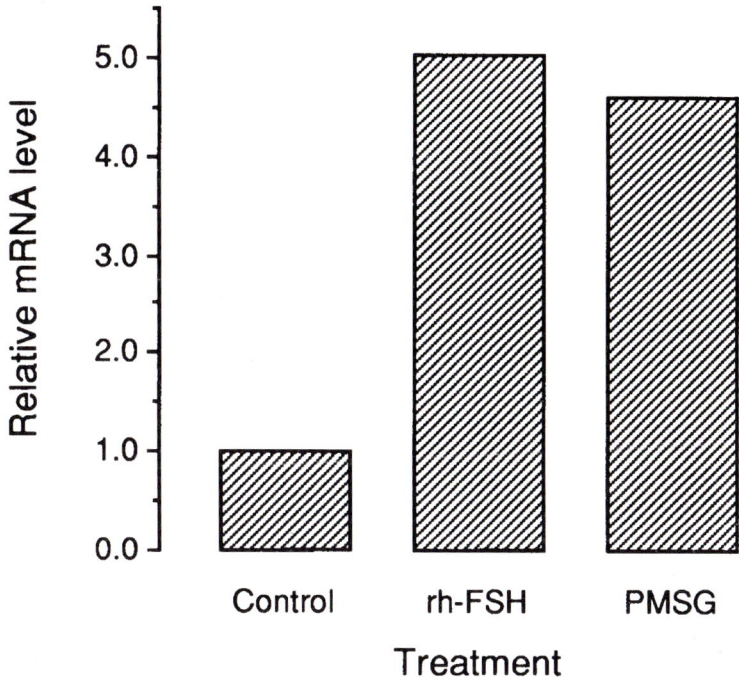

FIG. 1. Stimulation of ovarian cytochrome P450c17 mRNA expression by recombinant human FSH. 25-Day old immature female Wistar rats received four 12-hourly subcutaneous injections of recombinant human FSH (total dose 72 IU) (FSH); the negative control (C) was animals receiving injection vehicle; the positive control was animals receiving a single injection (15 IU) of pregnant mares' serum gonadotrophin (PMSG). Ovaries were removed 48 h after the first FSH injection. Total ovarian RNA was size-fractionated (25 µg/track) by electrophoresis on a 1.5% agarose-formaldehyde gel and blotted on to a nylon membrane. Northern analysis was carried out using a ^{32}P-labelled (random priming) bovine cytochrome P450c17 cDNA generously donated by Dr. Ian Mason. Exposure of the autoradiogram to Kodak XAR-5 film was overnight at -70°C using an intensifying screen. The relative abundance of the ~2.0 kb-sized cytochrome P450c17 transcript was determined by video densitometry. (Smyth, C.D. et al., in preparation.)

CONCLUDING REMARKS

Cytochrome P450c17 is expressed mainly in thecal cells and those ovarian cell-types derived from the theca interna such as thecal/interstitial or theca-lutein cells, and thecal cells do not express FSH receptors. We therefore interpret these data as direct evidence that FSH activates granulosa→theca signalling in the ovary. A previous study from this laboratory demonstrated that androgen synthesis by thecal interstitial cells isolated from animals treated with 'pure' FSH showed increased responsiveness to LH *in vitro* (6). The present finding that treatment with pure FSH directly stimulates P450c17 mRNA expression provides further evidence that one or more factors produced by FSH stimulated granulosa cells is likely to function as a paracrine modulator of androgen synthesis in the ovary. Further research is required to determine which granulosa-derived factor(s) mediates this action of FSH.

ACKNOWLEDGEMENTS

Supported by the MRC and Serono Laboratories UK Ltd. We thank Dr Ian Mason (Cecil H. and Ida Green Center for Reproductive Biology Sciences, University of Texas Soutwestern Medical Center, 5323 Harry Hines Boulevard, Dallas, Texas 75235, USA) for providing the P450c17 cDNA used in this work.

REFERENCES

1. Armstrong, D.T. and Dorrington, J.H. (1979) Estrogen biosynthesis in the ovaries and testes. In: Regulatory Mechanisms Affecting Gonadal Hormone Action, Vol. 2, edited by Thomas, J.A., Singhal, R.L., pp 217-258. University Park Press, Baltimore.
2. Franchimont, P. (1986) Foreword. Bailleré's Clinical Endocrinology, 15: ix-xiii.
3. Hillier, S.G. (1991) Cellular basis of follicular endocrine function. In: Ovarian Endocrinology, edited by Hillier, S.G., pp 73-106. Blackwell Scientific Publications, Oxford.
4. Hsueh, A.J.W., Adashi, E.Y., Jones, P.B.C. and Welsh, T.J. Jr. (1984) Hormonal regulation of the differentiation of cultured granulosa cells. Endocr. Rev., 5:76-126.
5. Richards, J.S., Jahnsen, T., Hedin, L., Lifka, J., Ratoosh, S.L., Durica, J.M. and Goldring, N.B. (1987) Ovarian follicular development: from physiology to molecular biology. Recent Prog. Horm. Res., 43:231-270.
6. Smyth, C.D., Mirø, F., Howles, C.M. and Hillier, S.G. (1992) Modulation by inhibin and insulin-like growth factor I (IGF-I) of LH-responsive androgen synthesis in rat ovarian theca/interstitial cell cultures. J. Endocrinol., 132 (supplement): abstract no. 46.
7. Tonetta, S.T. and DiZerega, G.S. (1989) Intragonadal regulation of follicular maturation. Endocr. Rev. 10:205-229.
8. Van Noorden, S. and Polak, J.M. (1979) Hormones of the alimentary tract. In: Hormones and Evolution, Vol. 2, edited by Barrington, E.J.W., pp 791-828. Academic Press, London.

Development-related Gene Expression in Granulosa Cells

J.S. Richards, J.W. Clemens, S.L. Fitzpatrick and J. Sirois

*Department of Cell Biology, Baylor College of Medicine,
One Baylor Plaza, Houston, Texas 77030, USA*

The LH/FSH surge is the physiological trigger which stimulates ovulation and luteinization of preovulatory follicles. Ovulation brings about structural reorganization and remodelling of the follicle (7). Luteinization establishes structural and functional changes within granulosa and theca cells, most notable of which are the cessation of cell division, cellular hypertrophy and the marked accumulation of lipid droplets. Specific biochemical changes associated with ovulation are the rapid but transient increase in a novel, distinct isoform of prostaglandin endoperoxide synthase, PGS-2 (17,-26,44,45,50-53), tissue plasminogen activator, tPA (1,2,11) and progesterone receptor, PR (21,32). Luteinization is characterized by the marked and sustained induction of P450scc as well as the dramatic and rapid decreases in mRNA for LH-R, RIIβ, aromatase and $P450_{17\alpha}$ (Fig. 1; 37). Once

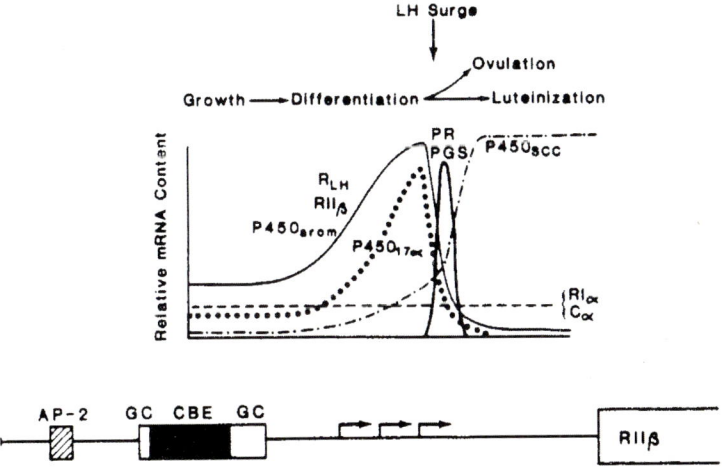

luteinization has occurred, genes regulated by FSH/LH/cAMP in the follicle are no longer regulated by these agonists in the corpus luteum. This apparent transition from cAMP-dependent regulation to cAMP-independent regulation of these genes has prompted us to ask the following questions.

1. Do genes regulated by the FSH/LH-cAMP-A-kinase pathway in the follicle respond to other signalling pathways in the corpus luteum?

2. Do low and high concentrations of gonadotropins (cAMP) regulate gene expression by the same signalling pathways and transcription factors or by different mechanisms?

3. Are the pathway(s) and transcription factors which mediate ovulation in response to high LH the same as those which stimulate the cellular processes of luteinization?

4. If pathways other than cAMP-A-kinase are involved in dictating ovulation and luteinization, what are they (C-kinases, tyrosine kinases) in what cells are they activated and what agonists are involved?

Evidence that cAMP plays a leading role in mediating the effects of low and ovulatory concentrations of gonadotropins in ovarian cell differentiation is well-documented and hard to dispute (36,38). Hormone binding to cell surface receptors (36,42) activates adenylyl cyclase (20,23) leading to the production of cAMP. Low levels of hormone stimulate increases in cAMP whereas ovulatory doses of hormone stimulate elevated production of the nucleotide. Forskolin directly activates the catalytic subunit of adenylyl cyclase and has been used successfully to mimic many (all?) of the effects of FSH and LH observed in granulosa cell cultures. For example, when granulosa cells obtained from small antral follicles are cultured in the presence of steroid (testosterone/estradiol) and either forskolin or FSH, they acquire a phenotype indistinguishable from that observed in granulosa cells of preovulatory follicles: e.g. elevated levels of aromatase, LH-R and RIIβ (8,38,42). Furthermore, if these differentiated granulosa cells are then exposed to ovulatory concentrations of FSH or LH or high levels of forskolin, changes in gene expression mimic those observed *in vivo* as a consequence of the LH/FSH surge: induction of PGS-2 (44,45,51,52), P450scc (30,31), α_2-macroglobulin (10) and suppression of aromatase, LH-R and RIIβ (8,38,42).

Despite the exhaustive litany supporting a primary role of cAMP mediating granulosa cell differentiation, there is also evidence that other pathways may be utilized. For example, gonadotropin receptors have been shown to be directly coupled to the phospholipase $C/Ca^{++}/C$-kinase pathway (5,14). Thus, the differential effects of basal versus ovulatory levels of gonadotropins cannot be associated unequivocally with activation of either (or both) pathways. Furthermore, the promoters of genes expressed in granulosa cells in response to hormones exhibit markedly different structural features. Some of the genes (aromatase, P450scc) contain TATA- and CAAT-box motifs and initiate transcription at a single site (9,18,31,34,35). Other genes (PGS-2, RIIβ, LH-R and activin βB) lack TATA- and CAAT-box motifs and initiate transcription at multiple sites (26-28,46-49). Thus, although changes in mRNA for aromatase, RIIβ and LH-R exhibit similar temporal changes in response to FSH and forskolin, the structure of their promoters differs markedly. Furthermore, none of these genes contains a consensus cAMP regulatory element (CRE : TGACGTCA) to which the well-characterized CREB protein, as well as members of the CREB family (DCREB ATFs, C/EBP, CREMs) bind (15,40). Promoters such as aromatase and P450scc contain an (CC)AGGTCA motif which appears to confer hormone/tissue specific inducibility in gonadal (aromatase and P450scc) cells (3,9) and adrenal (P450scc) cells (34,35) yet the pattern of expression of these two genes in granulosa cells is markedly different. As noted, aromatase is induced by low but increasing levels of hormone and is turned off by the ovulatory hormone surge (8) whereas P450scc is only increased marginally in granulosa cells of preovulatory follicles and appears to require the LH surge for maximal induction and subsequent constitutive maintenance (12,30,31). Thus, if the AGGTCA motif and surrounding contextual sequences are involved in regulating the expression of each of these genes, one would predict that multiple factors are capable of binding this sequence and/or transcription is regulated by differential modification (phosphorylation) of a limited number of factors. Genes, such as RIIβ (27), LH-R (24,48,49), PR (22) and activin βB (28) have promoters that are highly GC rich, whereas the promoter for the novel, distinct isoform of PGS (PGS-2) not only lacks the TATA-CAAT motifs but also lacks GC rich domains (46; preliminary data). Yet the pattern of expression of PGS-2 (17,44,45,50-51) and PR (21,29,32) are highly similar. Taken together these observations suggest that sequences unique to genes turned on and transiently expressed (PGS, PR) in response to the LH surge must be different from genes turned off by the LH surge (aromatase LH-R, RIIβ) or those turned on constitutively P450scc (37). These different patterns suggest that these genes are not only expressed in a cell-specific manner in the ovary but appear to be regulated by different *cis*-acting DNA motifs which recognize specific *trans*-acting factors. Thus, these DNA: protein regulatory units which do not appear to involve CRE/CREB need to be identified. Furthermore, the intracellular pathways leading to their activation/suppression need to be defined.

Evidence that pathways other than, or in addition to, the cAMP/A-kinase pathway are involved in gonadotropin action is indirect but based on the foregoing discussion requires special attention. First, it is known that GnRH (16,33) as well as FSH and LH (36,38) bind to ligand specific receptors in rat granulosa cells and can induce ovulation (6,25) and meiosis (13) *in vitro*. Second, GnRH, like FSH and LH at ovulatory concentrations can induce the expression of enzymes presumed to play key roles in ovulation; namely, PGS-2 (17,44,45,50-52) and tPA (1,2,11). Third, GnRH induces these enzymes (mRNA and protein) without stimulating marked increases in cAMP or progesterone (52), thus, suggesting that GnRH activates (shares) some, but not all, of the same pathways as elevated gonadotropins. Substantial evidence has accumulated to suggest that GnRH acts on pituitary gonadotropes primarily by increasing intracellular Ca^{++} and protein kinase C. However, the restriction of GnRH action to the C-kinase pathway has been challenged (4). Some of the inconsistencies in documenting an unequivocal role for C-kinase results from several factors. The GnRH receptor(s) has (have) not yet been cloned. Furthermore, there are multiple forms of C-kinase, with varying requirements for Ca^{++} and diacyl glycerol (DAG) as well as selective activation responses to phorbol esters. For example, phorbol myristate acid (PMA) will activate C-kinase a but not C-kinase bII whereas bryostatin will selectively activate C-kinase βII (19). Thus, use of PMA as the sole indicator of C-kinase activity in cells does not necessarily mimic the complexity of the C-kinase signalling pathway and specific cellular responses to this pathway. Attempts to mimic the effects of GnRH on preovulatory follicles by substituting PMA or bryostatin have not been successful (52). Induction of PGS-2 was not observed in the presence of increasing doses of either C-kinase activator. Nor did PMA/bryostatin cause the small increases in cAMP and progesterone observed when preovulatory follicles were incubated with GnRH. Thus, any explanation of the effects of GnRH in ovarian function suffer from these same problems as mentioned above. In addition, it is not known if the GnRH receptor in the ovary is the same as, or different from, that in the pituitary, despite similar binding affinities. Splice variants of receptors are common (41,47,48) and provide receptors with different intracellular, cytoplasmic domains such as exhibited by the PRL receptor (43,54). Lastly, there is no solid evidence yet for an ovarian GnRH-like peptide which might be involved in the ovulatory process. Nonetheless, use of GnRH in the foregoing studies has provided an analytic way to compare and dissect what may be multiple pathways involved in cAMP action in the preovulatory follicle.

In addition to GnRH, epidermal growth factor (EGF), acting via the EGF receptor-associated tyrosine kinase, also induces PGS-2 (52) and tPA (11), albeit less effectively. That tyrosine kinases might be involved in mediating some of the actions of ovulatory doses of FSH/LH or GnRH have been supported by experiments using tyrphostins such as genistein (an ATP binding inhibitor) and AG18 (a substrate binding inhibitor) of tyrosine kinases (52). Specifically, both of these tyrphostins block induction of PGS-2 by LH, FSH, forskolin, GnRH and EGF (52; preliminary results). Additionally, the induction of the chicken homologue of PGS-2 (CEF-147; 53) has been observed in chicken embryo fibroblasts transformed by the Rous sarcoma virus thus implicating the tyrosine kinase $pp60^{v-src}$ as a potential regulator of this enzyme. Thus, one possible way to link the cAMP/A-kinase pathway with a tyrosine-kinase pathway in granulosa cells is to suggest that cAMP (at elevated concentrations) leads to the phosphorylation and activation of pp60$^{c\text{-}src}$. It is known that cAMP/A-kinase can activate pp60$^{c\text{-}src}$ in other systems (39).

REFERENCES

1. Beers, W.H., Strickland, S. and Reich, E. (1975) Ovarian plasminogen activator: relationship to ovulation and hormonal regulation. Cell, 6:387.
2. Canipari, R., O'Connell, M.L., Meyer, G. and Strickland, S. (1987) Mouse ovarian granulosa cells produce urokinase-type plasminogen activator, whereas the corresponding rat cells produce tissue-type plasminogen activator. J. Cell Biol., 105:977-981.
3. Clemens, J.W. and Richards, J.S. (in preparation).
4. Conn, P.M. (1989) Does protein kinase C mediate pituitary actions of gonadotropin-releasing hormone? Mol. Endocrinol., 3:755-757.
5. Davis, J.S., Weakland, L., Farese, R. and West, L. (1987) Luteinizing hormone increases inositol triphosphate and cytosolic free Ca^{++} in isolated bovine luteal cells. J. Biol. Chem., 262:8515-8521.
6. Ekholm, C., Hillensjo, T. and Isaksson, O. (1981) Gonadotropin-releasing hormone agonists stimulate oocyte meiosis and ovulation in hypophysectomized rats. Endocrinology, 108:2022-2024.
7. Espey, L.L. (1980) Ovulation as an inflammatory reaction - a hypothesis. Biol. Reprod., 22:73-106.
8. Fitzpatrick, S.L. and Richards, J.S. (1991) Regulation of cytochrome P450 aromatase mRNA and activity by steroids and gonadotropins in rat granulosa cells. Endocrinology, 129:1452-1462.
9. Fitzpatrick, S.L. and Richards, J.S. Characterization of the aromatase promoter (in preparation).
10. Gaddy-Kurten, D. and Richards, J.S. (1991) Regulation of α_2-macroglobulin by luteinizing hormone and prolactin during cell differentiation in the rat ovary. Mol. Endocrinol., 5:1280-1291.
11. Galway, A.B., Oikawa, M., Ny, T. and Hsueh, A.J.W. (1989) Epidermal growth factor induction stimulates tissue plasminogen activator activity and messenger RNA levels in cultured rat granulosa cells: mediation by pathways independent of protein kinase-A and -C. Endocrinology, 125:126-135.
12. Goldring, N.B., Durica, J.M., Lifka, J., Hedin, L., Ratoosh, S.L., Miller, W.L., Orly, J. and Richards, J.S. (1987) Hormonal regulation of cholesterol side-chain cleavage P450 messenger RNA in rat ovarian follicles and constitutive expression in corpora lutea. Endocrinology, 120:1942-1950.
13. Goren, S., Oron, Y. and Dekel, N. (1991) GnRH-induced maturation of rat oocytes: a calcium-dependent process. In: Growth Factors and Fertility Regulation edited by Haseltine, F.P., Findlay, J.K., pp 13-22. Cambridge University Press, Cambridge.
14. Gudermann, T., Birnbaumer, M. Birnbaumer, L. (1992) Evidence for dual coupling of the murine luteinizing hormone receptor to adenylyl cyclase and phosphoinositide breakdown and Ca^{++} mobilization. J. Biol. Chem., 267:4479-4488
15. Habener, J.F. (1990) Cyclic AMP response element binding proteins: a cornucopia of transcription factors. Mol. Endocrinol., 4:1087-1094.
16. Harwood, J.P., Clayton, R.N., Chen, T.C., Knox, G. and Catt, K.J. (1980) Ovarian gonadotropin-releasing hormone receptors. II. Regulation and effects on ovarian development. Endocrinology, 107:414-421.
17. Hedin, L., Gaddy-Kurten, D., Kurten, R. and Richards, J.S. (1987) Prostaglandin endoperoxide synthase in rat ovarian follicles: content, cellular distribution, and evidence for hormonal induction preceding ovulation. Endocrinology, 121:722-731.
18. Hickey, G.J., Krasnow, J.S., Beattie, W.G.,and Richards, J.S. (1990) Aromatase cytochrome P450 in rat ovarian granulosa cells before and after luteinization: cAMP-dependent and independent regulation, cloning and sequencing of rat aromatase cDNA and 5' genomic DNA. Mol. Endocrinol., 4:3-12.
19. Hocevar, B.A. and Fields, A.P. (1991) Selective translocation of bII-protein kinase C to the nucleus of human promyelocytic (HL60) leukemia cells. J. Biol. Chem., 266:28-33.

20. Hunzicker-Dunn, M. and Birnbaumer, L. (1976) Adenylyl cyclase activities in ovarian tissues. III. Regulation of responsiveness to LH, FSH and PGE_1 in prepubertal, cycling, pregnant and pseudopregnant rats. Endocrinology, 99:198-234.
21. Iwai, M., Yasuda, K., Fukuoka, M., Iwai, T., Takakura, K., Taii, S., Nakanishii, S. and Mori, T. (1991) Luteinizing hormone induces progesterone receptor gene expression in cultured porcine granulosa cells. Endocrinology, 129:1621-1627.
22. Jeltsch, J., Turcotte, B., Garnier, J., LeRouge, T., Krozowski, Z., Gronemeyer, H. and Chambon, P. (1990) Characterization of multiple mRNAs originating from the chicken progesterone receptor gene. J. Biol. Chem., 265:3967-3974.
23. Jonassen, J.A., Bose, K. and Richards, J.S. (1982) Enhancement and desensitization of hormone-responsive adenylyl cyclase in granulosa cells of preantral and antral ovarian follicles: effects of estradiol and FSH. Endocrinology, 111:74-79.
24. Koo, Y., Ji, I., Slaughter, R.G. and Ji, T.H. (1991) Structure of the luteinizing hormone receptor gene and multiple exons of the coding sequence. Endocrinology, 128:2297-2308.
25. Koos, R.D. and LeMaire, W.J. (1985) The effects of a gonadotropin-releasing hormone agonist on ovulation and steroidogenesis during perfusion of rabbit and rat ovaries *in vitro*. Endocrinology, 116:628-632.
26. Kujubu, D., Fletcher, B., Varnam, B., Lim, R. and Hershmann, H. (1991) TIS 10, a phorbol ester tumor promoter-inducible mRNA from Swiss 3T3 cells, encodes a novel prostaglandin synthase/cyclo-oxygenase homologue. J. Biol. Chem., 266:12866-12872.
27. Kurten, R.C., Levy, L., Shey, J., Durica, J. and Richards, J.S. (1992) Identification and characterization of the GC-rich and cAMP-inducible promoter of the type IIb cAMP-dependent protein kinase regulatory subunit gene. Mol. Endocrinol., 6:536-550.
28. Mason, A.J., Berkemeier, L.M., Schmelzer, C.H. and Schwall, R.H. (1989) Activin B: precursor sequences, genomic structures and *in vitro* activities. Mol. Endocrinol., 3:1352-1358.
29. Natraj, U. and Richards, J.S. Hormonal regulation of the progesterone receptor in cultured granulosa cells. (in preparation).
30. Oonk, R.B., Krasnow, J.S., Beattie, W.G. and Richards, J.S. (1989) Cyclic AMP-dependent and -independent regulation of cholesterol side-chain cleavage cytochrome P450 (P450scc) in rat ovarian granulosa cells and corpora lutea. J. Biol. Chem., 264:21934-21942.
31. Oonk, R.B., Parker, K.L., Gibson, J.L. and Richards, J.S. (1990) Rat cholesterol side-chain cleavage cytochrome P450 (P450scc) gene. Structure and regulation by cAMP *in vitro*. J. Biol. Chem., 265:22392-22401.
32. Park, O.-K. and Mayo, K.E. (1991) Transient expression of progesterone receptor messenger RNA in ovarian granulosa cells after the preovulatory luteinizing hormone surge. Mol. Endocrinol., 5:967-978.
33. Pieper, D., Richards, J.S. and Marshall, J. (1981) Ovarian gonadotropin-releasing hormone (GnRH) receptors: characterization, distribution and induction by GnRH. Endocrinology, 108:1144-1155.
34. Rice, D.A., Mouw, A.R., Bogerd, A.M. and Parker, K.L. (1991) A shared promoter element regulates the expression of three steroidogenic enzymes. Mol. Endocrinol., 5:1552-1561.
35. Rice, D.A., Kirkman, M.S., Aitken, L.D., Mouw, A.R., Schimmer, B.P. and Parker, K.L. (1990) Analysis of the promoter region of the gene encoding mouse cholesterol side-chain cleavage enzyme. J. Biol. Chem., 265:11713-11720.
36. Richards, J.S. (1980) Maturation of ovarian follicles: actions and interactions of pituitary hormones on follicular cell differentiation. Physiol. Rev., 60:51-89.
37. Richards, J.S., Clemens, J.W., Sirois, J., Fitzpatrick, S.L., Wong, W.Y.L. and Kurten, R.C.(1991) Hormonal control of gene expression during ovarian cell differentiation. Serono Symposia USA: Molecular Basis of Reproductive Endocrinology, Vancouver, BC, July (in press).
38. Richards, J.S., Jahnsen, T., Hedin, L., Lifka, J., Ratoosh, S.L., Durica, J.M. and Goldring, N.B. (1987) Ovarian follicular development: from physiology to molecular biology. Recent Prog. Horm. Res., 43:231-276.
39. Roach, P. (1991) Multisite and hierarchal protein phosphorylation. J. Biol. Chem., 266:14139-14142.
40. Roesler, W.J., Vandenbark, G.R. and Hanson, R.W. (1988) Cyclic AMP and the induction of eukaryotic gene expression. J. Biol. Chem., 263:9063-9066.
41. Segaloff, D.L., Sprengel, R., Nikolics, K. and Ascoli, M. (1990) The structure of the lutropin/chorionic gonadotropin receptor. Recent. Prog. Horm. Res., 46:261-303.
42. Segaloff, D.L., Wang, H. and Richards, J.S. (1990) Hormonal regulation of luteinizing

hormone/chorionic gonadotropin receptor mRNA in rat ovarian cells during follicular development and luteinization. Mol. Endocrinol., 4:1856-1865.
43. Shirota, M., Banville, D., Ali, S., Jolicoeur, C., Boutin, J.-M., Edery, M., Djiane, J. and Kelly, P.A. (1990) Expression of two forms of prolactin receptor in rat ovary and liver. Mol. Endocrinol., 4:1136-1143.
44. Sirois, J. and Richards, J.S. (1991) Identification and characterization of a novel distinct isoform of prostaglandin endoperoxide synthase. J. Biol. Chem., 267:6382-6388.
45. Sirois, J., Simmons, D.L. and Richards, J.S. (1992) Hormonal regulation of messenger ribonucleic acid encoding a novel isoform of prostaglandin endoperoxide H synthase in rat preovulatory follicles. J. Biol. Chem., 267:11586-11592.
46. Sirois, J. and Richards, J.S. Characterization of the rat PGS-2 gene and its promoter. (in preparation).
47. Sprengel, R., Braun, T., Nikolics, K., Segaloff, D.L. and Seeburg, P.H. (1990) The testicular receptor for follicle stimulating hormone: structure and functional expression of the cloned cDNA. Mol. Endocrinol., 4:525-530.
48. Tsai-Morris, C., Buck, O.E., Wang, W., Xie, X. and Dufau, M. (1991) Structural organization of the rat luteinizing hormone (LH) receptor gene. J. Biol. Chem., 266:11355-11359.
49. Wang, H., Nelson, S., Ascoli, M. Segaloff, D.L. (1992) The 5' flanking region of the rat lutropin/chorionic gonadotropin receptor gene confers Leydig cell expression and negative regulation of gene transcription by cAMP. Mol. Endocrinol., 6:320-326.
50. Wong, W.Y.L., DeWitt, D.L., Smith, W.L. and Richards, J.S. (1989) Rapid induction of prostaglandin endoperoxide synthase in rat preovulatory follicles by luteinizing hormone and cAMP is blocked by inhibitors of transcription and translation. Mol. Endocrinol., 3:1714-1723.
51. Wong, W.Y.L. and Richards, J.S. (1991) Evidence for two antigenically distinct, molecular weight variants of prostaglandin H synthase in the rat ovary. Mol. Endocrinol., 5:1269-1279.
52. Wong, W.Y.L. and Richards, J.S. (1992) Induction of prostaglandin H synthase in rat preovulatory follicles by gonadotropin-releasing hormone. Endocrinology, 130:3512-3521.
53. Xie, W., Chapman, J.G., Robertson, D.L., Erickson, R.L. and Simmons, D.L. (1991) Expression of a mitogen-responsive gene encoding prostaglandin synthase is regulated by mRNA splicing. Proc. Natl. Acad. Sci. USA, 88:2692-2696.
54. Zhang, R., Bucko, E., Tsai-Morris, C.-H., Hu, Z.-Z. and Dufau, M.L. (1990) Isolation and characterization of two novel rat ovarian lactogen receptor cDNA species. Biochem. Biophys. Res. Commun., 168:415-422.

Apoptosis as the Basis of Ovarian Follicular Atresia

J.L. Tilly and A.J.W. Hsueh

Division of Reproductive Biology, Department of GYN/OB
Stanford University School of Medicine
Stanford, CA 94305-5317, USA

INTRODUCTION

It is well-established that the vast majority of follicles present in the ovary at birth are destined to degenerate during life. For instance, less than 400 of the more than 400,000 follicles present in the pubertal human ovary will actually ovulate whereas the remaining follicles (>99%) are irrevocably committed to undergo atresia. Despite its critical role during the recruitment of follicles for ovulation, the mechanisms underlying the onset and progression of atresia remain poorly understood (41,24). Although evaluation of the cellular and molecular events associated with follicular degeneration have been limited, previous reports have demonstrated that several morphological features associated with atresia resemble those observed during apoptosis or 'programmed cell death' (52,1). As a basis for elucidating the possible role of apoptosis in ovarian follicular atresia, the characteristic features of apoptosis will be discussed relative to our current understanding of follicular degeneration.

FOLLICULAR ATRESIA: MORPHOLOGY AND HORMONAL CORRELATES

Morphology. In general, follicles in advanced stages of atresia can be identified by several histological features, including detachment of the granulosa cell layer from the basement membrane (30), fragmentation of the basal lamina (3), and the presence of pyknotic nuclei within degenerating granulosa cells (21,26,8). These characteristics would suggest that atresia is temporally correlated with granulosa cell death, although a large number of granulosa cells found in follicles in the early stages of atresia appear to be morphologically normal (24). A reduction of DNA turnover within granulosa cells of atretic follicles has also been reported (17,24), although other studies have indicated that follicles in the early stages of atresia paradoxically incorporate more [^{3}H]-thymidine than healthy follicles (7). It has been postulated that the increased labeling of DNA during this period results from a re-utilization of DNA fragments released by granulosa cells undergoing nuclear condensation.

The fate of the theca layer during atresia has not been clearly established although species-specific differences have been reported. In the ovine ovary, theca cells derived from atretic follicles undergo nuclear condensation and degeneration similar to that observed for granulosa cells, albeit this process appears to be restricted to the more advanced stages of atresia (38). In contrast, theca cells of hamster follicles do not exhibit marked morphological changes in spite of sharply reduced follicular vascularity and total collapse of the granulosa layer (28,17), whereas human and rat theca cells undergo extensive hypertrophy during follicle atresia (5,15). In those instances where hypertrophy of the theca layer is observed, it is believed that these theca cells may form steroidogenically-active secondary interstitial cells in the stromal area (15). Regardless of species differences, however, it is generally accepted that the earlier stages of follicular demise are correlated with disorganization and degeneration of granulosa cells.

Ovarian Steroids. It is known that steroids normally present in the ovary can modulate follicular gonadotropin responsiveness (16,39) as well as affect the number of atretic follicles present in the ovary (19,32). Thus, changes in serum and follicular fluid steroid levels during follicle growth and degeneration have been extensively studied to establish the role, if any, of ovarian steroids in the onset and progression of atresia. In all species examined, atresia is highly correlated with increased progesterone production concomitant with a decline in estrogen synthesis (48,45,12,37,34). However, the basis for this shift in the progesterone-to-estrogen ratio appears to be species-specific and has been attributed to both a decrease in C17,20-lyase activity leading to a loss of substrate for granulosa cell aromatization (rat: 48; hamster: 44) as well as a loss of aromatase activity (sheep: 12, 47; pig: 34). Thus, decreased estrogen production in some species may result in a concomitant accumulation of androgens in the follicular fluid, suggesting a possible role for androgens in the progression of the atresia process. Several studies have reported that non-aromatizable androgens (e.g. 5α-dihydrotestosterone, DHT) not only inhibit aromatase activity (23) and stimulate progesterone production (43) in granulosa cells, but also induce preantral and antral rat follicles to undergo atresia (32,54,2). Considering the dependence of antral follicle development on estrogens (39, 40), and the relatively high levels of DHT reportedly present in follicular fluid of atretic follicles (36), changes in follicular steroid levels are likely involved in the progression of atresia, although their role in the onset of follicle degeneration remains unclear.

Gonadotropins and Their Receptors. Follicular atresia can be identified in essentially all stages of the reproductive cycle (4,9), including the prepubertal human infant ovary (5). Thus, the general process of atresia does not appear to be temporally related to marked changes in serum levels of pituitary gonadotropins, although a decrease in FSH and LH binding to ovarian cells in more advanced stages of atresia has been documented (11, 48,6). It has been suggested that 'rescue' of degenerating follicles can be achieved by administration of exogenous gonadotropins (22,6), although the viability and functional capacity of granulosa cells in 'rescued' follicles may be suspect (24). In any case, it has been postulated that changes in gonadotropin responsiveness of granulosa and theca cells are most likely secondary, but not primary, causes of follicle degeneration (11).

APOPTOSIS VERSUS NECROSIS

Based on morphological and biochemical differences, there are essentially two pathways by which cells die: necrosis and apoptosis (50, 51) (Table 1). In general, tissue necrosis is a consequence of cell injury or other traumatization characterized by a haphazard loss of cell structure, swelling and ultimately cell rupture that can damage adjacent cells, leading to immune cell infiltration. In contrast, apoptosis is an active orderly process which affects scattered single cells undergoing developmental changes or responding to alterations in physiological stimuli. The stepwise or 'programmed' process of cell death by apoptosis involves cell shrinkage, chromatin condensation and the formation of small spherical bits of membrane, referred to as apoptotic bodies, which contain the nuclear fragments and are usually phagocytized by neighboring cells. The most striking feature of apoptosis is the activation of calcium/magnesium-

Table 1. *Cellular and molecular parameters which distinguish apoptosis from necrosis*[1]

Apoptosis	Necrosis
Affects scattered individual cells	Affects tracts of contiguous cells.
Chromatin and cytoplasmic condensation, cell shrinkage	Cell swelling and rupture of plasma membrane.
May require mRNA and protein synthesis	Not dependent upon new mRNA or protein synthesis
Normal ATP level.	Decreased ATP level
Endonuclease activation and internucleosomal DNA cleavage (ladder pattern).	Activation of nonspecific DNases with generalized DNA breakdown (smearing).

[1] For review, see Arends *et al.*, 1990 (1); Wyllie *et al.*, 1980 (52); Wyllie, 1981 (51).

dependent endonuclease activity which specifically cleaves cellular DNA between regularly-spaced nucleosomal units. The end result is the generation of DNA fragments in size multiples of 185-200 basepair which can be visualized as a distinct ladder of DNA bands following agarose gel electrophoresis and ethidium bromide staining (50,1). This characteristic feature, which is the hallmark of cells undergoing apoptosis, is markedly different than the haphazard breakdown of DNA which occurs during necrosis that produces a generalized smear of DNA following analysis by ethidium bromide staining.

HORMONAL CONTROL OF APOPTOSIS

The factors which trigger apoptosis appear to be tissue-specific, although it is believed that different cell types may follow a series of diverse early steps that ultimately lead to a common pathway which locks all cells into the irrevocable progression of apoptotic cell death (Table 2). Exerting either suppressive or stimulatory actions, steroid hormones regulate apoptosis in several systems including the thymus gland (glucocorticoids: 50,14), prostate (androgens: 42,31) and mammary gland (estrogens: 13), apparently acting through their specific receptors (17). Recent studies have also ascribed a predominant role for diverse 'growth factors' in the control of apoptosis during embryogenesis (20), hematopoietic stem cell development (49), B-cell selection (27) and neuronal cell survival (33). In each case, the removal of growth factor from the culture triggers a rapid and irreversible progression of apoptotic cell death.

The mechanisms by which hormonal factors regulate apoptosis are not well-understood, although apoptosis can be rapidly initiated by pharma-

Table 2. *Hormonal regulation of apoptosis in various tissues*[1]

Hormone	Effect	Target	Reference
Glucocorticoids	↑	Thymus	Willie, 1980 (50)
Androgens	↓	Prostate	Sanford et al., 1984 (42)
Estrogens	↓	Mammary	Cho-Chung, 1978 (13)
EGF	↓	Palate	Hassell and Pratt, 1978 (20)
NGF	↓	Neurons	Marti et al., 1988 (33)
CSF's	↓	Stem Cells	Williams et al., 1990 (49)
Bcl-2 (27)	↓	B-cells	Hockenberry et al., 1990
ACTH	↓	Adrenal	Wyllie et al., 1973 (53)

[1] Abbreviations used are: EGF, epidermal growth factor; NGF, nerve growth factor; CSF's.

cological elevation of intracellular calcium levels (35,10) and blocked by protein kinase C activation (35). Furthermore, there is indirect evidence that the progression of apoptosis in some systems (33) but not others (18) is dependent upon the synthesis of new messenger RNA and/or protein.

APOPTOSIS DURING FOLLICULAR ATRESIA

Progress towards understanding the mechanisms underlying atresia has been hindered by the heterogeneity of follicles present in the ovary at any given time, as well as the limited numbers of cells present in individual follicles which limit in-depth biochemical analysis. Furthermore, establishment of a correlation between follicular atresia and apoptosis has proved difficult because of the large amounts of tissue required to conduct ethidium bromide staining analysis for the presence of internucleosomal DNA fragmentation, the hallmark feature of apoptosis.

Several investigators have previously suggested a role for apoptosis in the degeneration of follicles during atresia based on histological evaluation (7,38), although direct biochemical evidence for the presence of apoptotic endonuclease activity or the characteristic DNA fragmentation in ovarian cells was not demonstrated until recently. Using gonadotropin-primed immature rats, the existence of calcium- and magnesium-dependent endonuclease activity was identified in nuclei isolated from ovarian granulosa and luteal cells (55), although its relationship to follicle atresia was not addressed.

To begin analysis of the role of apoptosis in follicle degeneration, we established a sensitive autoradiographic method for the detection of apoptotic DNA fragments. This technique possesses 100- to 1000-fold greater sensitivity over that obtained with ethidium bromide staining (46). Using this procedure, we demonstrated a correlation between apoptosis and follicular atresia in individual avian and porcine follicles (46). Because these experimental models allow accurate morphological identification of healthy versus atretic follicles of the same developmental state, we were able to provide firm evidence indicating that apoptosis is essentially restricted to only those follicles identified as degenerative (Fig. 1). Furthermore, internucleosomal DNA fragmentation was observed in both the granulosa and theca layers of atretic follicles in these species, suggesting that apoptosis is not confined to one cell type during follicle degeneration (46).

Our findings of apoptotic DNA fragmentation in ovarian granulosa cells was consistent with a recent report showing a temporal correlation of DNA cleavage with morphological signs of atresia in gonadotropin-primed immature rats (29). However, interpretation of the data were complicated by the finding of DNA fragmentation in cells collected from control animals, which may have resulted from the extremely large numbers of cells needed to generate sufficient amounts of DNA for the ethidium bromide staining

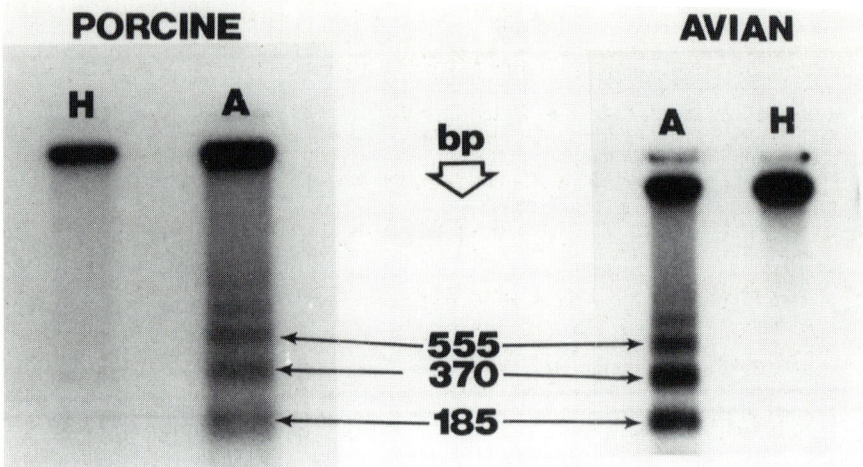

FIG. 1. Autoradiographic identification of internucleosomal DNA cleavage (400 ng/lane) in morphologically healthy (H) or atretic (A) porcine and avian ovarian follicles[1] (see Reference 41).

technique. Additionally, analysis of cells pooled from a heterogenous population of follicles did not permit a direct correlation of apoptosis to individual follicles identified as atretic.

In summary, our findings have provided a basis and as well as a sensitive methodology for studies on the role of apoptosis in the onset of follicular atresia. Additionally, the ability to detect and quantitate radiolabeled apoptotic DNA fragments in limited numbers of cultured cells will enable future analysis of the endocrine and paracrine regulation of apoptosis, and consequently follicle atresia, in the ovary. Results from these studies will provide a greater understanding of the atresia mechanism, and its relationship to the depletion of follicles found during menopause and premature ovarian failure.

ACKNOWLEDGEMENTS

The authors gratefully acknowledge Ms. Kim I. Kowalski for excellent technical assistance. Studies described herein were supported by NIH grant HD-23273 (AJWH). J.L. Tilly is a Postdoctoral Fellow supported by National Research Service Award HD-07556 and the Lalor Foundation.

REFERENCES

1. Arends, M.J., Morris, R.G. and Wyllie, A.H. (1990) Apoptosis: the role of the endonuclease. Am. J. Pathol., 136:593-608.
2. Azzolin, G.C. and Saiduddin, S. (1983) Effect of androgens on the ovarian morphology of the hypophysectomized rat. Proc. Soc. Exp. Biol. Med., 172:70-73.
3. Bagavandoss, P., Midgley Jr., A.R. and Wicha, M. (1983) Developmental changes in the ovarian follicular basal lamina detected by immunofluorescence and electron microscopy. J. Histochem. Cytochem., 31:633-640.
4. Brand, A. and de Jong, W.H.R. (1973) Qualitative and quantitative micromorphological investigations of the tertiary follicle population during the oestrous cycle of the sheep. J. Reprod. Fertil., 33:431-439.
5. Braw, R.H., Byskov, A.G., Peters, H. and Faber, M. (1976) Follicular atresia in the human infant ovary. J. Reprod. Fertil., 46:55-59.
6. Braw, R.H. and Tsafriri, A. (1980) Effect of PMSG on follicular atresia in the immature rat ovary. J. Reprod. Fertil., 59:267- 272.
7. Byskov, A.G.S. (1974) Cell kinetic studies of follicular atresia in the mouse ovary. J. Reprod. Fertil., 37:277-285.
8. Byskov, A.G.S. (1978) Follicular atresia. In: The vertebrate ovary, edited by Jones, R.E., pp 533-562. Plenum Press, New York.
9. Byskov, A.G.S. (1979) Atresia. In: Ovarian follicular development and function, edited by Midgley, A.R. and Sadler, W.A., pp 41-57. Raven Press, New York.
10. Caron-Leslie, L.-A.M., Cidlowski, J.A. (1991) Similar actions of glucocorticoids and calcium on the regulation of apoptosis in S49 cells. Mol. Endocrinol., 5:1169-1179.
11. Carson, R.S., Findlay, J.K., Burger, H.G. and Trounson, A.O. (1979) Gonadotropin receptors of the ovine ovarian follicle during follicular growth and atresia. Biol. Reprod., 21:75-87.
12. Carson, R.S., Findlay, J.K., Clarke, I.J. and Burger, H.G. (1981) Estradiol, testosterone, and androstenedione in ovine follicular fluid during growth and atresia of ovarian follicles. Biol. Reprod., 24:105-113.
13. Cho-Chung, Y.S. (1978) Interaction of cyclic AMP and estrogen in tumor growth control. In: Endocrine control of neoplasia, edited by Sharma, R. and Criss, W.E., pp. 335-346. Raven Press, New York.
14. Compton, M.M. and Cidlowski, J.A. (1986) Rapid in vivo effects of glucocorticoids on the integrity of rat lymphocyte genomic deoxyribonucleic acid. Endocrinology, 118:38-45.
15. Erickson, G.F., Magoffin, D.A., Dyer, C.A. and Hofeditz, C. (1985) The ovarian androgen producing cells: a review of structure/function relationships. Endocrine Rev., 6:371-399.
16. Goldenberg, R.L., Vaitukaitus, J.L. and Ross, G.T. (1972) Estrogen and follicle-stimulating hormone interactions on follicle growth in rats. Endocrinology, 90:1492-1498.
17. Greenwald, G.S. (1989) Temporal and topographic changes in DNA synthesis after induced follicular atresia. Biol. Reprod., 40:175-181.
18. Guillano, P.M., Cho-Chung, Y.S., Losonczy, I. and Grantham, F.H. (1974) Increase in RNA synthesis during mammary tumor regression. Cancer Res., 34:751-757.
19. Harman, S.M., Louvet, J.-P. and Ross, G.T. (1975) Interaction of estrogen and gonadotropins on follicular atresia. Endocrinology, 96:1145-1152.
20. Hassell, J.R. and Pratt, R.M. (1977) Elevated levels of cAMP alters the effect of epidermal growth factor in vitro on programmed cell death in the secondary palatal epithelium. Exp. Cell Res., 106:55-62.
21. Hay, M.F., Cran, D.G. and Moor, R.M. (1976) Structural changes occurring during atresia in sheep ovarian follicles. Cell Tissue Res., 169:515-529.
22. Hay, M.F., Moor, R.M., Cran, D.G. and Dott, H.M. (1979) Regeneration of atretic sheep ovarian follicles in vitro. J. Reprod. Fertil., 55:195-207.
23. Hillier, S.G., van den Boogaard, A.M.J., Reichert Jr., L.E. and van Hall, E.V. (1980) Alterations in granulosa cell aromatase activity accompanying preovulatory follicular development in the rat ovary with evidence that 5α-reduced C_{19} steroids inhibit the aromatase reaction in vitro. J. Endocrinol., 84:409-419.
24. Hirshfield, A.N. (1989) Rescue of atretic follicles in vitro and in vivo. Biol. Reprod., 40:181-190.
25. Hirshfield, A.N. (1991) Development of follicles in the mammalian ovary. Int. Rev. Cytol., 124:43-101.

26. Hirshfield, A.N. and Midgley Jr., A.R. (1978) Morphometric analysis of follicular development in the rat. Biol. Reprod., 19:606-611.
27. Hockenberry, D., Nunez, G., Milliman, C., Schreiber, R.D. and Korsmeyer, S.J. (1990) Bcl-2 is an inner mitochondrial membrane that blocks programmed cell death. Nature, 348:334-338.
28. Hubbard, C.J. and Greenwald, G.S. (1985) Morphological changes in atretic Graafian follicles during induced atresia in the hamster. Anat. Rec., 212:353-357.
29. Hughes Jr, F.M. and Gorospe, W.C. (1991) Biochemical identification of apoptosis (programmed cell death) in granulosa cells: evidence for a potential mechanism underlying follicular atresia. Endocrinology, 129:2415-2422.
30. Junquiera, L.C., Carneiro, J. and Kelly, R.O. (1989) Basic histology, pp 443-444. Appleton and Lange, Norwalk.
31. Kyprianou, N. and Isaacs, J.T. (1988) Activation of programmed cell death in the rat ventral prostate after castration. Endocrinology, 122:552-562.
32. Louvet, J.-P., Harman, S.M., Schreiber, J.R. and Ross, G.T. (1975) Evidence for a role of androgens in follicular maturation. Endocrinology, 97:336-372.
33. Martin, D.P., Schmidt, R.E., DiStefano, P.S., Lowry, O.H., Carter, J.G. and Johnson Jr, E.M. (1988) Inhibitors of protein synthesis and RNA synthesis prevent neuronal cell death caused by nerve growth factor deprivation. J. Cell. Biol., 106:829-844.
34. Mason, W.S., Haney, A.F. and Schomberg, D.W. (1985) Steroidogenesis in porcine atretic follicles: loss of aromatase activity in isolated granulosa and theca. Biol. Reprod., 33:495-501.
35. McConkey, D.J., Hartzell, P., Jondal, M. and Orrenius, S. (1989) Inhibition of DNA fragmentation in thymocytes and isolated thymocyte nuclei by agents that stimulate protein kinase C. J. Biol. Chem., 264:13399-13402.
36. McNatty, K.P. (1980) Regulation of follicle maturation in the human ovary: a role for 5α-reduced androgens. In: Endocrinology, edited by Cumming, I.A., Funder, J.W. and Mendelsohn, F.A.O. Australian Academy of Sciences, Canberra.
37. McNatty, K.P., Lun, S., Heath, D.A., Kieboom, L.E. and Henderson, K.M. (1985) Influence of follicular atresia on LH-induced cAMP and steroid synthesis by bovine thecae interna. Mol. Cell. Endocrinol., 39:209-215.
38. O'Shea, J.D., Hay, M.F. and Cran, D.G. (1978) Ultrastructural changes in the theca interna during follicular atresia in sheep. J. Reprod. Fertil. 54:183-187.
39. Richards, J.S., Ireland, J.J., Rao, M.C., Bernath, G.A., Midgley, A.R. and Reichert Jr., L.E. (1976) Ovarian follicular development in the rat: hormone receptor regulation by estradiol, FSH and LH. Endocrinology, 99:1562-1570.
40. Richards, J.S. and Kersey, K.A. (1979) Changes in theca and granulosa cell function in antral follicles developing during pregnancy in the rat: gonadotropin receptors, cyclic AMP and estradiol-17·. Biol. Reprod., 21:1185-1201.
41. Ryan, R. (1981) Follicular atresia: some speculations of biochemical markers and mechanisms. In: Dynamics of ovarian function, edited by Schwartz, N.B. and Hunzicker-Dunn, M., pp 1-11. Raven Press, New York.
42. Sanford, N.L., Searle, J.W. and Kerr, J.F.R. (1984) Successive waves of apoptosis in the rat prostate after repeated withdrawal of testosterone stimulation. Pathology, 16:406-410.
43. Schomberg, D.W. (1979) Steroid modulation of steroid secretion in vitro: an experimental approach to intra-follicular regulatory mechanisms. In: Ovarian follicular and corpus luteum function, edited by Channing, C.P., Marsh, J.M. and Sadler, W.A., pp 155-168. Plenum Press, New York.
44. Silavin, S.L. and Greenwald, G.S. (1984) Steroid production by isolated theca and granulosa cells after initiation of atresia in the hamster. J. Reprod. Fertil., 71:387-392.
45. Terranova, P.F. (1981) Steroidogenesis in experimentally induced atretic follicles of the hamster: a shift from estradiol to progesterone synthesis. Endocrinology, 108:1855-1890.
46. Tilly, J.L., Kowalski, K.I., Johnson, A.L. and Hsueh, A.J.W. (1991) Involvement of apoptosis in ovarian follicular atresia and postovulatory regression. Endocrinology, 129:2799-2801.
47. Tsonis, C.G., Carson, R.S. and Findlay, J.K. Relationships between aromatase activity, follicular fluid oestradiol-17 and testosterone concentrations, and diameter and atresia of individual ovine follicles. J. Reprod. Fertil., 72:153-163.
48. Uilenbroek, J.T.J., Woutersen, P.J.A. and van der Schoot, P. (1980) Atresia of preovulatory follicles: gonadotropin binding and steroidogenic activity. Biol. Reprod., 23:219-229.
49. Williams, G.T., Smith, C.A., Spooncer, E., Dexter, T.M. and Taylor, D.R. (1990)

Haemopoietic colony stimulating factors promote cell survival by suppressing apoptosis. Nature, 343:76- 79.
50. Wyllie, A.H. (1980) Glucocorticoid-induced thymocyte apoptosis is associated with endogenous endonuclease activation. Nature, 284:555-556.
51. Wyllie, A.H. (1981) Cell death: a new classification separating apoptosis from necrosis. In: Cell death in biology and pathology, edited by Bowen, I.D. and Lockshin, R.A., pp 9-34. Chapman and Hall Press, New York.
52. Wyllie, A.H., Kerr, J.F.R. and Currie, A.R. (1980) Cell death: the significance of apoptosis. Int. Rev. Cytol., 68:251-306.
53. Wyllie, A.H., Kerr, J.R.F., Macaskill, I.A.M. and Currie, A.R. (1973) Adrenocortical cell deletion: the role of ACTH. J. Pathol., 111:85-94.
54. Zeleznik, A.J., Hillier, S.G. and Ross, G.T. (1979) Follicle stimulating hormone-induced follicular development: an examination of the role of androgens. Biol. Reprod., 21:673-681.
55. Zeleznik, A.J., Little-Ihrig, L.L. and Bassett, S.G. (1989) Developmental expression of Ca^{++}/Mg^{++}-dependent endonuclease activity in rat granulosa and luteal cells. Endocrinology, 125:2218-2220.

The Regulation of Ovarian Proteolysis and its Role in Follicular Rupture

A. Tsafriri[1], S-Y. Chun[1] and R. Reich[2]

[1]*Department of Hormone Research, The Bernhard Zondek Hormone Research Laboratory, The Weizmann Institute of Science, Rehovot, 76100;*
[2]*Department of Pharmacology, Faculty of Medicine, Hebrew University of Jerusalem, Jerusalem, 91010, Israel*

INTRODUCTION

The preovulatory surge of gonadotropins induces a multitude of biochemical and morphological changes in the mature Graafian follicle, culminating with the rupture of its wall and the release of a fertilizable ovum. In view of the dense perifollicular meshwork of interstitial collagen fibers in the theca externa and tunica albuginea, it is clear that collagen degradation is a prerequisite for follicle rupture during ovulation. Indeed, considerable thinning of the perifollicular collagenous layers was observed during the preovulatory period (4,13,14).

The involvement of proteolytic processes in ovulation was suggested already by Schochet (33). More recent studies have demonstrated the role of a proteolytic cascade in follicular rupture. It was shown that granulosa cell secretion of plasminogen activator (PA) increases as ovulation approaches (3) and that plasmin, the product of PA acting on plasminogen, decreases the tensile strength of the follicle wall (2). Later studies demonstrated that tissue type (t-) PA is the major species stimulated by LH/hCG in the rat (30,31) and urokinase (u-PA) is the stimulated type in the mouse (7). A gonadotropin-stimulated increase in collagenolytic activity (32) and of activatable collagenase (11) were observed in rat ovaries. Plasminogen activators have been associated with the activation of procollagenases via plasmin (18,20,32). The essential role of proteolytic enzymes in ovulation was confirmed by pharmacologic inhibition of ovulation. Inhibitors of serine proteinases (30), antibodies to t-PA and the plasma-derived plasmin inhibitor, α_2-antiplasmin, reduced the ovulation rate in rats (35). Likewise, ovulation was inhibited by cysteine (32), a metaloproteinase inhibitor, talopeptine (21) and specific inhibitors of interstitial collagenase (5,6, Tsafriri, et al., unpublished). A delayed administration of inhibitors of the plasmin activating system (≥4 h after hCG) was ineffective in blocking ovulation (30,35). Such limited efficacy supports the role of PA and plasmin in the activation of interstitial collagenase.

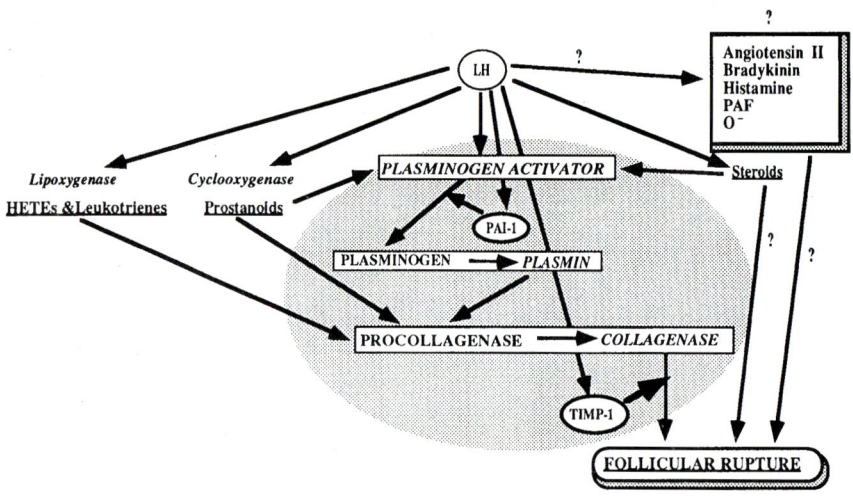

FIG 1. The proteolytic cascade involved in follicular rupture. Among the multitude of follicular responses triggered by LH/hCG, it stimulates the enzymes plasminogen activator and collagenases as well as their respective local inhibitors plasminogen activator inhibitor (PAI-1) and tissue inhibitor of metalloproteinases (TIMP-1). Other details in the text.

The activity of proteolytic enzymes is regulated locally by a series of inhibitors, such as PA inhibitors, α_2-antiplasmin, tissue inhibitor of metalloproteinases (TIMP) and α_2-macroglobulin (1). Among PA inhibitors, PA inhibitor type-1 (PAI-1) appears to be the primary physiologic inhibitor of both t-PA and u-PA (39). TIMP type 1 (TIMP-1) inactivates preferentially interstitial collagenase (16,40). Our studies on the preovulatory changes in ovarian interstitial collagenase activity and regulation of collagenase and TIMP-1 ovarian mRNA expression will be reviewed here. The proteolytic cascade plays an essential role in follicular rupture, nevertheless it is clear that multiple processes and regulatory mechanisms are required for normal ovulation. Some of these are represented in Fig. 1 and were recently reviewed (15,23,34,36,37). Therefore, the present review centering on the regulation of preovulatory ovarian collagenolysis gives only a partial account of follicular rupture.

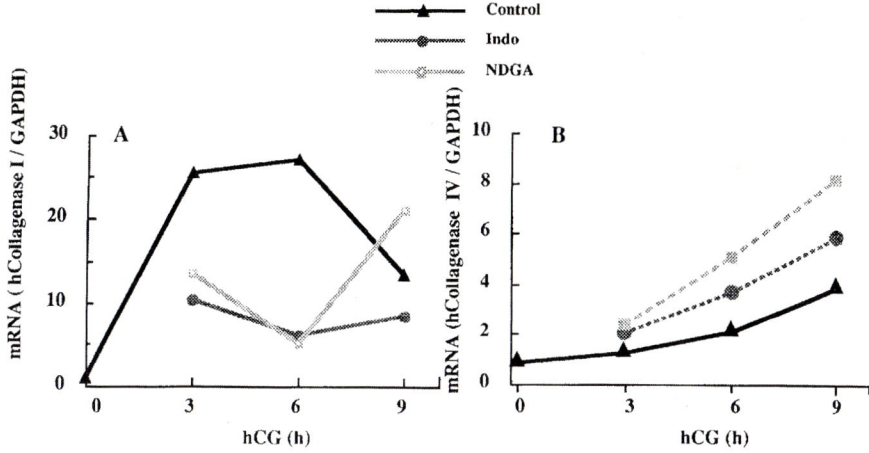

FIG. 2. Effect of hCG stimulation of ovulation on ovarian interstitial collagenase (A) and collagenase IV (B) mRNA. Ovarian mRNA was extracted at the indicated time-intervals after hCG stimulation of ovulation.The eicosanoid synthesis inhibitors were administered bilaterally into the ovarian bursae approx. 30 min prior to hCG. Five µg mRNA were analyzed by Northern blotting using a cDNA probe of human interstitial collagenase (17) or human collagenase IV (10). GAPDH cDNA probe was used as an internal standard (22). From Reich et al., 1991 (29), with permission of *Endocrinology*.

STIMULATION OF OVULATION AND EXPRESSION OF INTERSTITIAL AND TYPE IV COLLAGENASE mRNAs IN THE OVARY

Ovarian mRNA was isolated from immature, PMSG-treated rats at 3, 6 and 9 h after stimulation of ovulation by hCG. Northern-blot analysis of RNA revealed a band hybridizing with human interstitial (type I) collagenase cDNA probe (17). The steady-state levels of this mRNA were stimulated by hCG administration, reaching maximal increase between 3 and 6 h after the treatment (Fig. 2a). It should be noted that a suggested rat interstitial collagenase gene cloned recently (28) differs markedly from that of the human, rabbit and porcine (less than 47% homology at the amino acid level) and has a mRNA of 2.9-3.1 kb in size, higher than the mRNA band detected by us using the human interstitial collagenase cDNA probe (1.7 kb). Nevertheless, in several experiments, repeated under relaxed and stringent conditions, we were unable to obtain any rat ovarian mRNA band hybridizing with this rat collagenase cDNA probe. Therefore, while the final characterization of rat interstitial collagenase mRNA should be completed, we assume that the band of rat ovarian mRNA hybridizing with the human interstitial collagenase cDNA probe represents mRNA of interstitial collagenase or of a very closely related enzyme.

The human cDNA probe of collagenase IV (10) hybridized consistently with a mRNA of 3.1 kb, most probably corresponding to rat collagenase IV. The steady-state levels of this mRNA showed only slight but steady increase after hCG stimulation, reaching a maximum (4-fold as compared to zero time) at 9 h after hCG (Fig. 2b).

Separation of granulosa cells of the Graafian follicles and the residual ovarian tissue, which contains interstitial and theca tissues, as well as growing follicles and possibly some contaminating granulosa cells of Graafian follicles, revealed in both compartments a mRNA hybridizing with the human interstitial collagenase cDNA probe. By contrast, screening with the human collagenase IV cDNA probe revealed a hybridizing mRNA only in the residual tissue and not in the granulosa cells of the Graafian follicles (29).

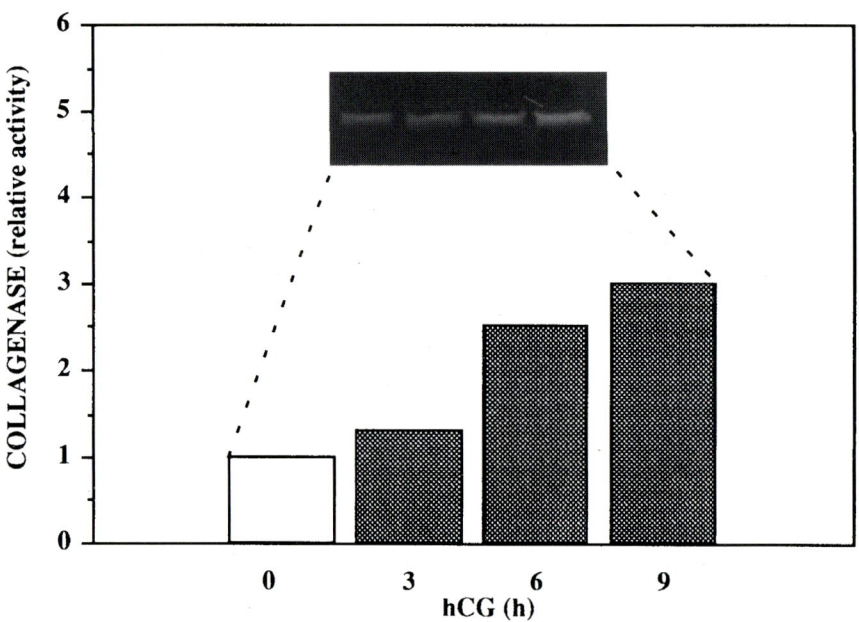

FIG. 3. Effect of hCG on follicular collagenase. Collagenase activity was measured by densitometry on a reversed-zymography gelatin gel. The preovulatory follicles were isolated at the indicated time-intervals after hCG stimulation of ovulation on the morning of proestrus. The visualized band (insert) is of about 52 kDa, corresponding to interstitial collagenase found in other mammalian species.

Zymographic analysis, using gelatin as a substrate, revealed a collagenolytic activity corresponding to interstitial collagenase in whole ovarian extracts or follicles (Fig. 3). This activity was stimulated by LH/hCG *in vivo* or in explanted rat follicles *in vitro* in a temporal pattern similar to that of interstitial collagenase mRNA.

EFFECT OF EICOSANOID INHIBITORS ON COLLAGENASE mRNA EXPRESSION

Interstitial Collagenase. As described above, the steady-state levels of interstitial collagenase mRNA were markedly increased by hCG stimulation. This effect of hCG was considerably attenuated by the administration of inhibitors of eicosanoid synthesis (29). In Fig. 2a the relative values of steady-state levels of interstitial collagenase mRNA in 4 different preparations of mRNA (for control and hCG-stimulated rats) or of 2 batches (for each of the eicosanoid inhibitors) are summarized.

Collagenase IV. The mRNA hybridizing with the human collagenase IV cDNA probe, exhibited only modest stimulation after hCG-treatment during the time-interval examined. The inhibitors of eicosanoids slightly stimulated, rather than attenuated, the expression of collagenase IV mRNA. The summary of the relative values of collagenase IV mRNA is given in Fig. 2b.

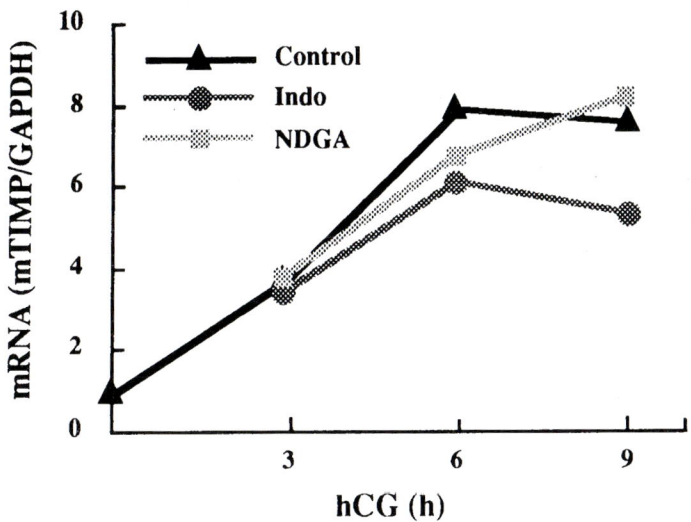

FIG. 4. Effect of hCG stimulation of ovulation and inhibition of eicosanoid synthesis on ovarian TIMP mRNA expression. Five µg mRNA were analyzed by Northern blotting using a cDNA probe of mouse TIMP (22). Other details as in Fig. 2. From Reich et al., 1991 (29), with permission of *Endocrinology*.

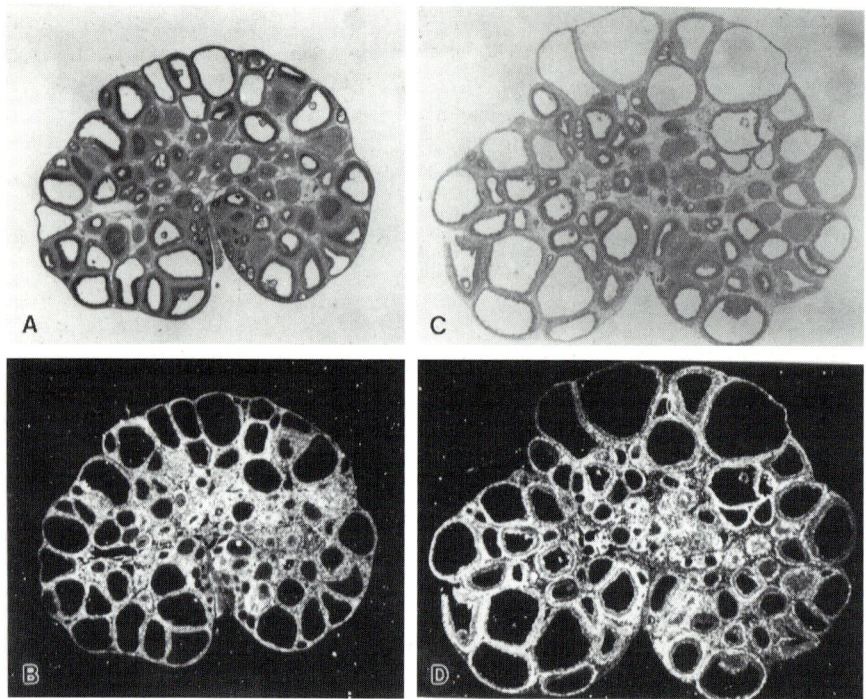

FIG 5. Expression of TIMP-1 mRNA in whole ovarian sections. **A** and **B** before hCG stimulation; **C** and **D** 9h after hCG. **A,C**-bright field micrographs, **B,D**-dark field micrographs. x11. From Chun et al., (8).

OVARIAN EXPRESSION OF TIMP mRNA

The mouse TIMP cDNA probe (22) hybridized with a 0.9 kb ovarian mRNA. The steady state levels of this mRNA were stimulated by hCG to reach a maximum (7-8 fold increase) at 6 and 9 h after the treatment. Administration of inhibitors of eicosanoid synthesis did not much affect the levels of TIMP mRNA (Fig. 4). When the cDNA probe of human TIMP was used, essentially, the same results were obtained (data not shown). TIMP mRNA was expressed in both, the granulosa cells of Graafian follicles and the residual tissue. Its levels in both compartments increased within 4 h of hCG stimulation (29).

PREOVULATORY EXPRESSION OF TIMP-1 mRNA AND ITS CELLULAR LOCALIZATION

To determine the ovarian cell types responding to hCG, we analyzed the expression of TIMP-1 mRNA by *in situ* hybridization in PMSG-primed ovaries collected before hCG and 9 h after hCG treatment. This time-interval was chosen on basis of Northern blot analyses, showing maximal expression of TIMP-1 mRNA around 9 h after hCG stimulation of ovulation (Fig. 4). As seen in the whole ovarian section of Fig. 5, TIMP-1 mRNA was expressed in interstitial cells of antral follicles as well as in the more distant stromal cells. Control experiments with sense RNA probes showed no hybridization (not shown).

Before hCG stimulation of ovulation, TIMP-1 mRNA was expressed in theca cells, but not in granulosa cells of healthy follicles (Fig. 5a,b). hCG stimulation greatly increased theca cell expression of TIMP-1 mRNA in most antral follicles. The pattern of TIMP-1 mRNA expression in granulosa cells after hCG treatment depended on follicular size. hCG induced TIMP-1 mRNA in granulosa cells of preovulatory and large antral follicles, but not in granulosa cells of medium-sized antral follicles (Fig. 6). In addition, surface epithelium of ovaries collected before hCG treatment expressed TIMP-1 mRNA, but this labeling disappeared after hCG stimulation. The increased theca cell expression of TIMP-1 mRNA by hCG stimulation is similar to that of PAI-1 mRNA (8).

DISCUSSION

The plasmin activating system appears to play an essential role in the rupture of the follicle during ovulation. Nevertheless, its primary role seems to be limited to early stages of the follicular response leading to the breaching of follicle wall and involves the activation of collagenase. Thus, ovulation may be blocked even when follicular PA production was not affected, while collagenase activity or production were suppressed. This may be achieved by inhibitors of eicosanoid synthesis or by inhibitors of metalloproteinases (5,32,37).

In the rat, it seems that t-PA is the major PA activity stimulated by the ovulatory hormone-LH, but in a closely related species, the mouse, u-PA seems to be the activity stimulated. While these findings seem to indicate that both types of PA can equally well participate in ovulation, detailed investigation of additional mammalian species is required for establishing the role of these two PA types in ovulation (reviewed in Reference 37).

In contradistinction to the plasminogen-activating system, collagenolytic activity is required throughout most of the time-interval between the stimulation of ovulation by the gonadotropin and the rupture of the follicle (32). Likewise, the gonadotropic stimulation of ovarian collagenolysis seems to be mediated by eicosanoids, while that of PA is not (37).

The expression of interstitial collagenase mRNA is stimulated by LH/hCG and this effect was suppressed by inhibitors of eicosanoid synthesis. Thus the stimulatory effect of the gonadotropin on both, collagenolytic activity and interstitial collagenase mRNA levels seems to be mediated by ovarian

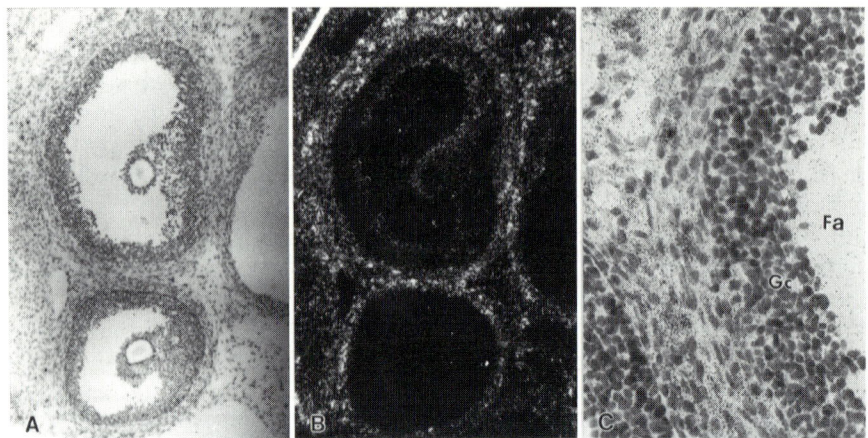

FIG. 6. TIMP mRNA expression in granulosa cells of preovulatory follicles after stimulation of ovulation by hCG. TIMP mRNA is expressed in granulosa cells of preovulatory (upper follicle), but not younger antral follicles (lower follicle), while it is expressed in the theca-interstitial cells of most antral follicles. x79. From Chun et al., (8).

eicosanoids. In contrast, the expression of collagenase IV mRNA was not suppressed by inhibitors of eicosanoids.

Seemingly paradoxical, but reflecting a common biological phenomenon, in parallel to stimulation of proteolytic enzymes gonadotropin also stimulates ovarian coexpression of protease inhibitors. Thus, LH/hCG also stimulated the ovarian expression of TIMP mRNA. Nevertheless, this activity of the gonadotropin was not blocked by inhibitors of eicosanoids.

The finding that inhibition of ovarian eicosanoid synthesis suppresses only the expression of interstitial collagenase, but not that of collagenase IV, may explain the observed 'intraovarian ovulation' in indomethacin- (26) or NDGA-treated rats (Reich and Tsafriri, unpublished observations). In such cases, the basal membrane disintegrates, probably due to undisturbed action of collagenase IV, but breaking of apical theca externa and tunica albuginea, constituted of interstitial collagen, is prevented due to blockage of interstitial collagenase production. Furthermore, the inhibition of interstitial collagenase, but not of LH/hCG stimulation of TIMP expression, by inhibitors of eicosanoid synthesis provide two complementary mechanisms by which follicle rupture is blocked by these drugs.

In our *in situ* hybridization studies constitutive expression of TIMP-1 mRNA was detected in theca-interstitial cells of antral follicles and in ovarian stromal cells. hCG stimulation of ovulation in PMSG-primed immature rats resulted in a marked increase in theca-interstitial cell expression of TIMP-1 mRNA and its induction in granulosa cells of preovulatory follicles. This gonadotropic stimulation of inhibitor mRNA expression corresponds with other studies demonstrating an increase in ovarian TIMP activity observed in ovulating rat ovaries (24,41). The simultaneous synthesis of enzymes and inhibitors was also demonstrated in other cells and tissues. Rat alveolar epithelial cells concomitantly expressed both PAI-1 and u-PA in response to inflammatory mediators *in vitro* (19), and PAI-1 and t-PA were parallelly increased upon infusion of tumor necrosis factor-α (TNFα) in patients with active malignancies (38). Concomitant increase in collagenase and TIMP activity have been found in avascular cartilage (12), fibroblasts (9) and osteoblasts (27). Such concurrent production and secretion of proteinases and their inhibitors allows strict regulation and localization of proteolytic activity. Thus, there is strict regulation of proteinase synthesis, which occurs only at moments of need, activation of the latent forms, and there are multiple inhibitors to check proteolysis before it goes too far (40). In the proteolytic degradation of follicular wall during ovulation, the increased secretion of proteinase inhibitors by gonadotropic stimulation might block proteinase activity diffusing away from the site of action, and thus provide localized control of extracellular matrix remodeling. Indeed, Zhu and Woessner (41) proposed that metalloproteinases escape the control of TIMP only in focal regions of the follicle, since the increase in rat ovarian TIMP is approximately one half of the increase in collagenase after gonadotropic stimulation of ovulation. TIMP-1 seems to be the major inhibitor that regulates matrix remodeling of perifollicular tissues, and is expressed constitutively in theca-interstitial cells even before hCG treatment. The hCG-stimulated expression of TIMP-1 mRNA in theca cells of small antral follicles probably assures their integrity in face of collagenolytic activity diffusing from preovulatory follicles.

The LH/hCG stimulated expression of TIMP-1 mRNA in granulosa cells is limited to the preovulatory follicles. This is in contrast to its expression in the theca of most antral follicles. The expression of TIMP-1 is uniform in the adluminal cells of the membrana granulosa of large antral follicles. Our present finding that hCG-stimulated TIMP-1 mRNA induction in granulosa cells is dependent on follicular size, may be related to the appearance of LH receptors. Mann *et al.* (24) demonstrated that hCG-induced expression of TIMP mRNA is independent of *de novo* protein synthesis, and that neither prostaglandins nor estrogens appear to play a role in stimulating the production of inhibitor. TIMP mRNA is also expressed in luteal cells of granulosa origin, suggesting that inhibitors may be required to prevent premature destruction of the corpora lutea (25). The exposure of granulosa cells to LH/hCG sets into motion the process of luteinization. It is likely that hCG-stimulated expression of PAI-1 and TIMP-1 mRNAs in follicular cells is associated with the extensive vascularization of the avascular membrana granulosa during formation of the corpus luteum, in addition to their regulation of proteolytic processes of follicular rupture. Indeed, proteinases and inhibitors are necessary to allow capillary endothelial cells to form new sprouts and to start angiogenesis (38).

In summary, the theca cells of most antral follicles express higher level of TIMP-1 mRNA after LH/hCG stimulation of ovulation. This enhanced expression of inhibitors in theca cells may be required for strict regulation of follicular connective tissue remodeling associated with ovulation, luteinization and with the preservation of younger follicles. On the other hand, only the granulosa cells of preovulatory follicles respond to LH/hCG with enhanced mRNA expression of TIMP-1 in membrana granulosa. The LH/hCG stimulated expression of TIMP-1 mRNA in the theca of nonovulatory follicles seems to protect them from proteolytic degradation and allows them to reach the ovulatory stage in subsequent cycles.

ACKNOWLEDGEMENTS

We thank Mrs. M. Kopelowitz for secretarial help. Our studies were supported in part by grants from the German-Israel Foundation for Scientific Research and Development (GIF), Jerusalem, Israel, and the Basic Science Research Foundation of the Israel Academy of Sciences and Humanities, Jerusalem, Israel.

REFERENCES

1. Alexander, C.M. and Werb, Z. (1989) Proteinases and extracellular matrix remodeling. Current Opinion in Cell Biology, 1:974-982.
2. Beers, W.H. (1975) Follicular plasminogen and plasminogen activator and the effect of plasmin on ovarian follicular wall. Cell, 6:379-386.
3. Beers, W.H., Strickland, S. and Reich, E. (1975) Ovarian plasminogen activator: Relationship to ovulation and hormonal regulation. Cell, 6:387-394.
4. Bjersing, L. and Cajander, S. (1974) Ovulation and the mechanism of follicular rupture. VI. Ultrastructure of theca interna and the inner vascular network surrounding rabbit Graafian follicles prior to induced ovulation. Cell and Tissue Res., 153:31-44.
5. Brännström, M., Woessner, J.F., Koos, R.D., Sear, C.H.J. and LeMaire, W.J. (1988) Inhibitors of mammalian tissue collagenase and metaloproteinases suppress ovulation in the perfused rat ovary. Endocrinology, 122:1715-1721.
6. Butler, T.A., Zhu, C., Mueller, R.A., Fuller, G.C., LeMaire, W.J. and Woessner Jr, J.F. (1991) Inhibition of ovulation in the perfused rat ovary by the synthetic collagenase inhibitor SC 44463. Biol. Reprod., 44:1183-1188.
7. Canipari, R., O'Connell, M.L., Meyer, G. and Strickland, S. (1987) Mouse ovarian granulosa cells produce urokinase-type plasminogen activator, whereas the corresponding rat cells produce tissue-type plasminogen activator. J. Cell Biol., 205:977-981.
8. Chun, S.Y., Popliker, M., Reich, R. and Tsafriri, A. (1992) Localization of preovulatory expression of plasminogen activator inhibitor type-1 and tissue inhibitor of metalloproteinase type-1 mRNAs in the rat ovary. Biol. Reprod. (in press).
9. Clark, S.D., Wilhelm, S.M., Stricklin, G.P. and Welgus, H.G. (1985) Coregulation of collagenase and collagenase inhibitor production by phorbol myristate acetate in human skin fibroblasts. Arch. Bioch. Biophys., 241:36-41.
10. Collier, I.E., Wilhelm, S.M., Eisen, A.Z., Marmer, B.L., Grant, G.A., Seltzer, J.L., Kronberger, A., He, C., Bauer, E.A. and Goldberg, G.I. (1988) H-ras oncogene-transformed human bronchial epithelial cells (TBE-1) secrete a single metalloprotease capable of degrading basement membrane collagen. J. Biol. Chem., 263:5679-5687.
11. Curry, T.E.J., Clark, M.R., Dean, D.D., Woessner, J.F.J. and LeMaire, W.J.J. (1986) The preovulatory increase in ovarian collagenase activity in the rat is independent of prostaglandin production. Endocrinology, 118:1823-1828.

12. Dean, D.D., Martel-Pelletier, J., Pelletier, J-P., Howell, D.S. and Woessner Jr, J.F. (1989) Evidence for metalloproteinase and metalloproteinase inhibitor imbalance in human osteoarthritic cartilage. J. Clin. Invest., 84:678-685.
13. Espey, L.L. (1978) Ovulation. In: The Vertebrate Ovary, edited by Jones, R.E., pp 503-532. Plenum Press, New York.
14. Espey, L.L., Coons, P.J., Marsh, J.M. and LeMaire, W.J. (1981) Effect of indomethacin on preovulatory changes in the ultrastructure of rabbit Graafian follicles. Endocrinology, 108:1040-1048.
15. Goetz, F.W., Berndtson, A.K. and Ranjan, M. (1991) Ovulation: mediators at the ovarian level. In: Vertebrate Endocrinology: Fundamentals and Biomedical Implications, edited by Pang, P.T.K., Schreibman, M.P. and Jones, R. pp 127-203. Academic Press, Inc., New York.
16. Goldberg, G.I., Marmer, B.L., Grant, G.A., Eisen, A.Z., Wilhelm, S. and He, C. (1989) Human 72-kilodalton type IV collagenase forms a complex with a tissue inhibitor of metalloproteases designated TIMP-1. Proc. Natl. Acad. Sci. USA, 86:8207-8211.
17. Goldberg, G.I., Wilhelm, S.M., Kronbey, A., Bower, F.A., Grant, G.A. and Eisen, A.Z. (1986) Human fibroblast collagenase. J. Biol. Chem., 261:6600-6605.
18. Grant, G.A., Eisen, A.Z., Marmer, B.C., Roswil, W.T., and Goldberg, G.I. (1987) The activation of human skin fibroblast procollagenase. J. Biol. Chem., 262:5886-5889.
19. Gross, T.J., Simon, R.H., Kelly, C.J. and Sitrin, R.G. (1991) Rat alveolar epithelial cells concomitantly express plasminogen activator inhibitor-1 and urokinase. Am. J. Physiol., 260:L286-L295.
20. He, C., Wilhelm, S.M., Pentland, A.P., Marmer, B.L., Grant, G.A., Eisen, A.Z. and Goldberg, G.I. (1989) Tissue cooperation in proteolytic cascade activity human interstitial collagenase. Proc. Natl. Acad. Sci. USA, 86:2632-2636.
21. Ichikawa, S., Ohta, M., Morioka, H. and Murao, S. (1983) Blockage of ovulation in the explanted hamster ovary by a collagenase inhibitor. J. Reprod. Fertil., 68:17-19.
22. Khokha, R., and Denhart, D.T. (1989) Matrix metalloproteinases and tissue inhibitor of metalloproteinases: A review of their role in tumorigenesis and tissue invasion. Invasion and Metastasis, 9:391-405.
23. Lipner, H. (1988) Mechanism of mammalian ovulation. In: The Physiology of Reproduction, edited by Knobil, E. and Neill, J., pp 447-488. Raven Press, Ltd., New York.
24. Mann, J.S., Kindy, M.S., Edwards, D.R. and Curry, J.T.E.. (1991) Hormonal regulation of matrix metalloproteinase inhibitors in rat granulosa cells and ovaries. Endocrinology, 128:1825-1832.
25. Nomura, S., Hogan, B.L., Wills, A.J., Heath, I.K. and Edwards, D.R. (1989) Developmental expression of tissue inhibitor of metalloproteinase (TIMP) RNA. Development, 105:575-583.
26. Osman, P. and Dullaart, J. (1976) Intraovarian release of eggs in the rat after indomethacin treatment at pro-oestrus. J. Reprod. Fert., 47:101-103.
27. Otsuka, K., Sodek, J. and Limeback, H. (1984) Synthesis of collagenase inhibitors by osteoblast-like cells in culture. Eur. J. Biochem., 145:123-130.
28. Quinn, C.O., Scott, D.K., Brinckerhoff, C.E., Matrisian, L.M., Jeffrey, J.J. and Partridge, N.C. (1990) Rat collagenase. Cloning, amino acid sequence comparison, and parathyroid hormone regulation in osteoblastic cells. J. Biol. Chem., 265:22342-22347.
29. Reich, R., Daphna-Iken, D., Chun, S.Y., Popliker, M., Slager, R., Adelmann-Grill, B.C. and Tsafriri, A. (1991) Preovulatory changes in ovarian expression of collagenases and tissue metalloproteinase inhibitor mRNA: Role of eicosanoids. Endocrinology, 129:1869-1875.
30. Reich, R., Miskin, R. and Tsafriri, A. (1985) Follicular plasminogen activator: Involvement in ovulation. Endocrinology, 116:516-521.
31. Reich, R., Miskin, R. and Tsafriri, A. (1986) Intrafollicular distribution of plasminogen activators and their hormonal regulation *in vitro*. Endocrinology, 119:1588-1601.
32. Reich, R., Tsafriri, A. and Mechanic, G.L. (1985) The involvement of collagenolysis in ovulation in the rat. Endocrinology, 116:521-527.
33. Schochet, S.S. (1916) A suggestion as to the process of ovulation and ovarian cyst formation. Anat. Rec., 10:447-457.
34. Thibault, C. and Levasseur, M.C. (1988) Ovulation. Human Reprod., 3:513-523.
35. Tsafriri, A., Bicsak, T.A., Cajander, S.B., Ny, T. and Hsueh, A.J.W. (1989) Suppression of ovulation rate by antibodies to tissue type plasminogen activator and α_2-antiplasmin. Endocrinology, 124:415-421.

36. Tsafriri, A., Daphna-Iken, D., Abisogun, A.O. and Reich, R. (1991) Follicular rupture during ovulation: Activation of collagenolysis. In: Advances in Assisted Reproductive Technologies, edited by Mashiach, S., Ben-Rafael, Z., Laufer, N. and Schenker, J.G., pp 103-112. Plenum Press, New York.
37. Tsafriri, A. and Reich, R. (1991) Plasminogen activators in the preovulatory follicle: Role in ovulation. In: Plasminogen Activators: From Cloning to Therapy, edited by Abbate, R., Barni, T. and Tsafriri, A., pp 91-93. Raven Press, New York.
38. Van Hinsbergh, V.W.M., Kooistra, T., Emeis, J.J. and Koolwijk, P. (1991) Regulation of plasminogen activator production by endothelial cells: role in fibrinolysis and local proteolysis. Int. J. Radiat. Biol., 60:261-272.
39. Vassali, J.D., Sappino, A.P. and Belin, D. (1991) The plasminogen activator/plasmin system. J. Clin. Invest., 88:1067-1072.
40. Woessner Jr, J.F. (1991) Matrix metalloproteinases and their inhibitors in connective tissue remodeling. FASEB J, 5:2145-2154.
41. Zhu, C. and Woessner Jr, J.F. (1991) A tissue inhibitor of metalloproteinases and α-macroglobulins in the ovulating rat ovary: possible regulators of collagen matrix breakdown. Biol. Reprod., 45:334-342.

Luteinization and Luteolysis

A.J. Zeleznik

*Departments of Physiology and Obstetrics,
Gynecology and Reproductive Sciences
The University of Pittsburgh School of Medicine, Pittsburgh, PA 15213, USA*

INTRODUCTION

The corpus luteum is formed in response to the midcycle gonadotropin surge as the result of the actions of LH on the Graafian follicle. Following ovulation, the corpus luteum exhibits a finite life span, the duration of which is highly species specific. Not only is the life span of the corpus luteum species specific, there also appears to be substantial differences amongst species with respect to the requirements for the hormonal control of luteal function (1). The goal of this chapter is to summarize the extant knowledge regarding the maintenance of luteal function as they pertain to subhuman primates. A more detailed version of this chapter is presented elsewhere (2).

THE 'LIFE CYCLE' OF THE GRANULOSA-LUTEAL CELL

The newly ovulated corpus luteum is often referred to as the 'new' or 'young' corpus luteum while the corpus luteum present in ovaries near the expected time of ovulation is typically referred to as the 'old' corpus luteum. Clearly, these descriptive terms are accurate when discussing the chronological age of the corpus luteum as an entity, but do not adequately address the developmental history of the luteal cells *per se*.

Because the luteal cell is a direct descendent of the preovulatory follicle granulosa cell, the actual life span of the granulosa-luteal cell is far longer than the life span of the corpus luteum. From studies of rats, it has been estimated that from the time of recruitment of the primordial follicle, the granulosa cells undergo at least 10 population doubling during the passage of the follicle through the preantral stages to the preovulatory stage. During most of the their doublings, the granulosa cells are present in an undifferentiated state and lack the characteristics of the typical steroid producing cells. It is only during the final stages of preovulatory follicular growth that differentiation of the granulosa cells occur under the control of follicle stimulating hormone (FSH). In response to FSH stimulation, granulosa cells undergo a major cellular differentiation which includes the acquisition of LH receptors (3), acquisition of cholesterol side chain cleavage enzyme (P450scc) and 3β-hydroxysteroid dehydrogenase/Δ^{5-4} isomerase (3β-HSD) which are required for progesterone secretion as well as aromatase which is responsible for conversion of thecally produced androgens into estrogen (4,5). Significantly, the appearance of the LH receptor as well as the enzymes involved in progesterone secretion, each of which are fundamental for the adequate functioning of the corpus luteum, occur prior to its actual formation. In addition to the aforementioned, other proteins such as inhibin and vascular endothelial growth factor are also induced during preovulatory follicular development and their expressions are maintained in the functioning corpus luteum (6,7). In essence, therefore, the major differentiated functions of the corpus luteum are actually set during the process of preovulatory follicle growth and maintained by luteal cells following luteinization. The process of luteinization involves the terminal differentiation of the granulosa cell as there is no evidence that luteal cells undergo cellular replication (8). Accordingly, when speaking of the age of the corpus luteum, it must be remembered that a 'young' luteal cell is actually a very old granulosa cell and that, as a terminally differentiated cell, its next transition is cell death. Therefore, in, discussing the control of luteal function and life span, it is important to appreciate that the newly formed corpus luteum is in its final differentiated state and its ultimate fate is to die.

PHYSIOLOGICAL ASPECTS OF LUTEAL FUNCTION

The typical luteal phase of non-fertile menstrual cycles has a 14-16 day duration. For the first five to six days following ovulation, serum progesterone concentrations rise and reach a plateau approximately one week after ovulation and remain elevated for 3-4 days. On approximately day ten of the luteal phase, serum progesterone concentrations begin to fall and continue to do so for the next four to six days until progesterone concentrations become non-detectable and menses ensues. Morphological studies have shown that the luteinizing granulosa cells continue to expand in volume, accumulate mitochondria and smooth endoplasmic reticulum for the first five - six days after ovulation and reach their maximum volume by day seven of the luteal phase. Shortly thereafter, beginning on approximately day 10 of the luteal phase, luteal cells begin to exhibit degenerative changes which become more pronounced as the time of menses approaches (9). Accordingly, three developmental stages of the corpus luteum can be defined; the luteinization stage (days 1-6 following ovulation), the fully developed stage (days 7-10 following ovulation) and the regressing stage (days 11-15) following ovulation).

The extent to which pituitary gonadotropin secretion is involved in the control of progesterone production and the maintenance of luteal life span has been studied using models in which the secretion of LH by the pituitary gland is interrupted. One strategy has been to treat women and subhuman primates with GnRH antagonists that compete with endogenous GnRH for pituitary receptors (10). The second approach has been to use subhuman primates whose secretion of GnRH is compromised by the placement of radio-frequency lesions in the hypothalamus and in which ovulatory menstrual cycles can be restored by the pulsatile administration of synthetic GnRH (11). With the latter model, the pattern of LH secretion can be controlled directly by altering the infusion of GnRH. Both models have shown that the interruption of LH secretion at any time during the luteal phase is rapidly followed by a dramatic reduction in progesterone secretion and premature menstruation indicating that pituitary gonadotropin secretion is absolutely required for luteal progesterone production (10,11). The hypothalamic-lesioned, GnRH pulsed animal model has also provided useful information pertaining to the role of LH on the maintenance of luteal life span. Fig. 1 illustrates one such study. In this experiment, the pulsatile infusion of GnRH was interrupted for three days during the early luteal phase of the menstrual cycle (12). It can be seen that interruption of GnRH support to the pituitary gland on Day 3 of the luteal phase was followed by a prompt and sustained fall in plasma LH and progesterone concentrations.

Reinitiation of the GnRH infusion on Day 6 of the luteal phase resulted in the restoration of LH secretion and the reinitiation of luteal progesterone production. Moreover, the resultant duration of the luteal phase was indistinguishable from animals which maintained on an uninterrupted regimen of GnRH. These data illustrate that although progesterone production by the corpus luteum is absolutely dependent upon LH secretion, the maintenance of luteal life span is less dependent upon the secretion of LH because interruption of LH support for three days did not result in irreversible luteal regression and menses ensued at the expected time, 14-16 days after ovulation. Similar findings that the macaque corpus luteum can recover from a transient withdrawal of LH support has also been obtained from the GnRH-antagonist model (10).

The aforementioned data support the notion that changes in LH secretion may not be causal to the onset of luteal regression. That changes in LH secretion are not causal to the onset of luteal regression is also supported by the findings that reducing the LH pulse frequency on Day 3 of the luteal phase from one pulse per hour to a frequency seen at the time of luteal regression (one pulse per eight hours) did not result in premature luteolysis (13). Moreover, acute reduction of plasma LH concentrations by >50% during the early luteal phase did not result in luteolysis (14). The findings that changes in LH secretion are not likely responsible for luteal regression as well as other studies that have negated estrogen as a luteolytic agent (15) strongly indicate that the regression of the corpus luteum is due to intrinsic changes

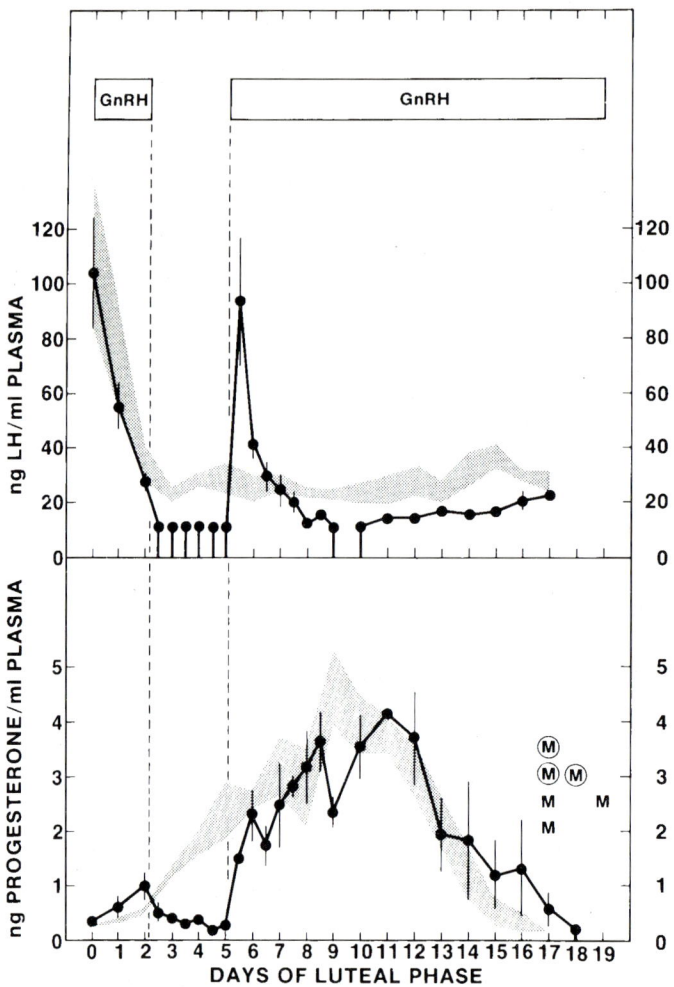

FIG.1. Effect of a transient withdrawal of LH upon progesterone secretion and life span of the corpus luteum. Rhesus monkeys with lesions of the medial-basal hypothalamus were treated with synthetic GnRH intravenously at a frequency of one pulse per hour to restore menstrual cyclicity. The shaded areas encompass one standard error about the mean of plasma LH concentrations (top panel) and progesterone concentrations (lower panel) in animals whose GnRH infusions were maintained at one pulse per hour throughout the entire menstrual cycle. The line graphs depict data from animals whose GnRH infusions were interrupted for three days (Days 3 through 5). Following interruption of GnRH infusion, plasma LH concentrations (top panel) and progesterone concentrations (lower panel) fell to non-detectable levels. Following reinitiation of the GnRH infusions, LH secretion resumed and the progesterone secretion by the corpus luteum returned to control values and luteal regression occurred at the expected time. Reproduced from Reference 12.

at the level of the corpus luteum itself rather than changes in the gonadotropic stimulus to the corpus luteum.

CELLULAR ASPECTS OF LUTEAL FUNCTION

Given that the regression of the corpus luteum does not appear to be caused directly by changes in LH secretion, attention must be given to the changes in luteal cell function which occur during the luteal phase of the menstrual cycle that may provide information on the cellular correlates of luteal regression. Studies using macaque luteal cells maintained in culture have shown that luteal cells isolated from corpora lutea collected during the early

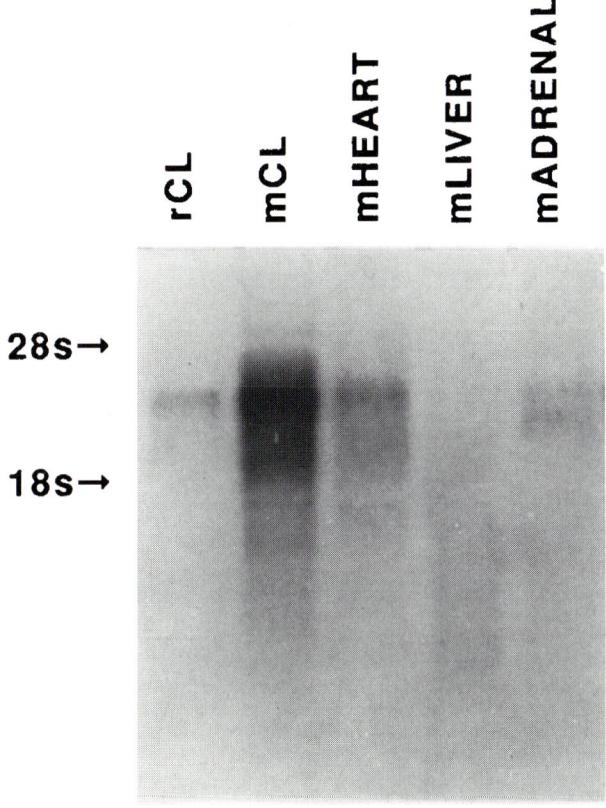

FIG. 2. Expression of messenger RNA for vascular endothelial growth factor in the primate corpus luteum. Five μg of total RNA from various sources were electrophoresed thorough a 1.2% agarose gel, transferred to a nylon membrane and probed with a ^{32}P-labeled cDNA for human vascular endothelial growth factor. The lower case **m** indicates tissues obtained from monkeys and the lower case **r**, tissue from rats. Reproduced from Reference 7.

luteal phase produce more progesterone *in vitro* than luteal cells isolated during the late luteal phase (16). More detailed studies of the biosynthetic capacity of isolated luteal cells have been obtained from human corpora lutea (17). In this study, it was shown that the absolute capacity of luteal cells to secrete progesterone was evident shortly after ovulation and luteinization and progressively declined throughout the remainder of the luteal phase. The divergence between the rate of progesterone production *in vitro* versus the rate of progesterone secretion *in vivo* is likely due to the fact that the newly formed corpus luteum has yet to become fully vascularized. Delivery of LDL-cholesterol to the luteal cells is thereby restricted and progesterone production by the highly active luteal cells is likely substrate limited. Recent findings reproduced in Fig. 2 illustrate that the monkey corpus luteum contains mRNA for the angiogenic factor, vascular endothelial growth factor (7). That the expression of this mRNA is high during the early luteal phase of the cycle and decreases at the time of menstruation provides suggestive evidence that VEGF may be responsible for the angiogenesis that accompanies the formation of the corpus luteum.

Recent studies on the patterns of expression of specific mRNAs by the corpus luteum have shed new light on the biology of the luteal cell. Using cDNA probes complementary to the major enzymes involves in steroid secretion, P450scc and 3β-HSD, we have shown that the newly formed corpus luteum exhibits maximal or near maximal levels of these mRNAs and their levels steadily decline throughout the luteal phase (Fig. 3). As can be seen in this figure, mRNA for 3β-HSD actually falls significantly during the mid-luteal phase of the menstrual cycle and is nearly undetectable 4-5 days before luteal regression occurs. Because the levels of these mRNAs appear to fall independently of the overall pattern of LH and progesterone secretion, it was originally speculated that LH may not be involved in the moment-to-moment control of these mRNAs (18). However, more recent preliminary data have revealed that interruption of LH support during the luteal phase of the monkey menstrual cycle by a GnRH-antagonist results in a more rapid fall in these mRNAs (19). Given that the 'steady-state' concentration of any mRNA is a function both of the rate of transcription and the rate of degradation, these data would therefore appear to indicate that overall the predominant pathway is one of degradation, especially for 3β-HSD mRNA because its level progressively declines during the luteal phase. The role of LH in the maintenance of this mRNA cannot be deduced from these studies because a fall in the mRNA levels after reducing LH secretion could either be due to diminished transcription or enhanced degradation. It is noteworthy that all luteal mRNAs do not appear to be controlled identically because mRNA for the LH receptor follows an inverse pattern to those of P450scc and 3β-HSD in that levels progressively rise throughout the luteal phase and fall to undetectable near the onset of luteal regression (20). Thus, while there appears to be a concordant regulation of induction of specific mRNAs in granulosa cells during preovulatory follicular development, it appears that following ovu-

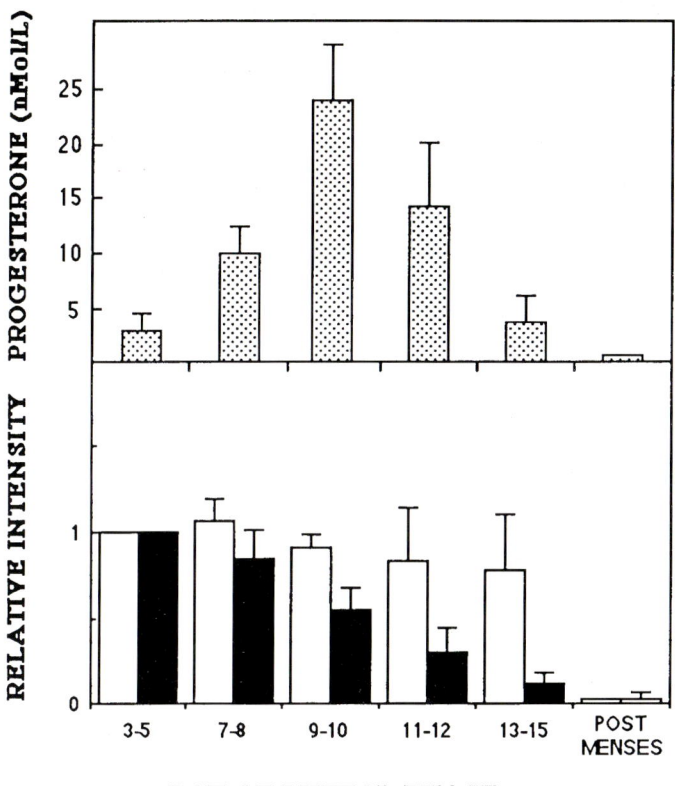

FIG. 3. Expression of mRNA for cholesterol side chain cleavage enzyme and 3β-hydroxysteroid dehydrogenase during the luteal phase of the primate menstrual cycle. The top panel shows serum progesterone concentrations at specified times of the luteal phase. The bottom panel illustrates the relative amounts of mRNA for cholesterol side chain cleavage enzyme (solid bars) and 3β-hydroxysteroid dehydrogenase (open bars) at defined times of the luteal phase. Note that mRNA for 3β-hydroxysteroid dehydrogenase declined well before the fall in progesterone concentrations. Reproduced form Reference 18.

lation and luteinization, steady state levels of these mRNAs appear to be differentially regulated.

While Northern analyses have provided useful information on the levels of luteal cell-specific mRNAs throughout the luteal phase of the menstrual cycle and will likely yield important information in hormonal manipulation studies, it must be reinforced that the overall utility of these analyses is somewhat limited. As is the case for any procedure that requires homogenization of an entire tissue, results obtained provide information regarding the average contents of mRNA per mass of tissue. In cases where the tissue is uniform throughout, results can be extrapolated to the single cell level.

However, in cases where the tissue is composed of heterogeneous cell types, results obtained cannot be equated to absolute changes at the single cell level. Is well established that the corpus luteum is not composed of a morphological uniform cell population but rather subpopulations of cells that likely differ in structure and function. Besides containing fibroblasts and endothelial cells, the corpus luteum contains subpopulations of steroidogenic cells that differ in their functional capacity and gonadotropin responsiveness.

In the primate corpus luteum, two different steroidogenic cell types can be identified; small cells with a diameter of ≤15 μm and large cells with a diameter of ≥15 μm (21). Because small luteal cells are less responsive to gonadotropin and produce far less progesterone per cell than do larage luteal cells, potential shifts in the luteal cell population during the luteal phase could account for changes in mRNA levels as shown in Fig. 3. Indeed, evidence from collagenase dissociated corpora lutea have demonstrated that the ratio of large:small cells decreases as the luteal phase progresses. Moreover, early histological studies on the morphology of the human corpus luteum during the menstrual cycle showed an increase in the number of small cells beginning on about Day 10 of the luteal phase, an the ratio of small:large cells continued to increase as the duration of the luteal phase progressed (22). Because cell shrinkage may be an early event in the process of cell death and luteal regression, it will be important to determine whether the changes in mRNA expression seen during the luteal phase are confined to subsets of luteal cells or whether the changes represent the entire luteal cell population and more importantly whether the changes are associated with the initiation of cell death. Such analyses will greatly enhance our knowledge in defining the cellular mechanisms responsible for luteal regression at the termination of non-fertile menstrual cycles as well as the cellular mechanisms responsible for the extension of the functional life span of the corpus luteum by human chorionic gonadotropin when pregnancy ensues.

REFERENCES

1. Niswender, G.D. and Nett, T.M. (1988) The corpus luteum and its control. In: The physiology of reproduction, edited by Knobil E., Neill J.D., pp 489-525. Raven Press, New York.
2. Zeleznik, A.J. (1990) Control of luteal endocrine function. In: Ovarian endocrinology, edited by Hillier S.G., pp 167-189. Blackwell Scientific, London.
3. Segaloff, D.L., Wang H. and Richards J.S. (1990) Hormonal regulation of luteinizing hormone /chorionic gonadotropin receptor mRNA in rat ovarian cells during follicular development and luteinization. Mol. Endocrinol., 4:1856-1865.
4. Doody, K.J., Lorence, M.C., Mason, J.I. and Simpson, E.R. (1990) Expression of messenger ribonucleic acid species encoding steroidogenic enzymes in human follicles and corpora lutea throughout the menstrual cycle. J. Clin. Endocrinol. Metab., 70:141-145.
5. Steinkampf, M.P., Mendelson, C.R. and Simpson, E.R. (1987) Regulation by follicle stimulating hormone of the synthesis of aromatase cytochrome P-450 in human granulosa cells. Mol. Endocrinol., 1:465-471.
6. Schwall, R.H., Mason, A.J., Wilcox, J.N., Bassett, S.G. and Zeleznik, A.J., (1989) Localization of inhibin/activin subunit mRNAs within the primate ovary. Mol Endocrinol., 4:75-79.

7. Ravindranath, N., Little-Ihrig, L., Phillips, H.S., Ferrara, N. and Zeleznik, A.J. (1992) Vascular endothelial growth factor expression in the primate ovary. Endocrinology (in press).
8. Hirshfield, A.N., (1984) Continuous [^{3}H] thymidine infusion: a method for the study of follicular dynamics. Biol. Reprod., 28:2712-2720.
9. Adams, E.C. and Hertig, A.T. (1969) Studies on the human corpus luteum I. Observations on the utltrastructure of development and regression of the luteal cells during the menstrual cycle. J. Cell. Biol., 41:696-715 .
10 Fraser, H.M., Nestor, J.J. and Vickery, B.H., (1987) Suppression of luteal function by a luteinizing hormone-releasing hormone antagonist during the early luteal phase in the stumptailed macaque monkey and the effects of subsequent administration of human chorionic gonadotropin. Endocrinology, 121: 612-618.
11. Hutchison, J.S. and Zeleznik, A.J. (1984). The rhesus monkey corpus luteum is dependent upon pituitary gonadotropin secrtion throughout the luteal phase of the menstrual cycle. Endocrinology, 115:1780-1786.
12. Hutchison, J.S. and Zeleznik, A.J. (1985). The corpus luteum of the primate menstrual cycle is capable of recovering from a transient withdrawal of pituitary gonadotropic support. Endocrinology, 117:1043-1049.
13. Hutchison, J.S., Nelson, P.B. and Zeleznik, A.J. (1986) Effects of different gonadotropin pulse frequencies on corpus luteum function during the menstrual cycle of rhesus moonkeys. Endocrinology, 119: 1964-1971.
14. Zeleznik, A.J. and Little-Ihrig, L.L. (1990) Effect of reduced luteinizing hormone concentrations on corpus luteum function during the menstrual cycle of rhesus monkeys. Endocrinology, 126:2237-2244.
15. Hutchison, J.S., Kubik, C.J., Nelson, P.B. and Zeleznik, A.J. (1987) Estrogen induces premataure luteal regression in rhesus monkeys during spontaneous menstrual cycles but not in cycles driven by exogenous gonadotropin releasing hormone. Endocrinology, 121:466-474.
16. Stouffer, R.L. Nixon, W.E., Gulyas, B. and Hodgen, G.D. (1977) Gonadotropin-sensitive progesterone production by rhesus monkey luteal cells in vitro: a function of age of the corpus lueum during the menstrual cycle. Endocrinology, 100: 506-512.
17. Fisch, B., Margara, R.A., Winston, R.M.L. and Hillier, S.G. (1989) Cellular basis of luteal steroidogenesis in the human ovary. J. Endocrinol., 122:303-311.
18. Bassett, S.G., Little-ihrig, L.L., Mason J.I. and Zeleznik, A.J. (1991) Expression of messenger ribonucleic acids that encode for 3β-hydroxysteroid dehydrogenase and cholesterol side-chain cleavage enzyme throughout the luteal phase of the macaque menstrual cycle. J. Clin. Endocrinol. Metab., 72:362-366.
19. Ravindranath, N., Little-Ihrig, L.L. and Zeleznik, A,J. (1991). Gonadotropic regulation of mRNA levels in corpora lutea during the primate menstrual cycle. Proceedings of the seventy-third annual meeting of the Endocrine Society, Washington DC, abstract 348.
20. Ravindranath, N., Little-Ihrig, L.L. and Zeleznik, A.J. (1992) Characterization of the levels of messenger ribonucleic acid that encode for luteinizing hormone receptor during the luteal phase of the primate menstrual cycle. J. Clin. Endocrinol. Metab., 74:779-785.
21. Brannian, J.D., Shigi, S.M. and Stouffer, R.L. (1991) Differential uptake of fluorescent-tagged low deensity lipoprotein by cells from the primate corpus luteum; isolation and characterization of subtypes of small and large luteal cells. Endocrinology, 129:3247-3253.
22. Corner, G.W. Jr., (1956) The histological dating of the human corpus luteum of menstruation. Am. J. Anat., 98:37-65.

Transgenic Manipulation of Reproduction

D.W. Lincoln

MRC Reproductive Biology Unit, University of Edinburgh Centre for Reproductive Biology, 37 Chalmers Street, Edinburgh EH3 9EW, UK

Mammalian reproduction, through the process of meiosis and the subsequent fusion of haploid gametes, including the interchange of material between sister chromatids and mutation, allows for some restructuring of the genome between one generation and the next. When projected over a time frame that might encapsulate a thousand or more generations, these reproductive processes have permited, when combined with natural selection, the development of great biological diversity. Far more rapid changes in the genetic constitution of animals have been established by man, first by selective breeding and more recently by the development of assisted reproduction (artificial insemination, embryo transfer, and cloning). Thus modern breeds of domestic and laboratory animals now exhibit only a general resemblance to the wild ancestors from which they were derived, combined with a reduction in genetic diversity. Indeed, steps are now required to prevent many of the traits enhanced by selective breeding over the past two hundred years from being lost in the near future, possibly through the long-term cryopreservation of embryos. The rigorous selection that has been applied in the breeding of domestic species has also served to minimise the expression of deleterious genes. Thus inherited diseases are a relatively minor concern in the veterinary field. One positive by-product of this rigorous selection process has been the discovery of a number of genetic anomalies, usually involving point mutations or small deletions in the genome of laboratory species, that reveal information regarding physiological processes - the experiments of nature. These include, in a reproductive context, the hypogonadal mouse with its inability to produce GnRH (5).

The human species, by contrast, has maintained most of its genetic diversity, save for the loss of some primitive tribes. Furthermore, the increased mobility of people within the past half century and the intermarrying of different races has perhaps served to broaden the genetic diversity of the individual. Many of the medical advances of the past century have, in addition, served to counter some aspects of natural selection. The incidence of some of the less dehabilitating inherited diseases, for example, is now rising due to medical treatments that allow affected individuals to survive to reproductive age and beyond. There are some 2500 inherited diseases related to the human genome; each is rare, but collectively these diseases are expressed in about 2% of the population. Infertility now afflicts 10-15% of all couples, a rate without parallel in the world of animal husbandry. Indeed, most men, if selected on the standards of semen quality applied in animal breeding, would find themselves on the way to the abbatoir. The many approaches to assisted conception introduced in the past decade are also allowing some couples to reproduce who in the past would not have been able to do so. Man has now to be regarded as a relatively poor reproductive specimen despite the global population explosion, and the situation is not improving.

Transgenic procedures, centred on the insertion of new genetic material into the genome, bypass the natural process of genetic recombination, and permit one to achieve in a single step changes in genomic structure, either by chance or design, that far exceed anything observed in nature. The microinjection of naked DNA into the pronuclei of fertilised eggs is the most widely used technique. Alternative techniques are under development, notably the use of retroviral vectors and embryonic stem cells. These techniques have been extensively reviewed in several recent publications (3,10).

Transgenic technology was wide application. Scientists involved in fundamental research stand to benefit enormously from the ability to manipulate gene structure in order to study the regulation of molecular and cellular processes, and endocrinological, immunological, reproductive and neurological mechanisms etc. Central to this research will be the design of cell lines and animal models within which biological processes have been modified for analytical purposes, and the production of animal models that simulate features of human disease (3). Those working in the field of animal production, on the other hand, have an interest in developing ever more elaborate ways to manipulate the genome in order to improve the efficiency of growth and feed conversion, to improve product characteristics, and to generate novel products of pharmaceutical importance in the medical world. The most striking achievement to date has perhaps been the production of human α_1-antitrypsin at high levels in the milk of sheep. Those working in the medical field, in contrast, have quite different goals and face major ethical obstacles regarding the manipulation of the human genome. More effective ways are required to monitor inherited diseases and to prevent deleterious genetic changes associated, for example, with ageing and environmental factors. Modern advances in the amplification of DNA have transformed the diagnostic perspective, and made it possible to probe for inherited disorders in just a few blastomeres of a still viable pre-embryo. Correcting those defects by transgenic procedures is out of the question for the moment at least, but the situation could change if reliable methods of homologous recombination were established. Somatic gene therapy is quite another matter. One practical application, now close to realisation, centres on the genetic manipulation of stem cells from bone marrow for the correction of haemopoietic diseases. Such technology could open a new medical era with somatic gene therapy being applied in a wide range of situations, which could include the treatment of post-menopausal osteoporosis and the long-term regulation of fertility.

Our ability to contemplate such radical steps, as those indicated above, relates to the breathtaking advances that have been made within the past decade in the ability 1) to analyse genomic structure and its regulation at the nucleotide level, 2) to selectively modify DNA structure and to synthesise new constructs, and 3) to introduce these constructs into the germ line of the gonads, thus allowing the modified genes to be passed to subsequent generations. There are still many bottlenecks and limitations to this technology.

Adding inserts to the genome is relatively straightforward. However, insertion is at random and the number of tandem repeats of the construct that are inserted at each site can range from 1-100. It is extremely rare for an insert to occupy its correct place in the genome. The mechanisms governing the process of insertion remain a matter of complete speculation. The random addition of multiple copies of a construct is a recipe for chaos, in some respects, with regard to regulation, level of expression, tissue specificity of expression, phenotypic development and physiological function. However, this first generation approach to transgenics produced many important observations, and some that were quite unexpected. The aberrant expression of genes in transgenic animals has been associated with a multitude of developmental and physiological abnormalities - the product of an unbalanced genome. The abnormal expression of factors regulating growth has produced both dwarf and giant animals, with muscle development in some cases exceeding skeletal adaptation. The uncontrolled expression of inserted genes, some generating analogues to regulatory peptides, have produced fascinating effects with regard to the down regulation of receptor mechanisms (1). Random inserts, irrespective of their genetic constitution, have themselves generated reproductive effects through the disruption of endogenous genes. Interestingly, many of these disruptive insertions appear to targeted genes involved in sperm function, generating impaired fertility in the offspring (2, 8). The expression of foreign genes in tissues other than those of interest is commonplace, and this placed a severe handicap on the first generation technology. Genetic ablation techniques, introduced below, have limited application if they destroy cells and tissues outwith those strategically targeted.

The heterogeneous nature of each transgenic insert continues to present the major logistic problem. Which line does one most actively pursue? Which lines should be stored as frozen embryos for later analysis? Which lines should be discarded? Work has been largely limited to the use of mice and is likely to remain so. These offer many advantages, including the ease of pronuclear injection, large litter size, rapid geneneration time, and low space requirements.

It is, for the moment, virtually impossible to redesign cells and tissues to a degree that they can assume complex biochemical processes, such as the synthesis of specific steroids or prostaglandins, where a requirement exists for the interaction of a cascade of enzymes - the products of many genes. Homologous recombination, where the objective is to replace one DNA sequence with another at a precise point within the genome, remains very much the target of current technical developments. However, a second generation of transgenic manipulations, within which these goals are now visible, is dramatically changing the picture, converting transgenic manipulations into a more predictable science.

Genes are being linked to different promotors to generate tissue specific expression, to generate immortalised cell lines and to permit genetic ablation, for example. The linking of a tissue specific regulatory element to a cellular toxin (toxigenes) permits the selective ablation of cells (4). Cell suicide occurs the moment that the gene is expressed. Alternatively, the inserts may be designed to express a precursor element, such that a cellular toxin is only produced at some later time through the administration of an exogenous agent. Genetic ablation has a multitude of applications in the reproductive field. Indeed, linking the GnRH gene to a precursor toxicant could be used in animal husbandry to procure endocrine castration. Linking the regulatory elements of endocrine genes to oncogenes (SV40 T-antigen) has allowed the production of immortalised transgenic tumour cell lines with specified properties (7,9). The αT3-1 pituitary cell line provides one example. This expresses the α-subunit of LH and the GnRH receptor (11). A similar approach has been used to produce GnRH-secreting, immortalised and, most important of all, well differentiated hypothalamic neurones (6,9). The tumours and tumour cells derived from these procedures are heterogeneous, and require clonal selection. Interestingly, many of these cell lines are far more differentiated than the cell lines that have been available hitherto - a feature of potential value.

Research in the reproductive field has been transformed in the past by technical advances, as in the development of immunological assays, the purification and sequencing of peptides, the production of monoclonal antibodies and immunohistochemistry, the cloning and synthesis of DNA for in situ hybridisation, and DNA sequencing for the structural analysis of complex hormones. Transgenic procedures promise to transform every aspect of biological research to an even greater degree, at times, turning science fiction into reality. In due course, these procedures could well generate fundamental and far reaching changes in both medical therapy and commercial animal production. Practical emphasis in the immediate future will undoubtedly centre on the controlled manipulation of genes for the evaluation of physiological processes, the generation of transgenic cell lines and animal models for the simulation of human diseases, and the use of farm species for the production of medically important proteins.

REFERENCES

1. Chen, W.Y., White, M.E., Wagner, T.E. and Kopchick, J.J. (1991) Functional antagonism between endogenous mouse growth hormone and a growth hormone analog results in dwarf transgenic mice. Endocrinology, 129:1402-1408.
2. Gordon, J.W., Pravicheva, D., Poorman, O.A., Moses, N.J., Brock, W.A. and Ruddle, F.H. (1989) Association of foreign DNA sequences with male sterility and translocation in a line of transgenic mice. Som. Cell Mol. Gen., 15:569-578.
3. Hooper, M.L. (1990) Genetically engineered animals: implications for the understanding and treatment of human disease. Biofuture, 86:30-35.
4. Kendall, S.K., Saunders, T.L., Jin, L., Lloyd, R.V., Glode, LK.M., Nett, T.M., Keri, R.A., Nilson, J.H. and Camper, S.A. (1991) Targeted ablation of pituitary gonadotropes in transgenic mice. Mol. Endocrinol., 5:2025-2036.
5. Mason, A.J., Pitts, S.L., Nikolics, K., Szonyi, E., Wilcox, J.N., Seeburg, P.H. and Stewart, T.A. (1986) The hypogonadal mouse: reproductive functions restored by gene therapy. Science, 234:1372-1378.
6. Mellon, P.L., Windle, J.J., Goldsmith, P.C., Pedula, C.A., Roberts, J.L. and Weiner, R.I. (1990) Immortalization of hypothalamic GnRH neurons by genetically targeted tumorigenesis. Neuron, 5:1-10.
7. Mellon, P., Windle, J.J. and Weiner, R. (1991) Immortalization of neuroendocrine cells by targeted oncogenesis. Rec. Prog. in Horm. Res., 47:69-96.
8. Merlino, G.T., Stahle, C., Jhappan, C., Linton, R., Mahon, K.A. and Willingham, M.C. (1991) Inactivation of a sperm motility gene by insertion of an epidermal growth factor receptor transgene whose product is overexpressed and compartmentalized during spermatogenesis. Genes Devel., 5:1395-1406.
9. Radovick, S., Wray, S., Lee, E., Nicols, D.K., Nakayama, Y., Weintraub, B.D., Westphal, H., Cutler, G.B. Jr. and Wondisford, F.E. (1991) Migratory arrest of gonadotropin-releasing hormone neurons in transgenic mice. Proc. Natl. Acad. Sci. USA, 88:3402-3406.
10. Wilmut, I, Hooper, M.L. and Simons, J.P. (1991) Genetic manipulation of mammals and its application in reproductive biology. J. Reprod. Fertil., 92:245-279.
11. Windle, J., Weiner, R. and Mellon, P. (1990) Cell lines of the pituitary gonadotrope lineage derived by targeted oncogenesis in transgenic mice. Mol. Endocrinol., 4:597-603.

Transgenesis and Infertility

R. Al-Shawi, J. Burke, J.O. Bishop, J.J. Mullins,
R.M. Sharpe[1], R. Lathe and L. Mullins

AFRC Centre for Genome Research, University of Edinburgh, King's Buildings, West Mains Road, Edinburgh EH9 3JQ. [1]MRC Reproductive Biology Unit, University of Edinburgh Centre for Reproductive Biology, 37 Chalmers Street, Edinburgh EH3 9EW, UK

INTRODUCTION

Infertility is a common problem, with possibly 10% of married couples remaining childless as a result. Although infertility can arise from a variety of causes, including developmental and endocrine disorders and infective agents, in many cases a substantial genetic component seems likely. However, the nature of the disease precludes easy assessment of the genetic component and a clear genetic etiology has only been demonstrated in diseases such as cystic fibrosis, myotonic dystrophy and familial male infertility. Because of the obvious selective disadvantage the finding that such a large proportion of the population is subfertile or infertile may argue that reproduction requires complex interplay between the products of a large number of genes. In support of this view, infertility is found at a surprisingly high frequency in transgenic rodents. Some 10% of transgenic insertion mutations are associated with infertility, although translocations associated with transgene insertion and consequent impairment of chromosomal synapsis at meiosis may play a role.

Transgenic intervention has not been widely used in the specific study of reproductive disorders. However, in a number of cases the analysis of transgenic animals has made an indirect contribution to the field. This paper introduces the topic of transgenic animals and reviews experiments in which transgenesis gives insights into the molecular mechanisms of infertility.

TRANSGENIC ANIMALS

Transgenic animals harbour new gene combinations and transmit them to their offspring. Gene constructs are most commonly introduced by microinjection of several hundreds of copies of the DNA construct into a pronucleus of the fertilised egg and, following reimplantation and development, 10 to 20% of the pups born carry between 1 and 100 copies of the transgene integrated at random into a single chromosomal location (31). Although little is known of the mechanism of integration, the transgene usually integrates as a tandem repeat and disrupts the chromosomal gene at the site of insertion. Although transgenesis has been achieved in a variety of species, including rabbit, sheep, goat and cattle, most work to date has been performed in mice and to a lesser extent in rats.

INFERTILITY AND GROWTH HORMONE

Some of the earliest transgenic animals were generated by injection of DNA constructs encoding growth hormone with a view to accelerating growth. As a recipient strain Hammer et al. (16) employed the dwarf little (*lit*) mouse strain which is deficient in growth hormone and shows reduced growth, delayed onset of puberty and male behavioural infertility. Transgenic animals were generated by injecting rat growth hormone (rGH) sequences, under the control of regulatory regions from the widely-expressed metallothionein II (MT) gene, into *lit/lit* eggs. These *lit/lit*, MT-rGH animals express large amounts of GH in their serum (1,400 to 30,000 ng/ml; normal values are usually considerably less than 250 ng/ml) and show a dramatic restoration of growth. However, mutant and normal females expressing GH were found to be infertile. In the male transgenics only 15 of 20 founder transgenics were fertile, nevertheless, their F1 progeny showed normal fertility even though GH over-expression was maintained.

To address the requirement for GH in normal fertility Behringer et al. (6) produced transgenic animals harbouring a fusion construct between GH regulatory regions and the cytotoxic diphtheria toxin A chain (DT-A). Expression of DT-A in pituitary somatotrophs was found to lead to specific destruction of GH-secreting cells and consequent dwarfism. Animals of both sexes displayed severely reduced fertility. However, the number of PRL-secreting cells in the pituitary was also reduced although the extent of the reduction was not as great as for GH cells (6). In contrast, Struthers et al. (1991) produced transgenic mice expressing a transcriptionally-inactive form of the cAMP response element binding protein, CREB, under the control of GH regulatory sequences. cAMP serves as a mitogenic signal in anterior pituitary somatotrope cells, and the overexpressed inactive CREB would be expected to compete with wild-type CREB activity and block the response to cAMP. As predicted, mice of both sexes showed a marked deficiency in pituitary somatropes (but not in other cell types) and pronounced dwarfism, demonstrating that the cAMP/CREB is involved in the proliferation of somatotropes in the pituitary. Surprisingly, however, infertility was not reported, although the extent of GH deficiency was not determined.

More recently we (5) generated transgenic mice harbouring human growth hormone (hGH) sequences under the control of the regulatory region of the ubiquitously-expressed gene encoding hydroxymethyl glutaryl CoA reductase (HMGCR). Peripheral blood hGH levels in HMGCR-hGH mice were typically in the range 1,000-4,400 ng/ml. and transgenic male mice expressing high levels of hGH were found to be of normal fertility. In contrast, all female transgenic mice were infertile, with one exception (a founder transgenic female which produced a single litter but was subsequently infertile).

The mechanism by which excess GH causes female infertility is unclear. It is of note that female patients with hyperprolactinaemia often present with amenorrhea and infertility. Because hGH can interact efficiently with the murine prolactin (PRL) receptor (9) many of the effects of excess hGH may be mediated through this receptor. This view is supported by the finding that transgenic mice over-expressing ovine GH, which does not react efficiently with the murine PRL receptor (9), have normal fertility (29). In addition, transgenic mice expressing growth hormone releasing factor (GRF) under MT control show increased growth rates and elevated serum levels of mouse GH (average mGH level 465 ng/ml). However, female fertility is normal (17). The infertility observed in mice expressing rat GH (above) may be attributed to the very high levels of circulating GH in these animals (1,400-30,000 ng/ml) and concentration-driven cross reaction with the PRL receptor.

GRF stimulation of pituitary somatotropes results in activation of receptor coupled Gs protein, activation of adenyl cyclase, and GH release. Burton *et al.* (13) constructed transgenic mice harbouring a construct in which an intracellular form of cholera toxin, a non-cytotoxic and irreversible activator of the Gs protein, was linked to the rat GH promoter. In such animals the toxin, expressed specifically in somatotropes, leads to constitutive secretion of GH. The average serum mGH level of F1 transgenics (558 ng/ml) was over 21-fold higher than that of controls (<26 ng/ml) with individual values as high as 2940 ng/ml, and marked growth enhancement was observed. However, no male or female infertility was reported (13).

These findings are to be contrasted with data with human patients where uncontrolled production of GH, as in gigantism and acromegaly, results in reproductive disorders in both females and males. Patients with acromegaly have circulating GH concentrations which rarely exceed 300 ng/ml (normal values are less than 5 ng/ml). However, in contrast to the situation in rodent, hGH seems to cross-react with the human prolactin receptor (10) and infertility may be mediated by this interaction.

In depth analysis of GH-mediated fertility has been performed by Bartke *et al.* (4) who showed that MT-hGH transgenic females exhibit cyclic changes in ovarian activity and produce fertilisable ova. However, PRL levels were markedly reduced from 6.9 ng/ml in controls to 3.8 ng/ml in transgenic females. Daily injections of progesterone, starting on day 1 post-coitum, led to maintenance of pregnancy in a number of animals, suggesting that inadequate luteal function may contribute to infertility. Naar *et al.* (28) examined animals transgenic for bovine GH (bGH) expressed under MT or phosphoenolpyruvate carboxykinase (PEPCK) control. Most MT-bGH or PEPCK-bGH females had changes in vaginal smears indicative of oestrous cycling but showed differing degrees of infertility including increased interval between pairing and conception, reduced number of litters, reduced fetal growth with increased fetal mortality, and sex ratio alterations. bGH, like ovine GH, is not lactogenic in rodents, but the high levels of bGH in these animals may also lead to cross-reaction with the PRL receptor and inhibition of luteal function.

PRL (and hence overexpression of GH) is thought to suppress LH and FSH secretion by inhibiting the activity of neurones secreting gonadotrophin releasing hormone (GnRH) in the hypothalamus. However, a direct inhibitory effect on gonadotrope function may also make a contribution (14). It is also of note that GH release in mammals is pulsatile rather than constant. Further, the pattern of pulsatility is sexually dimorphic in rodents. It cannot be excluded that some of the effects of constitutive GH secretion are related not only to the level of the hormone but also to the absence of a pulsatile release pattern.

GONADOTROPHIN TRANSGENES

Lutenising hormone (LH) and follicle stimulating hormone (FSH) play key roles in reproduction by stimulating the regulated production of sex steriods. LH and FSH are produced by pituitary gonadotropes in response to GnRH secretion from the hypothalamus, and hypogonadal (*hpg*) mice deficient in GnRH are sexually immature and display arrested germ cell development. Mason *et al.* (24) restored the normal phenotype by introducing an intact GnRH gene into homozygous *hpg* mice: females showed normal oestrus cyles and carried healthy litters to term while males displayed correct mating behaviour.

Conversely, Kendall *et al.* (20) were able to genetically ablate the pituitary gonadotropes of transgenic mice by injecting a construct in which the cytotoxic diphtheria toxin A chain was linked to regulatory regions from the bovine LH/FSH alpha subunit. Transgenic animals showed loss of pituitary gonadotropes, deficiency of both FSH and LH, marked reproductive deficit, and lack of gonadal differentiation. Despite the fact that the alpha subunit is normally also expressed in thyrotropes, no thyrotrope degeneration was observed and levels of circulating T4 were normal.

OTHER TRANSGENES CAUSING INFERTILITY

Overexpression of any of a number of genes can interfere with fertility. For instance, expression of Müllerian inhibiting substance is reported to block uterine and ovarian development (7) and expression of alpha interferon in the testes of transgenic mice leads to sterility (18). Similarly, inappropriate expression of oncogenes can lead to infertility - *int2* causes male infertility by inducing epithelial hyperplasia similar to prostatic hypertrophy (26,30) and expression of SV40 large T antigen under the control of the GnRH promoter arrests neuronal migration during development and may provide an animal model of human hypogonadotrophic hypogonadism (33).

INFERTILITY THROUGH GENE DISRUPTION IN HOMOZYGOTES

Infertility through transgene insertion provides a valuable tool to the dissection of molecular mechanisms of infertility: molecular cloning of the insertion mutation, using the transgene as a hybridisation probe, will permit the characterisation of the gene whose disruption leads to sterility.

There are a number of instances where transgene expression does not itself cause infertility but where insertion of the transgene has disrupted a locus necessary for fertility. Because transgene insertion only disrupts one copy of the resident gene backcrossing between transgenic animals is required to reveal the effect on fertility. Examples include disruptions of the the symplastic spermatids (*sys*) locus, leading to abnormal spermatid maturation (23), the germ-cell deficient (*gcd*) locus (32), and a sperm motility gene (25). This latter disruption, due to the insertion of a beta-actin/EGF receptor transgene, leads to a loss of sperm motility reminiscent of Kartagener's syndrome (see Reference 1).

Of particular interest are two reports where transgene insertion may have taken place into known loci linked to infertility. Kruwlewski *et al.* (21) report a mutation caused by insertion of a SV40-DHFR transgene. Heterozygous males and females of both genotypes were normally fertile while homozygous transgenic males were sterile. Inspection of homozygous males revealed testes devoid of late spermatids and epididymes containing no mature sperm. In view of similarities with mice mutant at the Purkinje cell degeneration (*pcd*) locus, crossing was performed between transgenic and *pcd* mice: heterozygous *pcd*/transgenic mice produced by crossing the two strains were shown to have sterility defects indicating that the transgene may disrupt the *pcd* locus.

Gordon *et al.* (15) report insertion of the same SV40-DHFR transgene into a second locus linked to infertility. Homozygous transgenic males, but not females, were sterile, while homozygous animals of both sexes showed ataxia. With the exception of one azoospermic animal, total and motile sperm counts were not significantly affected but the efficiency of in vitro fertilisation of intact oocytes was reduced 5-fold. The combination of ataxia with reduced fertilisation efficiency was thought to render males functionally sterile. Similarities with the hotfoot (*ho*) mutant strain of mice prompted crossing between the two strains, and the transgene insertion mutation failed to complement the *ho* mutation, indicating allelism.

DOMINANT GENE DISRUPTION AND INFERTILITY

Certain genetic disorders occur at elevated frequencies because they are X-linked (e.g. haemophilia). In view of the high frequency of male infertility, both X-linked and dominant mutations may play a role. An example of the latter is the insertional mutant mouse (*Lvs*; lacking vigorous sperm) of Magram and Bishop (22). No expression of the transgene was detected in this mutant, suggesting that it was indeed an insertional mutant. When the junction fragments containing DNA flanking the transgene insertion site were cloned, EcoRI polymorphisms were identified which represented the normal and disrupted locus. Interestingly, both male and female transgenics displayed the same pattern of EcoRI-generated bands, indicating an autosomal insertion site for the transgene. Light and electron microscopy revealed that spermatogenesis in this mouse line proceeds normally up to the point of nuclear condensation, when the nuclei become misshapen.

Following introduction of the mouse Ren-2 gene (as a 25 kb genomic fragment containing the entire renin structural gene, with 9 kb of upstream sequences and 5 kb downstream) into the rat genome (27) a number of different transgenic lines were generated. Several of these exhibited hypertension, and tissue surveys revealed that the transgene was expressed in a number of tissues including the kidney, adrenal glands, and the testis. One of these lines also demonstrated male infertility, suggesting that the phenotype might not be due to expression of the transgene per se, but rather to insertional inactivation of a gene important in the attainment of male fertility. The founder in TgRmRen2-26 was a female, and all female progeny carrying the transgene exhibit normal fertility. Transgenic males were found to be capable of mating (as measured by plug formation in the vagina) but were incapable of producing pregnant females.

Closer examination revealed that the sperm count was reduced. Light microscopic examination of sections taken from perfusion-fixed testes from control and transgenic littermates revealed no gross differences in spermatogenesis except in the final steps of spermiogenesis (steps 15-19). During this time period, normal elongate spermatids shed much of their cytoplasm (which is phagocytosed by the Sertoli cells) and are released finally at stage VIII of the spermiogenic cycle, leaving the final remnants of their cytoplasm behind in the form of structures called residual bodies. The latter are then drawn down through the seminiferous epithelium and are phagocytosed by the Sertoli cells. In the transgenic rats, this process of cytoplasmic elimination is abnormal in that 'blobs' of cytoplasm either remain attached to the sperm or are shed into the tubule lumen. Residual body formation and removal still occurs to some extent in the transgenics, and some spermatids are released normally from the epithelium. However, many of the spermatids are not released and remain attached up to at least stage XIV of the spermatogenic cycle. As a result, the epididymes of transgenic rats retain grossly subnormal numbers of spermatozoa, together with abundant 'blobs' of exfoliated spermatid cytoplasm. This presumably explains the infertility of the transgenic rats. At present it is not clear what events in the process of sperm release/cytoplasmic elimination are affected in the transgenics, although the deficiencies are clearly rather subtle. More detailed analysis at the electron microscopic level will be needed to pinpoint the adverse changes.

In an effort to characterise the site of insertion, we have undertaken short and long-range mapping using probes located within the transgene. Initially the transgene was estimated to be present at five copies. Short range mapping (using probes located at the extreme 5' and 3' of the transgene) has revealed that, rather than being a straightforward head-tail concatamer, the transgenes exhibit head-tail, head-head, tail-tail and truncated head-tail junctions. Additional bands, which cannot be accounted for from the above, suggest that the transgene complex is probably inserted at one site in the rat genome, but scrambling at the site of insertion cannot yet be ruled out.

Long-range mapping, using pulse-field gel electrophoresis and rare-cutting restriction enzymes such as NotI, SacII, SalI and BssHII, suggests that there is differential methylation of DNA, between males and females, over a 450 kb region spanning the insertion site (Southern blots were probed with a full length cDNA probe). For example, when high molecular weight DNA prepared from the spleens of male and female transgenics was subjected to such analysis, NotI digestion yielded a 450 kb male-specific fragment (in addition to the 500 kb fragment seen in control as well as transgenic DNA samples, and therefore presumed to be that of the endogenous renin gene). It should be noted that there are two NotI sites within each copy of the transgene. These sites are presumably completely methylated and are therefore not digested by NotI. SacII and BssHII digestions also yielded male and female-specific fragments.

We are at present attempting to determine whether or not the transgene is X-linked. Superficially, the phenotype of the rat line resembles that of the insertional mutant mouse line described by Magram and Bishop (22), but it also shares similarities, particularly regarding spermatid development, with the line described by Braun *et al.* (1990) which expresses thymidine kinase of herpes simplex virus in postmeiotic germ cells. It will obviously be important to analyse the site of expression of the transgene within the testis before the mechanism of its action can be determined fully and these studies are underway.

HETEROLOGOUS GENES AFFECTING FERTILITY

The best example of a heterologous gene affecting fertility is afforded by transgenic mice carrying the thymidine kinase gene of herpes simplex virus type I (HSV1tk). The HSV1tk gene was one of the first reporter genes to be used in transgenic animal work (12,35,36). More recently, it has has been used as a means to achieve conditional and cell-specific ablation in transgenic mice (19,8,37). We and others have created transgenic mice carrying various constructs that include the HSV1tk gene as a reporter (2,3,11,37). In nearly all of the lines established, the males are sterile (2,3). Female mice have normal fertility, and transmit the transgenes with the expected frequency. In all lines, HSV1tk expression is found in the testes irrespective of the promoter to which the HSV1tk gene is linked, suggesting that the HSV1tk structural gene is capable of directing its own expression to this tissue. When a promoterless HSV1tk gene was introduced into the germ-line of mice, this too led to expression of HSV1tk in the testes confirming the above conclusion. Expression of HSV1tk in other tissues was found to be unique to each construct and was specified by the promoter to which the HSV1tk gene was linked.

Analysis of testis mRNA products from different transgenic lines showed that a number of common transcripts were generated, all of which initiated downstream of the normal cap site and the normal translation initiation codon. The transcripts initiate from a region between the first and second ATG codon, which has a high G+C content, and which is devoid of a TATA-box like motif. We therefore conclude that the HSV1tk gene contains a cryptic promoter similar to those of housekeeping genes, but which is testis-specific (3).

Analysis of protein extracts from transgenic testis shows that two predominant protein products of mol wt 39 kDa and 37 kDa react with an anti-HSVtk antibody. These products are both smaller than the normal HSVtk enzyme (43 kDa), and are consistent with transcription initiation downstream of the first ATG codon and translation from the two proximal downstream ATG codons (Met46 and Met60). Enzyme assays performed on transgenic testis extracts show that both nucleoside and nucleotide kinase activity is elevated, and therefore at least one of the truncated polypeptides is functional, with characteristics similar to those of the full-size enzyme.

Thymidine kinase assays on transgenic testis at various postnatal developmental stages show that activity is present at low levels in the testes of 7-day old mice, the earliest age at which the assay may be performed with confidence. At this stage of mouse development spermatogonia are the only germ-cells present in the testis. Between 10 and 19 days of age there is a moderate increase in the amount of HSV1tk activity, while at around day 21 of age, when the first haploid spermatids appear, there is an abrupt increase in the amount of HSV1tk activity. Immunohistochemistry on mature transgenic testis shows that expression is confined to the spermatids. Because expression is confined to the germ-cell lineage in adult mice, it is likely that the expression in young mice is due to expression in germ cells earlier in the lineage, the spermatogonia and spermatocytes.

The characteristics of the infertility differs with expression levels. Mice expressing high levels of HSV1tk in the testis have low testis weights and low sperm-counts. Sperm isolated from the vas deferens are structurally abnormal and non-motile. Histological examination of transgenic testes shows many abnormally staining spermatogonia and spermatocytes, and the numbers of spermatids and spermatozoa in the tubules are reduced. Large, abnormal cells with degenerate nuclei are present in many tubules, and these are thought to originate from the germinal epithelium. There is no evidence of vasculitis or inflammation, and the intertubular connective tissue contains normal numbers of Leydig cells. In contrast, mice with moderate levels of expression have normal sperm counts and histological sections of the testes do not appear different from those of control animals. Although the sperm appear to be morphologically normal, as determined by light and electron microscopy, they exhibit reduced motility and, unlike non-transgenic sperm, lose their motility after a short period of culture *in vitro*. Mice from moderately expressing lines are able to sire the occasional pup (2) and the sperm are able to fertilize eggs *in vitro* (11).

HSV1tk-mediated sterility does not appear to be restricted to mice since we have evidence that a male transgenic sheep and a male transgenic rat which carry constructs containing the HSV1tk gene as a reporter are also sterile (J.P. Simons, R.A.S., J.J.M., unpublished). Sperm from the transgenic sheep were found to express significant levels of HSV1tk, and had characteristics in common with transgenic mouse sperm (see above).

There are several cases reported where expression of different transgenes has been consistently found in the testis. In some cases expression in the testis was not predicted, whereas in others expression was directed to the germ-cells using the protamine promoter. Where histological examination has been carried out, expression is usually found to be confined to the spermatids. In only one case (18) has expression in the testis been associated with sterility. These results suggest that the sterility of HSV1tk transgenic mice is unlikely to be simply the result of over-expression of a foreign RNA or foreign protein and is more likely to be due to the properties of the HSV1tk enzyme itself. Non-transgenic testis extracts phosphorylate thymidine 2.5 to 10 times less efficiently than transgenic extracts. Unlike the cellular thymidine kinase, HSV1tk is not under tight cell-cycle regulation and has a low km for thymidine. This, together with the fact that the viral thymidine kinase has the ability to phosphorylate both purine and pyrimidine nucleosides, and is not subject to end product inhibition, suggests that nucleotide metabolism is perturbed. This itself could lead to infertility; for instance, a reduction in the level of ATP could give reduced sperm motility.

In high expressing lines, the more severe abnormality requires a different explanation. Expression of HSV1tk in spermatogonia may change the availability of deoxynucleoside triphosphates in these dividing cells. This could result from elevation of the dTTP pool due to the abnormal thymidine kinase activity; dTTP is a feedback inhibitor of both dTTP and dCTP synthesis. The spermatogonia could thus be starved of dCTP, interfering with DNA synthesis, cell division and ultimately, fertility.

CONCLUDING REMARKS

Genetic analysis of the common human condition of infertility is hindered by the lack of linkage data occasioned by restricted transmission of mutant alleles from affected individuals. Transgenic animals afford a means to introduce defined alterations into the mammalian genome and permit the physiological consequences to be determined even in cases where fertility is restricted. The use of transgenic animals may well give fresh insights into the causes of human infertility.

ACKNOWLEDGEMENTS

We wish to thank Dr. S. Bachman for perfusing line TgRmRen2-26 rats, Dr. U. Ganten for providing animals, and Drs. A. Chandley and D. Buxton for assistance with histology. We thank the AFRC for supporting our research.

REFERENCES

1. Aitken, J. (1991). A clue to Kartagener's. Nature, 353:306.
2. Al-Shawi, R., Burke J., Jones, C.T., Simons, J.P. and Bishop, J.O. (1988). A Mup promoter-thymidine kinase reporter gene shows relaxed tissue-specific expression and confers male sterility upon transgenic mice. Mol Cell. Biol., 8:4821-4828.
3. Al-Shawi, R., Burke J., Wallace, H., Jones, C.T., Harrison, S., Buxton, D., Maley, S., Chandley, A. and Bishop, J.O. (1991). The herpes simplex virus type 1 thymidine kinase is expressed in the testes of transgenic mice under the control of a cryptic promoter. Mol. Cell. Biol., 8:4207-4216.
4. Bartke, A., Steger, R.W., Hodges, S.L., Parkening, T.A., Collins, T.J., Yun, J.S. and Wagner, T.E. (1988). Infertility in transgenic female mice with human growth hormone expression: evidence for luteal failure. J. Exp. Zool., 248:121-124
5. Bchini, O., Mehtali, M. and Lathe, R. (1991). Abrogation of dominant glucose intolerance in SJL mice by a growth hormone transgene. J. Mol. Endocrinol., 6:129-135.
6. Behringer, R.R., Mathews, L.S., Palmiter, R.D. and Brinster, R.L. (1988). Dwarf mice produced by genetic ablation of growth hormone-expressing cells. Genes Dev., 2:453-461.
7. Behringer, R.R., Cate, R.L., Froelick, G.J., Palmiter, R.D. and Brinster, R.L. (1990). Abnormal sexual development in transgenic mice chronically expressing M,llerian inhibiting substance. Nature, 345:167-170.
8. Borrelli, E., Heyman, R.A., Adrias, C., Sawchenko, P.E., and Evans R.M. (1989). Transgenic mice with inducible dwarfism. Nature, 339:538-541.
9. Boutin, J-.M., Jolicoeur, C., Okamura, H., Gagnon, J., Edery, M., Shirota, M., Banville, D., Dusanter-Fourt, I., Djiane, J. and Kelly, P.A. (1988). Cloning and expression of the rat prolactin receptor, a member of the growth hormone/prolactin receptor gene family. Cell, 53: 69-77.
10. Boutin, J-.M., Edery, M., Shirota, M., Jolicoeur, C., Lesueur, L., Ali, S., Gould, D., Djiane, J. and Kelly, P.A. (1989). Identification of a cDNA encoding a long form of prolactin receptor in human hepatoma and breast cancer cells. Mol. Endocrinol., 3:1455-1461.
11. Braun, R.E., Lo, D., Pinkert, C.A., Widera, G., Flavell, R.A., Palmiter R.D. and Brinster, R.L., (1990). Infertility in male transgenic mice: disruption of sperm development by HSV-tk in postmeiotic germ cells. Biol. Reprod., 43:684-693.
12. Brinster, R.L., Chen, H.Y., Trumbauer, M., Senear, A.W., Warren, R. and Palmiter, R.D. (1981). Somatic expression of herpes thymidine kinase in mice following injection of a fusion gene into eggs. Cell, 27:223-231.

13. Burton, F.H., Hasel, K.W., Bloom, F.E. and Sutcliffe, J.G. (1991). Pituitary hyperplasia and gigantism in mice caused by a cholera toxin transgene. Nature, 350:74-77.
14. Cheung, C.Y. (1983). Prolactin suppresses lutenizing hormone secretion and pituitary responses to LHRH by a direct action at the anterior pituitary. Endocrinology., 113:632-638.
15. Gordon, J.W., Uehlinger, J., Dayani, N., Talansky, B.E., Gordon, M., Rudomen, G.S. and Neumann, P.E. (1990). Analysis of the hotfoot (ho) locus by creation of an insertional mutation in a transgenic mouse. Dev. Biol., 137:349-358.
16. Hammer, R.E., Palmiter, R.D. and Brinster, R.L. (1984). Partial correction of murine hereditary growth disorder by germ-line incorporation of a new gene. Nature, 311: 65-67.
17. Hammer, R.E., Brinster, R.L., Rosenfeld, M.G., Evans, R.M. and Mayo, K.E. (1990). Expression of human growth hormone-releasing factor in transgenic mice results in increased somatic growth. Nature, 315:413-416.
18. Heckman, A.C.P., Trapman J., Mulder, A.H., van Gaalen, J.L.M. and Zwarthoff, E.C. (1988). Interferon expression in the testes of transgenic mice leads to sterility. J. Biol. Chem., 263:12151-12155.
19. Heyman, R. A., Borelli, E., Lesley, J., Anderson, D., Richman, D.D., Baird, S.M., Hyman, R. and Evans R. M. (1989). Thymidine kinase obliteration: creation of transgenic mice with controlled immune deficiency. Proc. Natl. Acad. Sci. USA, 86:2698-2702.
20. Kendall, S.K., Saunders, T.L., Jin, L., Lloyd, R.V., Glode, L.M., Nett, T.M., Keri, R.A., Nilson, J.H. and Camper, S.A. (1991). Targeted ablation of pituitary gonadotropes in transgenic mice. Mol. Endocrinol., 5:2025-2036.
21. Krulewski, T.F., Neumann, P.E. and Gordon, J.W. (1989). Insertional mutation in a transgenic mouse allelic with Purkinje cell degeneration. Proc. Natl. Acad. Sci. USA, 86:3709-3712.
22. Magram, J. and Bishop, J.M. (1991). Dominant male sterility in mice caused by insertion of a transgene. Proc. Natl. Acad. Sci. USA, 88:10327-10331.
23. MacGregor, G.R., Russell, L.D., Van Beek, M.E.A.B., Hanten, G., Kovac, M.J., Kozak, C.A., Meistrich, M.L. and Overbeek, P.A. (1990). Symplastic spermatids (sys): A recessive insertional mutation in mice causing a defect in spermatogenesis. Proc. Natl. Acad. Sci. USA, 87:5016-5020.
24. Mason, A.J., Pitts, S.L., Nikolics, K., Szonyi, E., Wilcox, J.N., Seeberg, P.H. and Stewart, T.A. (1986). The hypogonadal mouse: reproductive functions restored by gene therapy. Science, 234:1372-1378
25. Merlino, G.T., Stahle, C., Jhappan, C., Linton, R., Mahon, K.A. and Willingham, M.C. (1991). Inactivation of a sperm motility gene by insertion of an epidermal growth factor receptor transgene whose product is overexpressed and compartmentalised during spermatogenesis. Genes Dev., 5:1395-1406.
26. Muller, W.J., Lee, F.S., Dickson, C., Peters, G., Pattengale, P. and Leder, P. (1990). The int-2 gene product acts as an epithelial growth factor in transgenic mice. EMBO J. 9: 907-913.
27. Mullins, J.J., Peters, J. and Ganten, D. (1990). Fulminant hypertension in transgenic rats harbouring the mouse Ren-2 gene. Nature, 344:541-544.
28. Naar, E.M., Bartke, A., Majumdar, S.S., Buonomo, F.C., Yun, J.S. and Wagner, T.E. (1991). Fertility of transgenic female mice expressing bovine growth hormone or human growth hormone variant genes. Biology Reprod., 45:178-187
29. Orian, J.M., Snibson, K., Stevenson, J.L., Brandon, M.R. and Herington, A.C. (1991). Elevation of growth hormone (GH) and prolactin receptors in transgenic mice expressing ovine GH. Endocrinology, 128:1238-1246.
30. Ornitz, D.M., Moreadith, R.W. and Leder, R. (1991). Binary system for regulating transgene expression in mice: Targeting int-2 gene expression with yeast GAL4/UAS control elements. Proc. Natl. Acad. Sci., USA, 88:698-702.
31. Palmiter, R.D. and Brinster, R.L. (1986). Germ-line transformation of mice. Annu. Rev. Genet., 20:465-499.
32. Pellas, T.C., Ramachandran, B., Duncan, M., Pan, S.S., Marone, M. and Chada, K. (1991). Germ-cell deficient (gcd), an insertional mutation manifested as infertility in transgenic mice. Proc. Natl. Acad. Sci. USA, 88:8787-8791.
33. Radovick, S., Wray, S., Lee, E., Nicols, D.K., Nakayama, Y., Weintraub, B.D., Westphal, H., Cutler, G.B. and Wondisford, F.E. (1991). Migratory arrest of gonadotrophin-releasing hormone neurons in transgenic mice. Proc. Natl. Acad. Sci. USA, 88:3402-3406.
34. Struthers, R.S., Vale, W.W., Arias, C., Sawchenko, P.E. and Montminy, M.R. (1991). Somatotroph hypoplasia and dwarfism in transgenic mice expressing a non-phosphorylatable CREB mutant. Nature, 350:622-624.

35. Wagner, E.F., Stewart, T.A. and Mintz, G. (1981). The human beta-globin gene and a functional viral thymidine kinase gene in developing mice. Proc. Natl. Acad. Sci. USA, 78:5016-5020.
36. Wagner, T.E., Hoppe, P.C., Jollick, J.D., Scholl, D.R., Holinka, R.L. and Gault, J.B. (1981). Microinjection of a rabbit beta-globin gene in zygotes and its subsequent expression in adult mice and their offspring. Proc. Natl. Acad. Sci. USA, 78: 6376-6380.
37. Wallace, H., Ledent, C., Vassart, G., Bishop, J.O. and Al-Shawi, R. (1991). Specific ablation of thyroid follicle cells in adult transgenic mice. Endocrinology, 129:3217-3226

Targeting the Expression of Gonadotrophin Genes

A.J. Clark[1], P. Brown[2], J.R. McNeilly[3], J. Mullins[2] and A.S. McNeilly[3]

[1] AFRC Institute of Animal Physiology and Genetics Research, Edinburgh Research Station, Roslin, Midlothian EH25 9PS
[2] Centre for Genome Research, King's Buildings, West Mains Road, Edinburgh EH9 3JQ
[3] MRC Reproductive Biology Unit, University of Edinburgh Centre for Reproductive Biology, 37 Chalmers Street, Edinburgh EH3 9EW, UK

INTRODUCTION

Growth and development of the preovulatory follicle is controlled by the gonadotrophin hormones, follicle stimulating hormone (FSH) and luteinising hormone (LH) (10,23). Both LH and FSH are heterodimers consisting of a common a subunit and a hormone specific β-subunit. The synthesis and release of these hormones from the gonadotrope cells in the anterior pituitary are positively driven by gonadotrophin releasing hormone (GnRH) released in pulses from the hypothalamus (10), and regulated by feed-back effects of gonadal steroids and inhibin acting at the pituitary and/or hypothalamus (17,11). The molecular and cellular mechanisms whereby these factors interact and control the synthesis and release of these hormones is still, however, unclear.

We have been studying the the control of expression of LH and FSH *in vivo* in sheep at both the hypothalamic and gonadal axes. As well as determining the pituitary and plasma concentrations of these hormones, we have also measured the corresponding mRNA levels in the pituitary using specific molecular probes for the α and β subunit genes. A key factor *in vivo* is the differential synthesis and release of these two hormones and this is reflected by the differential expression of the corresponding hormone-specific β subunit genes. To address the question of differential control we are developing an approach based on the use of transgenic animals in which LH and/or FSH producing cells are specifically ablated *in vivo*.

DIFFERENTIAL CONTROL OF GONADOTROPHINS

GnRH is released from the hypothalamus in a pulsatile manner (10). The amount and pattern of GnRH release is fundamental in the control of the secretion of LH and FSH. We have removed the effect of endogenous GnRH pulses on the pituitary in intact ewes by long term (6 weeks) treatment with a GnRH agonist ([D-Ser(But)^6]-GnRH (1-9) nonapeptide-ethylamine; Buserilin, obtained from Hoescht A.G. Frankfurt). This chronic treatment abolishes the responsiveness to GnRH pulses without effect on the other pituitary hormones (22,27).

The absence of GnRH pulses leads to a dramatic down regulation of LH-β gene expression. Thus following agonist treatment the steady-state LH-β mRNA levels were reduced to 5% of the control luteal values (Fig. 1). The absence of GnRH pulses also dramatically decreased the quantity of LH stored in the pituitary to 3% of the control luteal values (Table 1). The fact that LH-β mRNA was reduced but not abolished indicates that there is a basal level of subunit gene expression which is independent of GnRH. This basal level of expression is sufficient to maintain peripheral levels of LH to approximately 50% of the luteal values, although pulsatile release is abolished. Interestingly, the steady-state levels of α mRNA are increased significantly in agonist treated animals (Fig. 1). Despite this increase there is, overall, a dramatic reduction in a subunit levels (in terms of gonadotrophin and free α) in both pituitary and blood, suggesting that translational controls may, in part, be controlling synthesis.

Table 1. *Pituitary weight and concentrations of LH, FSH and free α subunit of pituitaries from ewes on day 14 of the luteal phase (n=4) and after 6 weeks of treatment with an implant of GnRH agonist (Buserilin; GnRHAg; n=5). Results are ± S.E.M. expressed as mg per pituitary protein (data from McNeilly et al., 1991) (23)*

	n	Pit. wt (mg)	Pit. LH (ng/mg)	Pit. FSH (ng/mg)	Pit. free α (ng/mg)
Treatment					
Luteal	4	879±147	3137±693	104±11	606±155
GnRHAg	5	670±43	112±4**	34±2*	171±37*

*$P < 0.05$, **$P<0.001$ compared with luteal control (Student's t-test).

In the absence of GnRH pulses the FSH-β subunit mRNA is decreased (Fig. 1) with a consequent reduction in both pituitary and circulating concentrations of the hormone. The effects of GnRH agonist on all aspects of FSH regulation is, however, much less dramatic than is seen with LH and the mRNA and pituitary levels are reduced to only about 30% of the control luteal values (Fig. 1; Table 1).

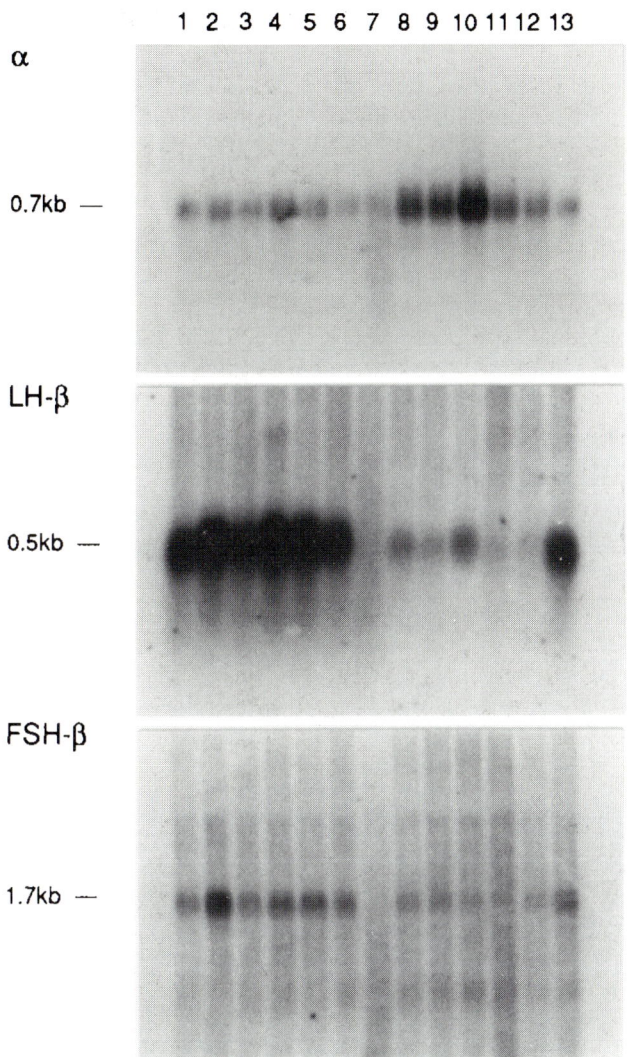

FIG. 1. Northern blotting analysis of sheep pituitary RNA from control (lanes 2-5) and gonodotrophin-releasing hormone agonist treated (lanes 7-12) ewes. Lanes 1,6 and 13 contain total RNA extracted from a pool of adult pituitaries. The hybridisation probes used were bovine α, ovine LH-β and bovine FSH-β cDNAs. The size of the hybridising bands are indicated (data from McNeilly et al., 1991) (23).

We have also begun an investigation on the role of gonadal factors in the control of FSH and LH using oestradiol implants and bovine follicular fluid (as a source of inhibin). Oestradiol implants induce a premature follicular phase and *in vivo* and this treatment leads to a significant increase in FSH-β mRNA, although no increase in circulating FSH is detected. By contrast only a small decrease in LH-β mRNA is observed. Treatment of intact and castrated ewes with inhibin showed that the plasma level of FSH is directly correlated with the corresponding FSH-β mRNA level. Injections of follicular fluid decrease FSH-β mRNA in a dose dependent manner and no effect is observed on LH-β or α-subunit mRNA levels (J.R. McNeilly, unpublished observations).

The control of gene expression, subunit synthesis and hormone secretion are complex but clearly inter-related and a variety of transcriptional and post-transcriptional mechanisms must be operating in the gonadotrope cells. Although the results presented here are limited to sheep it is clear that similar mechanisms are operating in other species (15, 30, 28). A key feature is the differential control of the two hormones. LH is expressed at far higher levels than FSH both in terms of β-subunit mRNA levels and overall pituitary content. In contrast to FSH a high proportion of synthesised LH is stored in the cell during most of the cycle, in what appears to be a highly GnRH-dependent process. Finally, the hormonal feedback controls acting on the two β-subunit genes are clearly different.

MONO-HORMONAL vs MULTI-HORMONAL CELLS

The simplest hypothesis to explain the differential regulation of FSH and LH is that they are produced in different cells. The evidence by *in situ* staining and hybridisation in some species indicates that this may not be the case. Thus in the pig, it is suggested that LH and FSH are present predominantly in the same cell (18). In the rat multi-hormonal LH/FSH producing cells have also been demonstrated and the proportion of these cells shown to vary throughout the reproductive life, apparently dependent on GnRH input. (7,8,9,20). A proportion of monohormonal LH and FSH cells do remain in the rat but it is not known whether these are differentially regulated. Such studies are based on isolating cells from the pituitary and staining *in vitro* and the biological significance is unclear. Furthermore, these results are based on terminally differentiated cells and so it is not possible to determine their developmental relationship. To resolve this issue it is important to understand the cellular origins of gonadotropes and so determine whether distinct FSH and LH cell lineages exist. If distinct cell lineages do exist it will be important to determine how these are regulated *in vivo* and how this contributes to the observed differential control of gonadotrophins. Finally, it should be noted that a recent study using immunocytochemical techniques on pituitary sections has suggested that LH and FSH are, indeed, produced in quite separate cells in the cow (2). This provocative report awaits confirmation.

CELL-SPECIFIC ABLATION

To understand the cellular origins of LH- and FSH- producing cells we are developing an approach that is based on using transgenic animals in which LH and/or FSH producing cells are specifically ablated. The approach involves the transfer of gene constructs comprising cell-specific regulatory elements linked to a DNA sequence encoding a DNA toxin. The toxin is expressed specifically in the cells targeted by the regulatory elements and destroys them. Transgenic mice have been produced in which the somatotropes of the pituitary, the exocrine cells of the pancreas and the lens cell of the eye have been ablated by targeting the A chain of Diptheria toxin (Dt-A) to these cells (3,26,4). In the studies on the somatotropes the Dt-A chain was targeted using the regulatory sequences derived from the rat GH gene. These animals were used to clarify the relationship between GH and prolactin (PRL) producing cells. In mice it had been suggested that PRL producing cells were derived from a GH-producing progenitor. The finding that animals in which the somatotropes were ablated still contained a substantial population of lactotropes showed that not all lactotropes were derived from a GH-expressing progenitor (3).

More recently gonadotrope cells have been ablated in transgenic mice using regulatory sequences from the bovine α-subunit promoter linked to the Dt-A chain (14). The phenotype of these transgenic mice is identical to mice homozygous for the spontaneous mutation *hpg* which is due to a deletion in the gene encoding GnRH. Radioimmunoassay and immunohistochemical staining showed that they lacked LH producing cells whereas the pituitary content of ACTH and GH was normal. This work demonstrates the feasibility of ablating gonadotrope cells and suggests that other pituitary cell types are able to differentiate independently of terminal gonadotrope differentiation and function in the absence of any paracrine signalling that they may provide. The use of regulatory sequences from the common α-subunit, of course, precludes any conclusion about the cellular origins or differential regulation of LH- and FSH-producing cells.

An alternative and elegant method for cell-specific ablation is to use the thymidine kinase (*tk*) gene of Herpes simplex. Under most normal circumstances *tk* is not toxic to the cells in which it is expressed (an exception to this is the testis: expression of the *tk* gene from a cryptic internal promoter in the testis dramatically reduces sperm viability and, hence, male fertility; see page 195). In the presence of specific anti-Herpes drugs such as FIAU and Ganciclovir, which are nucleoside analogues, *tk* expression will kill the cell (6). It is thought that cell killing is due to the phosphorylation of these nucleoside analogues by *tk* and their subsequent incorporation into host DNA. Because the mode of action of *tk* ablation appears to require DNA synthesis it was thought that only actively dividing cells would prove to be a suitable target. Recent work on the ablation of thyroid cells in transgenic mice (29) has suggested, however, that non-dividing tissues are also susceptible to this form of ablation. The *tk* approach enables the inducible ablation of a particular cell type at a chosen stage of development. Furthermore, the ablating agent can be subsequently removed allowing the regeneration of differentiated cell types to be studied.

GONADOTROPE-SPECIFIC EXPRESSION

The pre-requisite for genetic ablation is the appropriate regulatory sequences to target expression of the ablating agent to the desired cell type. As discussed above, a short promoter segment from the bovine α-subunit gene specifically targets the expression of Dt-A to gonadotrope cells (14). The human α-subunit gene promoter has also been shown to target the expression of SV40 T antigen to these cells in transgenic mice (31). Recently the tissue specific expression of the entire bovine FSH-β subunit gene in transgenic mice has been demonstrated (16).

To obtain the appropriate regulatory sequences for targeting expression to LH- and FSH-producing cells we have screened a sheep genomic library with LH-β and FSH-β specific probes. The LH-β subunit gene has been isolated and completely sequenced. The structural gene encompasses approximately 1 kb of chromosomal DNA, comprises 3 exons and shows strong homologies with the previously published bovine and human genes (P. Brown, unpublished observations). A 1.9 kb promoter segment has been isolated from this clone. We have also isolated and characterised clones corresponding to the ovine FSH-β subunit gene (Guzman *et al.*, 1991) and isolated a short promoter segment from this gene.

To test the function and specificity of the LH-β promoter we have fused it to the bacterial reporter gene chloramphenicol aceltyltransferase (CAT) (Fig. 2). This hybrid gene (oLHb-CAT) was excised from the plasmid vector and used to generate transgenic mice by pronuclear injection. Two out of three transgene positive lines were shown to express CAT in the pituitary.

To assess the tissue-specific pattern of expression in transgenic mice CAT activity was measured in a variety of tissues from these lines. High levels of CAT expression were detected in the pituitary but no detectable expression

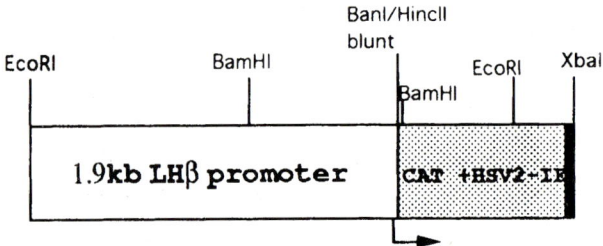

FIG. 2. Structure of oLHβ-CAT. The 1.9 kb promoter segment from the ovine LHβ gene was fused to a CAT reporter gene.

was observed in any other of the tissues examined (Fig. 3). This demonstrates that the sheep promoter segment can target expression specifically to the pituitary.

The levels of CAT expression were compared between males and females. In one line the levels of CAT were similar in males and females, whereas in the other the female levels were more than 5-fold higher than the males.

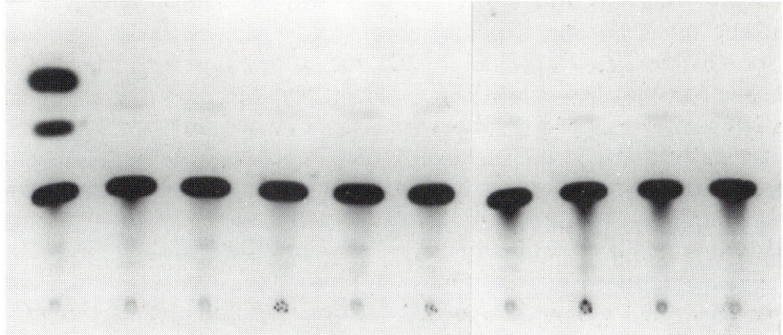

Pituitary Hypothal Salivary Thyroid   Lung   Spleen   Adrenal   Kidney   Liver   Repro Tract

FIG. 3. Tissue-specific expression of oLHβ-CAT in transgenic mice. Cell extracts from a variety of tissues were analysed for CAT expression. Detectable expression was observed only in pituitary extracts.

This contrasts with the levels of endogenous pituitary LH which was shown to to be approximately three times higher in males as compared to females. The reason for these differences are unknown at present, but may reflect 'position effects' acting at the site of transgene insertion.

To determine if the oLHβ-CAT transgene was under the appropriate feedback control from gonads the effects of castration were assessed. Castrated males showed a marked increase in the level of CAT expression showing that the transgene was under the anticipated feedback control. In female mice a smaller increase of CAT expression was observed after castration.

The above experiments demonstrated that the 1.9 kb ovine LH-β promoter contained the appropriate regulatory elements for targeting expression to the pituitary and, moreover, contained the sequences necessary to mediate negative hormonal feedback regulation by the gonads. To confirm that the promoter targeted expression to the correct cell type within the pituitary *in-situ* immunocytochemistry experiments were performed using anti-sera to CAT protein and to murine LH. The results showed that CAT expression was localised to a small proportion of gonadotrope-like cells in these pituitaries and, moreover, co-localisation experiments suggested these to be LH-producing cells.

From the above experiments we have concluded that the LHβ promoter targets expression to LH-producing cells in the pituitary. We have therefore utilised this segment to construct a hybrid gene designed to target the expression of Dt-A to these cells.

TRANSGENIC MODELS

In animals the vast majority of gene transfer experiments have been carried out in the mouse. It is a convenient laboratory model and the techniques for superovulation, pronuclear injection and surgical transfer are well established in this species. In experienced hands 3-5% of the injected and transferred eggs will give rise to a transgenic mouse. The mouse, however, is not a particularly suitable animal model for analysing the physiological consequences of cell ablation. For example, given that distinct populations of monohormonal and multihormonal gonadotropes do co-exist in the pituitary it would be important to investigate how these different populations of cells are regulated physiologically. The mouse is inappropriate for this type of study and for this reason we have chosen to carry out the ablation experiments in the rat.

The production of transgenic rats has been recently described (25,13). The procedures used are essentially the same as for transgenic mice although the superovulation regimen is somewhat different, requiring a continuous infusion of FSH. In appearance the fertilised eggs are similar to those of mouse; the pronuclei are readily visible and this facilitates microinjection. Overall, the frequency of generating transgenic rats is similar to that observed for mice (25,13). The use of rats will enable us to investigate the physiological consequences of cell ablation, both at the hypothalamic and gonadal axis. Furthermore, rats are a classic model for studying gonadotrope function (11) and hence the consequences of cell ablation can be interpreted in the light of a substantial body of knowledge.

CONCLUDING REMARKS

Studies in sheep and other animals have demonstrated the complex regulation of LH and FSH. Control is exerted from the hypothalamus by GnRH and from the gonads by steroids and inhibin. These various controls act directly at the level of the individual subunit genes to modulate mRNA abundance but also at other levels that control the assembly, storage and release of these hormones. LH and FSH are differentially regulated in the pituitary and an as yet unsolved question is to what degree this due is to specific LH-producing and FSH-producing gonadotrope cells. Cell separation and immunocytochemical approaches have yielded contradictory results, although this may in part be due to significant species differences. Nevertheless if discreet LH- and FSH-producing populations do exist these approaches will not elucidate the developmental relationship between these cells types or enable an investigation of their physiological behaviour *in vivo*. For these reasons we have chosen a transgenic approach which is based upon the specific ablation of LH and/or FSH producing cells. The genes encode ovine LH-β and FSH-β have been cloned and promoter segments isolated. The LH-β promoter has been linked to a CAT reporter gene and introduced into transgenic mice. Tissue-specific and hormonally regulated CAT expression was observed and *in-situ* immunocytochemistry confirms that the LH-β promoter targets expression to a discrete population of LH-producing cells. This promoter segment has been linked to the gene encoding the A chain from Diptheria toxin and is being introduced into transgenic rats. We have elected to use rats because they will enable a physiological assessment of the consequences of ablation. Ultimately, we anticipate that such animals will provide a unique resource to study the mechanisms of fertility.

REFERENCES

1. Al-Shawi, R., Burke, J., Jones, C., Harrison, S., Buxton, D., Maley, S., Chandley, A. and Bishop, J.O. (1991). The herpes simplex virus type 1 thymidine kinase is expressed in the testes of transgenic mice under the control of a cryptic promoter. Mol. Cell. Biol., 11:4207-4216.
2. Bastings, E., Beckers, A., Reznik, M. and Beckers, J-F. (1991). Immunocytochemical evidence for the production of luteinising hormone and follicle stimulating hormone in separate cells in the bovine. Biol. Reprod., 45:788-796.
3. Behringer, R.R., Mathais, L.S., Palmiter, R.D. and Brinster, R.L. (1988). Dwarf mice produced by genetic ablation of growth hormone expressing cells. Genes Dev., 2:453-461.
4. Breitman, M.L., Rombola, H., Maxwell, I.H., Klintworth, G.K. Bernstein, A., (1990). Genetic ablation in transgenic mice with an attenuated diptheria toxin A gene. Mol. Cell. Biol., 10:474-479.
5. Borrelli,E., Heyman, R., Hsi, M. and Evans, R.M. (1988). Targeting an inducible toxic phenotype in animal cells. Proc. Natl. Acad. Sci., 86:7572-7576.
6. Borrelli, E., Heyman, R., Arias, C., Sawchenko, P.E. and Evans, R.M. (1989). Transgenic mice with inducible dwarfism. Nature, 339:538-541
7. Childs, G., Ellison, D., Foster, L. and Ramaley, J.A. (1981). Endocrinology, 109:1683-1692.
8. Childs, G., Unabia, G., Tibolt, R. and Lloyd, J.M. (1987). Cytological factors that support non-parallel secretion of LH and FSH during the estrous cycle. Endocrinology, 121:1546-1558.
9. Childs, G.V., Unabia, G., Wierman, M.E., Shupnik, M.A. and Chin, W.W. (1990). Castration induces time-dependent changes in the follicle-stimulating hormone β-subunit messenger RNA ribonucleic acid-containing gonadotrope cell population. Endocrinology, 126:2205-2213.
10. Clarke, I. J. and Cummins, J.T. (1982). The temporal relationship between gonadotrophin releasing hormone (GnRH) and luteinising hormone (LH) in ovariectomised ewes. Endocrinology, 111:1737-1739.
11. Gharib, S.D. Wierman, M.E., Shupnik, M.A. and Chin, W.W. (1990). Molecular biology of the pituitary gonadotropins. Endocr. Rev., 111:177-199.
12. Guzman, K., Miller, C.D., Philippes, C.L. and Miller, W.L. (1991). The gene encoding ovine follicle-stimulating hormone β; Isolation, characterisation, and comparison of a related ovine genomic sequence. DNA and Cell Biol., 10:593-601.
13. Hammer, R.E., Maika, S.D., Richardson, J.A., Tang, J.P. and Taurog, (1990). Spontaneous inflammatory disease in transgenic rats expressing HLA-B27-associated human disorders. Cell, 63:1099-1112.

14. Kendall, S.K., Saunders, T.L., Jin, L., Lloyd, R.V., Glode, L.M., Nett, T.M., Keri, R.A., Nilson, J.H. and Camper, S.A. (1991). Targeted ablation of pituitary gonadotropes in transgenic mice. Mol. Endocrinol., 12:2025-2036.
15. Kim, W.H., Swerdloff, R.S. and Bhasin, S. (1988). Regulation of alpha and rat luteinising hormone beta messenger ribonucleic acids during gonadotropin-releasing hormone agonist treatment *in vivo* in the male rat. Endocrinology, 123:2111-2116.
16. Kumar, T.R., Fairchild-Huntress, V., Low, M.J. (1992). Gonadotrope-specific expression of the human follicle-stimulating hormone β-subunit gene in the pituitaries of transgenic mice. Mol. Endocrinol., 6:81-90.
17. Lincoln, D.W., Fraser, H.M., Lincoln, G.A., Martin, G.B. and McNeilly, A.S. (1985). Recent Prog. Horm. Res., 41:369-419.
18. Liu, Y.C., Kato,Y., Inoue, K., Tanaka,S. and Kurosumi, K. (1988). Co-localisation of LH-β and FSH-β mRNAs in the porcine anterior pituitary by *in situ* hybridisation with biotinylated probes. Biochem. Biophys Res. Commun., 251:291-299.
19. Lloyd, J.M. and Childs, G.V. (1988). Changes in the number of GnRH receptive cells during rat estrous cycle: biphasic effects of estradiol. Neuroendocrinology, 48:138-146.
20. McNeilly, A.S. (1988). The control of FSH secretion. Acta Endocrinol., 288:31-40.
21. McNeilly, A.S. and Fraser, H.M. (1987). Effect of gonadotrophin releasing hormone agonist-induced suppression of LH and FSH on follicle growth and corpus luteum functon in the ewe. J. Endocrinol., 115:273-282.
22. McNeilly, A.S., Picton, H.M., Campbell, B.K. and Baird, D.T. (1991). Gonadotrophic control of follicle growth in the ewe. J. Reprod. Fertil. Suppl. (in press).
23. McNeilly, J.R., Brown, P., Clark, A.J. and McNeilly, A.S. (1991). Gonadotrophin-releasing hormone modulation of gonadotrophins in the ewe: evidence for differential effects on gene expression and hormone secretion. J. Mol. Endocrinol., 7:35-43.
24. Mullins, J.J., Peters, J. and Ganten, D. (1990). Fulminant hypertension in transgenic rats harbouring the mouse Ren-2 gene. Nature, 344:541-543.
25. Palmiter, R.D., Behringer, R.R., Quaife, C.J., Maxwell, F., Maxwell, I.H. and Brinster, R.L. (1987). Cell lineage ablation in transgenic mice by cell-specific expression of a toxin gene. Cell, 50:435-443.
26. Picton, H.M., Tsonis, C.G. and McNeilly, A.S. (1990). FSH causes a time-dependent stimulation of pre-ovulatory follicle growth in the absence of pulsatile LH secretion in ewes chronically treated with gonadotrophin-releasing hormone. J. Endocrinol., 126:297-307.
27. Rodin, D.A., Lalloz, M.R.A. and Clayton, R.N. (1989). Gonadotropin releasing hormone regulates FSH-β subunit expression in the male rat. Endocrinology, 125:1282-1289.
28. Wallace, H., Ledent, C., Bishop, J.O. and Al-Shawi, R. (1991). Specific ablation of thyroid cells in adult transgenic mice. Endocrinology, 129:3217-3226.
28. Wierman, M.E., Rivier, J.E. and Want, C. (1989). Gonadotropin releasing hormone-dependent regulation of gonadotropin subunit messenger ribonucleic acid levels in the rat. Endocrinology, 124:272-278.
30. Windle, J.J., Weiner, R.I. and Mellon, P.L. (1990). Cell lines of the pituitary gonadotrope lineage derived by targeted oncogenesis in transgenic mice. Mol. Endocrinol., 4:597-603.

Dominant Negative Mutants of the Activin A Gene

A.J. Mason

*Department of Endocrine Research, Genentech, Inc.
460 Point San Bruno Boulevard
South San Francisco, CA 94080, USA*

INTRODUCTION

Activin A is a member of the transforming growth factor-β family, which was originally isolated based on the ability to stimulate follicle stimulating hormone (FSH) release from pituitary cells (12). Activin A is a homodimer of two $β_A$ subunits, whilst activin AB and activin B are a heterodimer and homodimer of the $β_A$ and $β_B$ subunits, respectively. Activin has diverse roles in reproduction, erythroid differentiation, and mesodermal differentiation in amphibians (2,10). During development activin induces different regions of dorsoventral tissues in a dose-dependent manner as well as anterior structures in axial pattern formation. Activin inhibits retinoic acid induced differentiation of P19 cells and some types of neuroblastoma cells (13,11, 4). Activin A and activin B have been shown to be equipotent in many of the above *in vitro* assays. Studies of the distribution and timing of activin A and B mRNA expression suggest further that activin A and B can have different roles, e.g. activin B mRNA is expressed earlier than activin A mRNA in embryogenesis (11).

Clearly, activin is involved in a large number of pleotrophic events. Techniques in molecular biology can be harnessed to analyze these in detail. Recent advances have made it possible to construct mice that are deficient in a particular gene product (1,5). Analysis of such animals can provide many clues to the role of the protein in development. The use of the gene 'knock out' technique to study the role of activin may yield some interesting results, but the deleterious effects of such a mutation could be lethal in the homozygote. We have chosen to use the alternative approach of dominant negative mutants in trying to discern the many effects of activin (6). By this technique the function of a gene can be blocked at the protein level. To achieve this the cloned gene is altered so that it encodes a mutant product capable of inhibiting the wild type gene product, thus causing the cell to be deficient in the function of the gene product. Such a mutation is both dominant and negative. We set out to generate such a mutant of the β_A subunit of activin A. Such a subunit could also be expected to form dimers with the α-inhibin subunit. Hence the presence of mRNA and protein for the α and β_B subunit complicate this scenario. For this reason we have decided to demonstrate the usefulness of a dominant negative mutant of activin A in the erythroid differentiation system since it has been shown that only the β_A mRNA is present (8). Furthermore the use of a dominant negative mutant of activin A targeted for bone marrow expression may provide clues as to how essential activin A is for erythroid differentiation. The following addresses the use of mutagenesis to find a dominant negative mutant of activin A which could be used in transgenic animals.

Since activin A is a homodimer of two β_A subunits, and dimerization is necessary for activity, we reasoned that mutants of one of the 9 cysteine residues in each subunits may interfere with intracellular dimerization. Mutants of each of the 9 cysteines were analyzed. An alternative approach of removing the Arg5 processing site from activin A was also used to try to generate a biologically inert dimer.

RESULTS

Mutagenesis of Human Activin A

The activin A molecule is synthesized as a 426 amino acid precursor. The pro-region contains four cysteine residues (Fig. 1). A mutant in which these four cysteines were changed to alanines was constructed by *in vitro* mutagenesis, to determine if these cysteines were essential for dimerization of pro-activin A

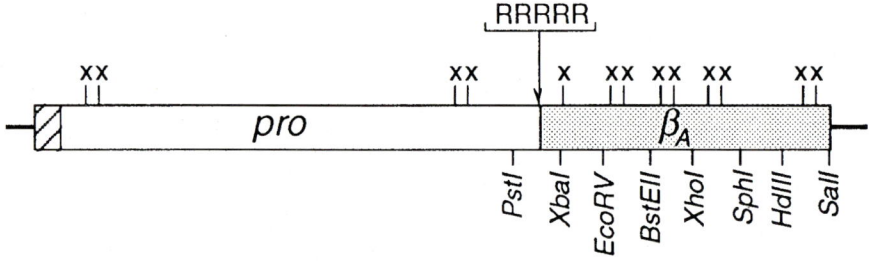

FIG. 1. Diagrammatic representation of pre-pro activin A protein. The position of the cysteine residues 1-13 are indicated by "X's". Position of unique six bp restriction sites used to construct pActA are as indicated. Mutants 1-4, 5, 6, 7, etc., have the corresponding cysteines replaced by alanine residues. The position of the five consecutive arginines is indicated by the arrow and 5R's.

The active region of activin A is 116 amino acids in length. To facilitate the generation of a large number of mutants a synthetic activin gene was constructed. The restriction map is shown in Fig. 1, along with the position of the nine cysteine residues. Unique six base-pair restriction sites were inserted into the activin A coding sequence to create plasmid pActA (3). These restriction sites did not change the reading frame and could be used to generate mutants. For example, to generate cysteine mutant number 5 a synthetic fragment with XbaI and EcoRV cohesive ends and the triplet coding for Cys5 changed to code for alanine was used to replace the native XbaI–EcoRV fragment. In this way each cysteine mutant could be quickly generated. Activin cDNAs in which each of the cysteine residues was substituted with an alanine (mutants Cys5 to 13) were constructed. Integrity of the clones was confirmed by DNA sequencing.

The mutant Δ5R, which is missing arginine residues 220 to 225, was generated by digesting pActA with PstI and XbaI and inserting a synthetic PstI–XbaI fragment in which the bases coding for Arg residues were deleted (see Fig. 1).

Expression of the Mutant Proteins in Transfected 293S Cells

The mutant activin cDNA constructs of cysteine mutants 1 to 13 were cloned into a cytomegalovirus expression vector (9). A human embryonic kidney cell line 293 was used to check the expression of the mutant protein (9). Thus, cysteine mutant 1-4 was transfected into 293 cells and the cells were metabolically labeled with [^{35}S]cysteine and methionine. In cells transfected with the wild type activin A cDNA construct a 40 to 50 kDa pro-region molecule and the 25 kDa activin A homodimer were secreted (see Fig. 2, lanes 13 and 14). As can be seen in Fig. 3 lane 2, the mutant Cys1-4 had the same bands as with the wild-type construct. This suggests that cysteine residues 1-4 are not necessary for dimer formation. In a similar

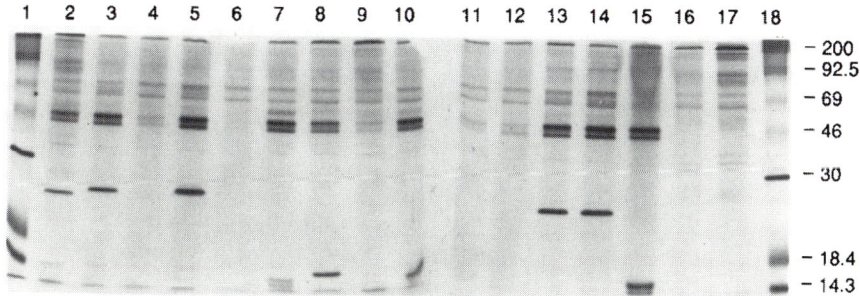

FIG. 2. 293 cell expression pattern of cysteine mutant proteins analyzed under non-reducing conditions. 293 cells were transfected with mutant constructs and pulse labeled with [^{35}S]cysteine and methionine. Lane 1, M.W. markers; lane 2, Cys1-4; lane 3, Cys5; lane 4, Cys6; lane 5, Cys7; lane 6, Cys8; lane 7, Cys9; lane 8, Cys10; lane 9, Cys11; lane 10, Cys12; lane 11, Cys13; lane 12, Cys12-13; lane 13, pActA; lane 14, wild-type β_A cDNA; lane 15, wild-type β_A cDNA reduced; lane 16, 17, mock transfected cells; lane 18, M.W. markers.

fashion cysteine mutants 5-13 were tested. With cysteine mutants 5 and 7 an activin A dimer was secreted (see Fig. 2, lanes 3 and 5). Interestingly the mutants 5 and 7 migrated at a higher molecular weight than wild type activin A. Activin dimers missing either cysteine 5 and 7 are still active in an FSH release assay (data not shown). Cysteine mutants 9, 10 and 12 were secreted as monomers (see Fig. 2, lanes 7, 8 and 10). They migrate at slightly different positions suggesting that they are folded in different fashions.

293 cells transfected with the Δ5R construct were found to secrete a molecule of ~100 kDa (see Fig. 3, lane 5). This corresponds to a dimer of two full length subunits. In repeated experiments antisera (both monoclonal and polyclonal) failed to recognize the Δ5R protein (data not shown). Heat treatment of the supernatant with heat enabled monoclonal 3D9 to recognize the Δ5R protein (Fig. 3, lane 6); this antibody is specific for recombinant activin A.

Biological Activities

Cysteine mutants that were secreted from tissue culture cells were tested for biological activity in the erythroid differentiation K562 assay. Dimers of Cys5 and Cys7 possess activin activity in the K562 assay. Specific

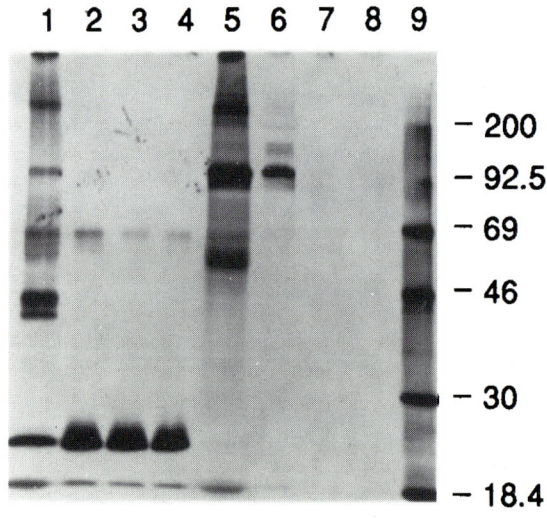

FIG. 3. Transfection of 293 cells with activin A and Δ5R protein. Lanes 1-4 are with β_A construct; lane 1, cell supernatant; lane 2, immunoprecipitate with MAb 3D9; lane 3, immunoprecipitate MAb 2E10, lane 4, immunoprecipitate with MAb mix: lane 5-8 are with the Δ5R construct; lane 1 cell supernatant, note the presence of a 100 kD protein; lane 6-8, immunoprecipitates of Δ5R supernatants with MAb 3D9; MAb 2E10 and MAb mix. Lane 9, molecular weight markers. MAb were generated against recombinant activin A.

activities were not determined. Mutants 9, 10, and 12 and the Δ5R protein possess undetectable levels of activin activity (data not shown). This Δ5R data would suggest that the processing event is an essential part in the activin biosynthetic pathway.

Expression of Cysteine 9 Mutant Decreases the Amount of Wild-type Activin A Secreted in Transfected 293 Cells

Cotransfection of Cys9 DNA with wild type activin A DNA resulted in decreasing amounts of wild type activin A being secreted. As shown in Fig. 4, transfection of a 10-fold excess of Cys9 decreased wild-type β_A dimers below detectable level (Fig. 4, lanes 1-3). Testing of an identical mutant of activin β_B designated β_BCys9 had a similar effect on activin β secretion (Fig. 4, lanes 4 and 5). A similar mutant of TGF-β had analogous effects on TGF-β secretion. At this stage it looked like Cys9 mutants could be used as a dominant negative mutant of activin A, but we were concerned that the overexpression of this protein may affect the secretion of other proteins. We chose to examine the effects of Cys9 mutants on human growth hormone (hGH) secretion. Our results indicate that although wild-type activin A, B, or TGF-β expression does not affect hGH secretion (Figs. 2-4), the cysteine

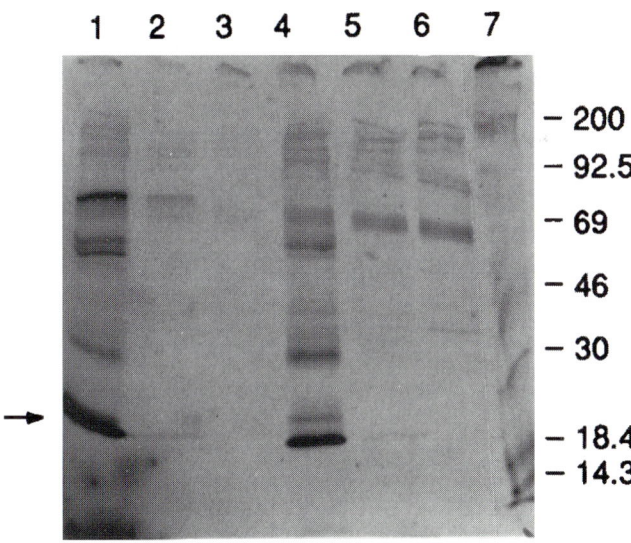

FIG. 4. Co-transfection of mutant cysteine constructs and wild-type activin constructs were transfected at 1:10 ratio with Cys9 constructs. Cell supernatants were immunoprecipitated with an activin A MAb or activin B MAb and analyzed under non-reducing conditions. Lane 1, wild-type activin A; lane 2, β_ACysA9 and wild-type activin A at ratio 10:1; lane 3, β_ACysA9; lane 4, wild-type activin B; lane 5, β_BCys9 and wild-type activin β at ratio 10:1; lane 6, mock transfected cells.

9 mutants interfere with hGH secretion (Fig. 5, lane 1). These results may be explained if the accumulation of misfolded Cys9 molecules interferes with the overall secretion process of the cell.

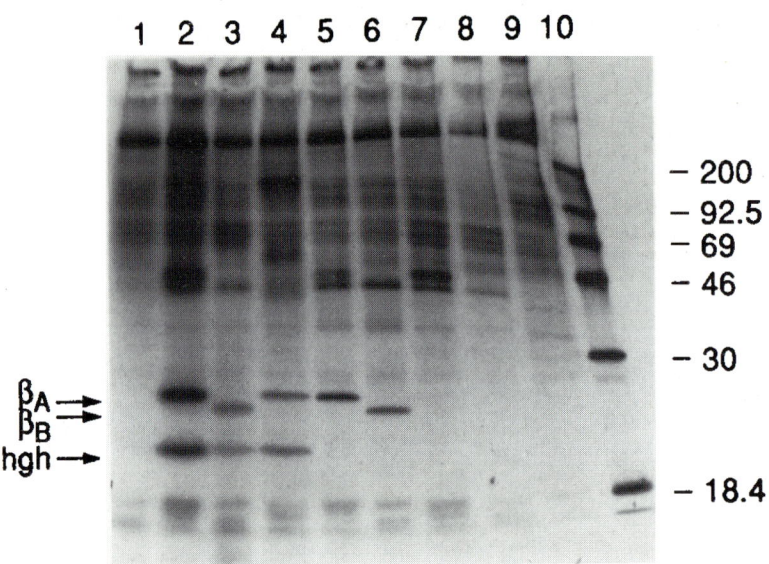

FIG. 5. Co-transfection of cysteine mutants and hGH. Cells were transfected as listed, labeled with [^{35}S]cysteine and methionine and analyzed by non-reducing gel electrophoresis. The migration position of activin A, activin B and hGH are indicated by arrows. Lane 1, hGH and β_BCys9; lane 2, hGH and β_A; lane 3, hGH and β_B; lane 4, hGH and TGF-β; lane 5, β_A; lane 6, β_B; lane 7, β_A and β_BCys9; lane 8, β_B and β_BCys9; lane 9, mock transfected cells; lane 10, molecular weight markers.

Overexpression of Δ5R Prevents the Accumulation of Activin A Dimers

As shown in Fig. 6, expression of Δ5R and wild-type activin construct at a 1:1 ratio results in decreased 25 kDa activin dimer secreted (lanes 7 and 8). The majority of the protein is present as partially processed 66 kDa protein and a ~100 kDa dimer (lane 7). Expression of Δ5R and activin A at a 10:1 level decreases the amount of activin A secreted to below detection (lanes 5, 6). No biological activity was found in the supernatants of cells expressing a 10-fold excess of Δ5R. This suggested that the overexpression of Δ5R in a cell producing activin A protein would nullify any activin produced. Experiments with hGH suggested that the expression of Δ5R didn't interfere with hGH secretion, as had been observed with the cysteine 9 mutants.

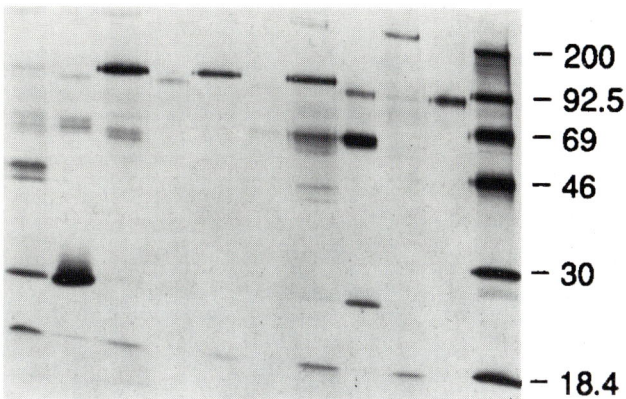

FIG. 6. Co-transfection of wild-type activin A and Δ5R protein. Lane 1, activin A; lane 2, immunoprecipitates of activin A; lane 3, Δ5R protein; lane 4, immunoprecipitate of Δ5R; N.B., Δ5R does not react with polyclonal Ab; lane 5, transfection of Δ5R and activin A at 10:1 ratio; lane 6, immunoprecipitate of same; lane 7, transfection of Δ5R and activin A at 1:1 ratio; lane 8, immunoprecipitate of same; lane 9, mock transfection; lane 10, immunoprecipitation of mock transfected cells.

Design of Transgenic Experiments

As outlined in the introduction we choose to test the Δ5R dominant negative mutant in a simple system in transgenic animals. We decided to express the Δ5R protein in a tissue in which only the β_A mRNA is detected, the bone marrow, though it is unclear which particular cell type expresses activin A in this tissue. Since activin is observed in developing erythroleukemia cells (7) it is possible that red blood cells may produce activin. We constructed vectors in which the human β-globin promoter and enhancer was fused to genomic β_A activin and Δ5R genomic constructs. It is hoped that the use of the human β globin protein will delay expression of the activin transgenic proteins until erythropoiesis switches from the yolk sac to the liver.

DISCUSSION

We have designed a mutant of activin A which can be used as a dominant negative mutation. This mutation (Δ5R) removes the arginines of the activin processing site, the resulting 100 kDa dimer produced is biologically inactive. More importantly hybrids of Δ5R and wild-type activin A appear to be biologically inactive in culture. Vectors designed to express the Δ5R protein in red blood cells have been constructed. It is hoped that mice transgenic for these constructs may demonstrate the usefulness of this approach in analysing the *in vivo* effects of activin and inhibin. If successful the effects of activin in reproduction, mesodermal differentiation and neurological development may be explored.

REFERENCES

1. Capecchi, M.R. (1989) Altering the genome by homologous recombination. Science, 244:1288-1292.
2. Eto, Y., Tsuji, T., Takezawa, M., Takano, S., Yokogawa, Y. and Shibai, H. (1987) Purification and characterization of erythroid differentiation factor (EDF) isolated from human leukemia cell line THP-1. Biochem. Biophys. Res. Commun., 142:1095-1103.
3. Gray, A. and Mason, A.J. (1990) Requirement for activin A and transforming growth factor-β1 pro-regions in homodimer assembly. Science, 247:1328-1330.
4. Hashimoto, M., Kondo, S., Sakurai, T., Etoh, Y., Shibai, H. and Muramatsu, M. (1990) Activin/EDF as an inhibitor of neural differentiation. Biochem. Biophys. Res. Commun., 173:193-200.
5. Hasty, P., Ramirez-Soles, R., Krumlauf, R. and Bradley, A. (1991) Introduction of a subtle mutation into the Hox-2.6 locus in embryonic stem cells. Nature, 350:243-246.
6. Hershowitz, I. (1987) Functional inactivation by dominant negative mutations. Nature, 329:219-222.
7. Murata, M., Eto, Y., Shibai, H., Sakai, M. and Muramatsu, M. (1988) Erythroid differentiation factor is encoded by the same mRNA as that of the inhibin β_A chain. Proc. Natl. Acad. Sci. USA, 85:2434-2438.
8. Meunier, H., Rivier, C., Evans, R., Vale, W. (1988) Gonadal and extragonadal expression of inhibin α, β_A and β_B subunits in various tissues predicts diverse functions. Proc. Natl. Acad. Sci. USA, 85:247-251.
9. Schwall, R.H., Nikolics, K., Szonyi, E., Gorman, C. and Mason, A.J. (1988) Recombinant expression and characterization of human activin A. Mol. Endocrinol., 2:1237-1242.
10. Smith, J.C., Price, B.M., Van Nimmen, K.V. and Huylebroeck, D. (1990) Identification of a potent *Xenopus* mesoderm-inducing factor as a homologue. Nature, 345:729-731.
11. Thomsen, G., Wool, T., Whiteman, M., Sokol, S., Vaughan, J., Vale, W. and Melton, D.A. (1990) Activins are expressed early in *Xenopus* embryogenesis and can induce axial mesoderm and anterior structures. Cell, 63:485-493.
12. Vale, W., Rivier, J., Vaughan, J., McClintock, R., Corrigan, R., Woo, W., Karr, D. and Spiess, J. (1986) Purification and characterization of an FSH releasing protein from porcine ovarian follicular fluid. Nature, 321:776-779.
13. Van den Eijnden-Van Raaij, A.J.M., Van Zoelent, E.J.J., Van Nimmen, K., Koster, C.H., Snoek, G.T., Durston, A. and Huylebroeck, P. (1990) Activin-like factor from a *Xenopus laevis* cell line responsible for mesoderm induction. Nature, 345:732-734.

Assisted Reproduction in Women

D.T. Baird

Department of Obstetrics and Gynaecology, University of Edinburgh, Centre for Reproductive Biology, 37 Chalmers Street, Edinburgh EH3 9EW, UK

INTRODUCTION

In spite of the dramatic increase in the population of the world, a significant proportion of couples remain infertile. Studies by James Y. Simpson and Matthews Duncan in the mid-19th century documented that 10-15 per cent of marriages remained childless. The prevalence of infertility in developed countries today remains very similar, although detailed population studies defining the incidence by specific diagnosis are lacking. In the last 35 years, increasing knowledge of the physiological mechanisms involved in the control of the reproductive system have led to the development of methods of treating certain types of infertility. Amongst the most successful is the treatment of anovulation with gonadotrophins and obstructive tubal disease by *in vitro* fertilisation and embryo transfer (IVF-ET). Although these methods of 'assisted reproduction' have provided hope for thousands of couples who would otherwise have remained childless, problems still remain.

INDUCTION OF OVULATION WITH GONADOTROPHINS

Induction of follicular development and ovulation with gonadotrophins was first described by Gemzell and Roos in 1938. With appropriate selection of hypogonadotrophic women, a pregnancy rate per cycle similar to that observed in normal fertile couples can be achieved. However, this high success rate conceals the fact that about 25 per cent of the pregnancies are multiple with a very high perinatal mortality and morbidity. Attempts have been made to reduce the number of follicles which are stimulated to develop, by adjusting the dose of follicle stimulating hormone (FSH) to simulate the changes in gonadotrophin secretion which occurs during a normal cycle. However, accurate and repeated adjustment of the dose of FSH is difficult due to the very long half-life of the human gonadotrophin (hMG) (~48 hours). It has been proposed that gonadotrophin molecules could be produced by recombinant techniques with much shorter half-lives (e.g. 4 hours) which is similar to that found in pituitary gonadotrophins. The role of luteinising hormone (LH) in the process of selecting a single follicle for ovulation, requires to be investigated further. The addition of LH significantly reduces the number of ovulatory follicles stimulated by injection of FSH in sheep and rats. Thus, the LH induced androgen production may be important in hastening atresia of non selected large antral follicles.

CONSTRAINTS TO SUCCESS IN IVF

In spite of extensive research over the last 14 years, IVF still remains a relatively inefficient procedure. The delivery rate per cycle remains at approximately 15 per cent even although 2-3 embryos are replaced into the uterus. It has been proposed that the in vitro culture system is sub-optimal, that the uterine environment is relatively unfavourable for implantation and that the endocrine environment associated with superovulation results in premature regression of the corpus luteum. However, the fact that the pregnancy rate per cycle is directly related to the number of embryos transferred, suggests strongly that the quality of the embryos is all important. Direct analysis of embryos formed in vitro has demonstrated that approximately 30 per cent show major chromosome abnormalities which are incompatible with normal development. These abnormalities, which include trisomies and monosomies, arise at the first or second meiotic division of the oocytes and are a consequence of the poor quality of the oocyte. The fact that the incidence of errors in meiosis rises with maternal age suggests strongly that the low pregnancy rate following IVF in women over the age of 40 years is due to defective oocytes. Further evidence for this hypothesis is provided by the results of studies involving donor oocytes. The pregnancy rate in older women given donor oocytes from younger women is very high and the implantation rate per embryo is similar whether they are placed in the uterus of the donor women or in that of the recipients. The cause of the decline in oocyte quality with age is unknown but it may reflect cumulative damage to the cytoskeleton of the egg or the chromosomes themselves by environmental factors. The possibility of treating agonadal women with transplants of oocytes from younger women is raised by the studies of Roger Gosden reported in this session (see page 237).

Superovulation Strategy

S. Franks and E.J. Owen

*Department of Obstetrics and Gynaecology
St Mary's Hospital Medical School
Imperial College of Science Technology and Medicine
London W2 1PG, UK*

INTRODUCTION

The normal human menstrual cycle is characterized by unifollicular ovulation, but the pregnancy rate following egg collection during natural cycles or in superovulated cycles where only one embryo is available after in vitro fertilisation (IVF), is considerably less than that observed after successful superovulation (9,4). This point is illustrated by the data shown in table 1. The pregnancy rate after transfer of two embryos was twice that observed when only one embryo was transferred. The pregnancy rate was even higher if the two 'best' embryos could be selected from a pool of three or more but, not surprisingly, the rate of twin pregnancy was higher in this group.

Table 1. *Outcome of IVF treatment according to number of embryos transferred (adapted from Dawson et al., 1991) (Reference 4)*

embryos	cycles	pregnancies	single	twin	triplet
1	160	22 (14%)	20		
2 (of 2)	160	45 (28%)	30	4	
2 (>2)	355	151(43%)	72	49	
3 (of 3)	174	63 (36%)	35	16	4
3 (>3)	485	211(44%)	99	62	22

The aim of ovarian stimulation for an IVF programme, therefore, is to achieve multiple oocytes. Induction of follicular maturation is normally dependent upon the inter-cycle rise in follicle-stimulating hormone (FSH); the principle of super-ovulation strategy is to amplify and/or prolong FSH stimulation of developing follicles (9).

CHOICE OF TREATMENT FOR SUPEROVULATION

Amplification and/or prolongation of the inter-cycle rise in FSH can be achieved by increasing and extending secretion of endogenous FSH (for example, by the use of clomiphene citrate or pulsed gonadotrophin releasing hormone [GnRH]), by the administration of exogenous gonadotrophins or by a combination of these methods. The use of clomiphene alone has the advantages of simplicity and low cost, but the follicular response is variable and it cannot be considered reliable enough for routine use. Treatment with clomiphene in the early part of the follicular phase (amplification of endogenous FSH) followed by administration of exogenous gonadotrophins from the mid-follicular phase cycle, has proved a popular and effective strategy for superovulation. It is, however, more difficult to control the ovarian response when compared to the use of gonadotrophins alone. In the latter case, the dose of gonadotrophin can be 'titrated' against the follicular number and oestradiol response. This is particularly desirable in women who either respond poorly to superovulation or, conversely, hyper-respond to treatment, as descibed below. There is no evidence that the use of 'pure' FSH (Metrodin, Serono) gives more favourable results than that of HMG; indeed, gonadotrophin preparations with minimal or no luteinising hormone (LH) activity may be *less* effective in stimulating folliculogenesis in subjects rendered functionally LH deficient by the use of GnRH analogues.

One of the most common reasons for cancellation of a superovulation cycle is the occurrence of a premature LH surge triggered by supra-physiological concentrations of oestradiol. Fleming and colleagues (7) introduced the use of a long-acting agonist analogue of GnRH for management of induction of ovulation in infertile patients. Following suppression of endogenous gonadotrophins, ovulation was subsequently induced by human menopausal gonadotrophin (HMG). A premature LH surge and 'premature luteinisation' can thereby be prevented. This strategy was applied to superovulation therapy for IVF by Porter *et al.* (24), and has subsequently been adopted by a large number of groups not only for the management of 'poor responders' (31, 27), but also as a first-line treatment (for review see Reference 12). The principal advantage of combined GnRH agonist and gonadotrophin therapy is that it allows more flexibility in the timing of egg collection. There remains controversy about whether combined treatment improves the chance of successful pregnancy. The results of the few controlled prospective studies will be discussed below.

Comparison of Superovulation Regimens

Despite the plethora of papers describing and comparing various methods of superovulation, there have been very few randomised, prospective controlled clinical trials. Most of these have focused on the use of GnRH analogues (GnRHa). Pregnancy rates were reported to be significantly higher following combined therapy when compared with gonadotrophin alone in two studies (22, 26), but four other studies revealed no significant difference in outcome between the two treatments (2,6,18,14).

More recently, simplified protocols have been employed for the combined use of GnRHa and gonadotrophins. Rather than waiting until the ovaries have been suppressed, GnRHa, usually delivered by a nasal insufflation, is started just before gonadotrophin injections at the beginning of the menstrual cycle. Treatment with analogue is then continued either until the time of chorionic gonadotrophin (HCG) administration (the so-called 'short protocol'), or simply for three days from day 1 or 2 of the cycle ('ultra-short protocol') (12). In both the long and short protocols a premature LH surge can be prevented, but this is not necessarily the case with the ultra-short protocol. Two recent controlled studies have compared the long and short methods of GnRHa administration. Tan and colleagues (32) retrieved a higher number of oocytes and observed a higher fertilisation rate in IVF cycles following the long, compared with the short, protocol. There was no significant difference, however, in the pregnancy rate per cycle or per embryo transfer. Achyra *et al.* (1992) were likewise unable to find a significant difference in pregnancy rates and, in this study, the number of oocytes and the fertilisation rates were similar in the two groups of subjects.

A useful, four-way comparative study was performed by Kingsland and colleagues (14), who examined a group of 308 patients undergoing their first attempt at IVF, who were randomised treatment with HMG alone, clomiphene citrate and HMG, an ultra-short course of GnRHa and HMG, or ovarian suppression by GnRHa followed by HMG. Interestingly, they could find no significant differences in outcome between any of the protocols used.

In summary, the available data from controlled studies are not in total agreement, but suggest that, overall, no one of the commonly used superovulation regimens confers a significant advantage in terms of successful pregnancy rate per cycle or per embryo transfer. Minor differences in outcome between the studies might be explained by differences in selection criteria for the subjects included. Many centres, however, adopt the pragmatic approach of using GnRH analogues, in the long protocol, so that the timing of egg collection can be more easily programmed for the convenience of patients and medical staff. It would also seem advisable to use GnRHa pretreatment in women who are at greater risk of inappropriate elevation of serum LH concentrations during follicular development, i.e. those with polycystic ovary syndrome (27).

Luteal Phase Support

It is probably not necessary to give hormonal support in the luteal phase if treatment with gonadotrophin alone or gonadotrophin with clomiphene has been used. In a randomised study Buvat *et al.* (3) observed no difference in the outcome of treatment between cycles supported with HCG and those for which no treatment was given during the luteal phase. Luteal phase insufficiency has been reported following combined GnRHa/HMG treatment and, in a randomised trial, the implantation rate was significantly higher in cycles in which the luteal phase was supported with HCG treatment. In practice, it appears to make little difference whether HCG or progesterone is used (34), although HCG therapy may increase the risk of ovarian hyperstimulation.

MONITORING SUPEROVULATION THERAPY

In most centres, superovulation therapy for IVF is monitored by a combination of pelvic ultrasonography and serial measurements of oestradiol and LH. It should also be noted that ultrasound and endocrine assessment before the start of therapy is important in predicting the outcome of treatment. In particular, a polycystic morphology of the ovaries, even in subjects without the typical clinical and endocrine features of polycystic ovary syndrome (8) are more likely to hyper-respond to treatment and may need lower doses of gonadotrophin (see below). Probably the most important pre-treatment endocrine investigation is measurement of serum FSH (see below). During superovulation therapy there is, overall, a good correlation between the number of potential ovulatory follicles and serum oestradiol measurements (9), but a combination of ultrasound scanning and serial oestradiol measurements allows the optimal timing of HCG administration. Serial measurements of LH are mandatory, except perhaps after the use of the long protocol of GnRHa/HMG treatment.

MANAGEMENT OF HYPO-RESPONSIVE PATIENTS

One of the major problems in attempting to assess the usefulness of super-ovulation regimens in the management of hypo-responsive patients is that there is no generally agreed definition of 'poor responders'. A simple and useful definition of poor response is 'inadequate follicular response resulting in cancellation of a cycle' (33). This is commonly a spurious event and may not necessarily recur in a subsequent treatment cycle but repeated hypo-responsiveness is a major problem in management. This is particularly likely to occur in patients greater than 35 years of age, those with elevated basal (or clomiphene stimulated) serum FSH values, with ovarian endometriosis and with extensive pelvic adhesions (33). An elevated serum FSH concentration is undoubtedly a poor prognostic index, and evaluation of pretreatment endocrine profiles in women being considered for IVF has shown that raised serum FSH values may be associated with regular and apparently ovulatory menstrual cycles (29,20,33). The use of a clomiphene stimulation test (i.e. measurement of the FSH following a 5-day course of treatment with clomiphene citrate 100 mg daily) may uncover abnormalities of FSH, predicting poor outcome of treatment in women whose basal FSH value is within the normal range (21,15,33).

GnRH analogues

There is limited evidence to suggest that GnRH analogues may be advantageous in the management of previously poor responders, but, again, data from appropriately controlled trials are difficult to find (17) and it remains unclear whether this is a useful strategy except perhaps when a previous cycle was cancelled due to the occurrence a premature LH surge. There is no evidence that any form of superovulation therapy is useful in women whose hyporesponsiveness is associated with persitently elevated pretreatment FSH concentrations.

Growth hormone

There has been a flurry of interest recently in the use of growth hormone as a co-gonadotrophin. Treatment with recombinant human growth hormone has been shown to reduce the requirements for gonadotrophin in hypogonadotrophic women who underwent induction of ovulation (11). This action of growth hormone may be mediated by insulin-like growth factor-1 (IGF-1), derived either from the circulation or the ovary, but may also be explained by a direct gonadotrophic effect of growth hormone on oestradiol production by granulosa cells of the human follicle (19). Preliminary data from Homburg et al. (10) suggested that the addition of growth hormone to gonadotrophin therapy improved the ovarian response during superovulation in previously poor responders.

Subsequently, Owen et al. (1991) were able to demonstrate, in a randomised prospective clinical trial, that co-treatment with growth hormone reduced the amount of gonadotrophin required and led to an increase in the number of oocytes retrieved in women who received superovulation after GnRHa pre-treatment. One notable feature of this study was an obvious placebo effect, in that poor responders to GnRHa/HMG therapy who had subsequently received the same treatment without growth hormone produced more oocytes than in the previous cycle. The effect was merely amplified in women who received growth hormone and was due mainly to an increased response in those women with polycystic ovaries (Fig. 1). There were insufficient numbers in this study to comment on the effect on pregnancy rate, and we currently await the outcome of larger randomised studies before it is possible to evaluate the place of growth hormone in superovulation treatment regimens.

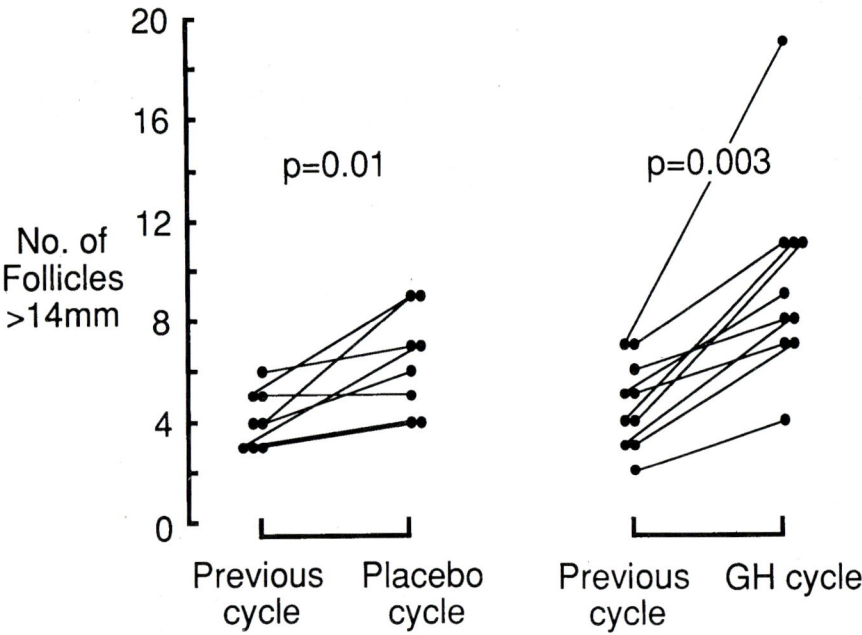

FIG 1. Number of follicles obtained after treatment with GnRHa/HMG +/- growth hormone (GH) in patients with polycystic ovaries who had a previously poor response to superovulation. Note the significant effect of placebo (i.e. GnRHa/HMG alone) but there were more follicles ($P = 0.04$) in the patients who also received GH (from Owen et al., 1991) (Reference 23).

HYPER-RESPONSIVE PATIENTS

Ovarian hyperstimulation syndrome (OHSS) is a well recognised risk associated with multiple follicle development following induction of ovulation or superovulation therapy. In a recent review, Rizk and Smitz (25) reported that the prevalence of moderate and severe hyperstimulation was between 0.6 and 8.4% of cycles. In the two series involving their own centres, and a total of some 3000 cycles, severe hyperstimulation occurred in approximately 1% of cycles, a figure which is probably not very different from that expected following induction of ovulation with gonadotrophins. Nevertheless, it is clear that certain patients are at increased risk of OHSS, notably those with polycystic ovaries. MacDougall and colleagues (16) also reported a prevalence of severe OHSS of around 1% (15 of 1302 cycles) and noted that of these cases of severe hyperstimulation, 11 (73%) occurred in women with the ultrasound appearance of polycystic ovaries. This emphasises the importance of investgating the ultrasound morphology of the ovaries before commencing superovulation. In subjects with polycystic ovaries, the risk of OHSS may be minimised by the combined use of GnRHa and HMG in a long protocol, and by starting gonadotrophin therapy at a relatively low dose (e.g. 1 ampoule per day). If there is an excessive number of follicles, HCG can be withheld and GnRHa continued until follicular activity subsides. It has also been suggested that in any patient from whom more than 10 oocytes have been collected, the use of HCG for luteal support should be avoided (25).

CONTROLLED SUPEROVULATION

The aim of controlled superovulation is to stimulate the development of two or three follicles to a preovulatory stage, a strategy which is particularly appropriate for the management of idiopathic infertility by ovulation induction and intrauterine insemination (IUI) (13).

The principle of this approach is to minimalise the chance of multiple pregnancy, which occurs in some 30% of superovulation/IUI pregnancies (28,5). A recent report of the outcome of multiple pregnancy in 629 IVF pregnancies from Norfolk, Virginia, emphasises the serious sequelae of twin and higher order gestations (30). The rationale for limiting the number of embryos transferred to two seems clear (4) but there may also be a case for reducing the number of follicles stimulated during superovulation for IVF. As shown in the Hammersmith Hospital series (Table 1), the pregnancy rate per embryo transfer was 28% and the twin pregnancy rate was a relatively modest 12% when only two embryos were available for transfer.

Controlled superovulation may seem desirable in theory but in practice it is likely to be difficult to achieve. An obvious approach is to 'titrate' the dose of gonadotrophin against the ovarian response, but the problem with currently available gonadotrophin preparations (including recombinant FSH) is that the half-life of FSH in the circulation is very long. The development of shorter acting isoforms of recombinant FSH would undoubtedly increase the flexibility of FSH treatment.

SUMMARY

Superovulation offers a better chance for pregnancy than natural cycle IVF and remains, therefore, an important part in the management of infertile couples who require assisted conception. Recent data suggest that it is rarely necessary to transfer more than two embryos, so that in future triplet and higher order pregnancies should be avoidable. An examination of the various superovulation regimens shows little difference in efficacy between methods but the use of gonadotrophin releasing hormone analogues in combination with gonadotrophins allows greater flexibility in the timing of egg retrieval. Patients who persistently have an inadequate follicular response to superovulation remain difficult to treat. A raised serum FSH is an important prognostic index of poor response and there is little point in repeated cycles of superovulation in women who have evidence of insipient ovarian failure. Co-treatment with human recombinant growth hormone may be useful in certain subjects with an inadequate follicular response, but, as yet, there are insufficient data from controlled clinical studies to advocate its routine use in the management of poor responders. Severe ovarian hyperstimulation syndrome is a serious complication of approximately 1% of superovulated cycles. Women with polycystic ovaries are at particular risk of OHSS. Modulation of the super-ovulation regimen in women with polycystic ovaries can reduce this risk considerably. The development of recombinant preparations of FSH and LH, particularly shorter acting forms of FSH, may provide further options for control of follicle development in superovulated cycles.

REFERENCES

1. Acharya, U., Hamilton, M., Small, J., Templeton, A. and Randall, J. (1992). Prospective study of short and long regimens of gonadotrophin-releasing hormone agonist in in vitro fertilization program. Fertil. Steril., 57:815-818.
2. Antoine, J.M., Salat-Baroux, J., Alvarez, S., Cornet, D., Tibi, Ch., Mandelbaum, J., et al., (1990). Ovarian stimulation using human menopausal gonadotrophins with or without LHRH analogues in a long protocol for in-vitro fertilization: a prospective randomised comparison. Hum. Reprod., 5:565-9.
3. Buvat, J., Dehaene, J.L., Marcolin, G., Verbecq, P., Herbaut, J-C. and Fourlinnie, J-C. (1988). A randomized trial of human chorionic gonadotrophin support following in vitro fertilization and embryo transfer. Fertil. Steril., 49:458-61.
4. Dawson, K.J., Rutherford, A.J., Margara, R.A. and Winston, R.M.L. (1991). Reducing triplet pregnancies following in vitro fertilisation. Lancet, 337:1543-4.
5. Dodson, W.C. and Haney, A.F. (1991). Controlled ovarian hyper-stimulation and intrauterine insemination for treatment of infertility. Fertil. Steril., 55:457-67.
6. Ferrier, A., Rasweiler, J.J., Bedford, J.M., Prey, K, and Berkeley, A.S. (1990). Evaluation of leuprolide acetate and gonadotropins versus clomiphene citrate and gonadotropins for in vitro fertilization or gamete intra-fallopian transfer. Fertil. Steril., 54:90-5.
7. Fleming, R., Adams, A.H., Barlow, D.H., Black, W.P., McNaughton, M.C. and Coutts, J.R.T. (1982). A new systematic treatment for infertile women with abnormal hormone profiles. Br. J. Obstet. Gynaecol., 80:80-5.
8. Franks, S. (1989). Polycystic ovary syndrome: a changing perspective. Clin. Endocrinol., 31:87-120.
9. Hillier, S.G., Afnan, A.M.M., Margara, R.A. and Winston, R.M.L. (1985). Super-ovulation strategy before in vitro fertilization. Clin. Obstet. Gynaecol., 12:687-723.
10. Homburg, R., Eshel, A., Abdulla, H.I. and Jacobs, H.S. (1988). Growth hormone facilitates ovulation induction by gonadotrophins. Clin. Endocrinol., 29:113-7.
11. Homburg, R., West, C., Torresani, T. and Jacobs, H.S. (1990). Cotreatment with human growth hormone and gonadotrophins for induction of ovulation: a controlled clinical trial. Fertil. Steril., 53:254-60.

12. Howles, C. (1990). GnRH analogues, past present and future uses in superovulation regimens. In: Clinical IVF Forum; Current views in assisted reproduction, edited by Matson, P.L. and Lieberman, B.A., pp 41-62. Manchester University Press, Manchester.
13. Kemmann, E., Bohrer, M., Shelden, R., Fiasconaro, G., Beardsley, L. (1987). Active ovulation management increases the monthly probability of pregnancy occurrence in ovulatory women who receive intrauterine insemination. Fertil. Steril., 48:916-20.
14. Kingsland, C., Mason, B., Tan, S.L., Campbell, S. and Bickerton, N. (1992). The routine use of gonadotrophin-releasing hormone agonists for all patients undergoing in vitro fertilization. Is there any medical advan- tage? A prospective randomized study. Fertil. Steril., 57:805-9.
15. Loumaye, E., Billion, J-M., Mine. J-M., Psalti, I., Pensis, M. and Thomas, K. (1990). Prediction of individual response to controlled ovarian hyper- stimulation by means of a clomiphene citrate challenge test. Fertil. Steril., 53:295-301.
16. MacDougall, M.J., Tan, S.L., Mills. C. and Jacobs, H.S. (1990). In vitro fertili- zation and the ovarian hyperstimulation syndrome. Hum. Reprod. 6 (suppl 1): abstr p90.
17. MacLachlan, V., Besanko, M., O'Shea, F., et al., (1989). A controlled study of luteinizing hormone-releasing hormone agonist (buserelin) for the induction of folliculogenesis before in vitro fertilization. N. Engl. J. Med., 320:1233-37.
18. Maroulis, G.B., Emery, M., Verkauf, B.S., Saphier, A., Bernhisel, M. and Yeko, T.R. (1991). Prospective randomized study of human menotrophin versus a follicular and a luteal phase gonadotropin-releasing hormone analog-human menotropin stimulation protocols for in vitro fertilization. Fertil. Steril., 55:1157-64.
19. Muasher, S.J., Oehninger, S., Simonetti, S., Matta, J., Ellis, L.M., Liu, H-C., et al., (1988). The value of basal and/or stimulated serum gonadotrophin levels in prediction of stimulation response and in vitro fertilization outcome. Fertil. Steril., 50:298-307.
20. Mason, H.D., Martikainen, H., Beard. R.W., Anyaoku, V. and Franks, S. (1990). Direct gonadotrophic effect of growth hormone on oestradiol production by human granulosa cells in vitro. J. Endocrinol., 126:R1-R4.
21. Navot, D., Rosenwaks, Z. and Margalioth, E.J. (1987). Prognostic assess- ment of female fecundity. Lancet., 2:645-7.
22. Neveu, S., Hedon, B., Bringer, J., Chinchole, J-M., Arnal, F., Humeau, C., et al., (1987). Ovarian stimulation by a combination of a gonadotropin- releasing hormone agonist and gonadotropins for in-vitro fertilization. Fertil. Steril., 47:639-43.
23. Owen, E.J., West, C., Mason, B.A. and Jacobs, H.S. (1991). Co-treatment with growth hormone of sub-optimal responders in IVF-ET. Hum. Reprod. 6:524-28.
24. Porter, R.N., Smith, W., Craft, I.L., Abdulwahid, N.A. and Jacobs, H.S. (1984). Induction of ovulation for in vitro fertilisation using buserelin and gonadotropins. Lancet, 2:1284-5.
25. Rizk, B. and Smitz, J. (1992). Ovarian hyperstimulation syndrome after superovulation using GnRH agonists for IVF and related procedures. Hum. Reprod., 7:320-7.
26. Ron-El, Herman, A., Golan, A., Nachum, H., Soffer, Y. and Caspi, E. (1991). Gonadotropins and combined gonadotropin-releasing hormone agonist - gonadotropins protocols in a randomised prospective study. Fertil. Steril. 55:574-8.
27. Rutherford, A.J., Subak-Sharpe, R.J., Dawson, K.J., Margara, R.A., Franks, S. and Winston, R.M.L. (1988). Improvement of in-vitro fertilisation after treatment with buserelin, an agonist of luteinising hormone releasing hormone. Br. Med. J., 296:1765-8.
28. Serhal, P.F., Katz, M., Little, V. and Woronowski, H. (1988). Unexplained infertility - the value of Pergonal superovulation combined with intrauterine insemination. Fertil Steril., 49:602-6.
29. Scott, R.T., Toner, J.P., Muasher, S.J., Oehninger, S., Robinson, S. and Rosenwaks, Z. (1989). Follicle-stimulating hormone levels on cycle day 3 are predictive of in vitro fertilization outcome. Fertil. Steril., 51:651-4.
30. Seoud, M.A-F., Toner, J.P., Kruithoff. C. and Muasher, S.J. (1992). Outcome of twin, triplet, and quadruplet in vitro fertilization pregnancies: the Norfolk experience. Fertil. Steril., 57:825-34.
31. Smitz, J., Devroey, P., Braeckmans, P., Camus, M., Khan, I., Staessen, C., et al., (1987). Management of failed cycles in an IVF/GIFT programme with the combination of a GnRH analogue and hMG. Hum. Reprod., 2:309-14.
32. Tan, S-L., Bradfield, J., Kingsland. C., Alexander, N., Campbell, S., Yovich, J., Mills, C. and Jacobs, H.S. (1992). The long protocol of administration of gonadotropin-releasing hormone agonist is superior to the short protocol for ovarian stimulation for in vitro fertilization. Fertil. Steril., 57:810-4.

33. Tanbo, T., Norman, N., Dale, P.O., Abyholm, T. and Lunde, O. (1992). Prediction of response to controlled ovarian hyperstimulation: a comparison of basal and clomiphene citrate-stimulated follicle-stimulating hormone levels. Fertil. Steril., 57:819-24.
34. Van Steirteghem, A.C., Smitz, J., Camus, M., Van Waesberghe, L., Deschacht, J., Khan, I., Staessen, C., Wisanto, A., Bourgain, C. and Devroey, P. (1992). The luteal phase after in-vitro fertilization and related procedures. Hum. Reprod., 3:161-4.

Transplantation of Follicle and Germ Cells

R.G. Gosden and A.A. Murray

*Department of Physiology, University Medical School
Teviot Place, Edinburgh EH8 9AG, UK*

Transplantation of gonadal tissue is not a novel technique, nor have its applications been confined to the treatment of hypogonadism. First, it was an experimental novelty that helped to launch the new science of endocrinology, then it was tested as a remedy for human sterility - it has even been used as a panacea for premature senility. Controversies surrounding the more sensational claims have discouraged serious clinical attention in recent decades, although gonadal transplantation continued to make important contributions to advancing biological science. The chequered history of transplanting gonadal cells will be briefly reviewed and potential applications will be considered in the light of recent research progress.

HISTORICAL BACKGROUND

The first attempt to transplant sex organs is attributed to the 18th Century Scottish surgeon-anatomist, John Hunter. He recorded a qualified success following some studies in chickens: "I had formerly transplanted the testicles of a cock into the abdomen of a hen, and they had sometimes taken root there, but not frequently, and then had never come to perfection..." (35). Full details of the experiments have not survived although his specimens are still preserved in the Hunterian Museum of the Royal College of Surgeons of England. His grafts were probably affected by the allograft reaction and credit for the first completely successful grafts should be given to a Gottingen biologist. Berthold (5) succeeded because he returned the extirpated organs of capons to the body cavity of the same bird and so maintained the state of the comb, plumage and courting behaviour. His discovery was a landmark in the history of endocrinology because it demonstrated that the gonadal influence on phenotype was blood-borne rather than dependent on innervation. It was another 70-80 years, however, before the sex hormones were recovered, purified and synthesized.

The implications of Berthold's discovery were not fully appreciated at the time and the virtues of grafting operations were largely overlooked until the end of the century. Confirmation of his results in mammals was forthcoming in 1896 when Knauer (26) reported that rabbit ovaries autografted to the broad ligaments restored both ovarian and uterine physiology. He too was lucky to have chosen autografting since the scientific community at large was ignorant of transplantation immunity at that time. Shortly afterwards, Foa (18) showed that immature ovaries begin functioning precociously after grafting to an adult environment. The earlier onset of follicular secretion and ovulation in these organs indicated that the gonads have to wait for gonadotrophic stimulation, and later studies showed that immature organ grafts generally performed better and for longer than adult gonads because they possess more follicles.

A New York surgeon, Robert Morris (34), was probably first to take the bold step of transplanting ovaries in sterile patients. While in some operations he transposed ovaries to the stump of a fallopian tube to by-pass an obstruction, in others he used allografts to overcome premature menopause. Both types of operation were claimed to be successful, but it is impossible after so long an interlude to properly verify whether pregnancies had become established from grafts rather than from regenerated traces of host tissue. Morris was also interested in using testicular transplantation to help anorchic patients, but this vain hope is now mainly remembered in connection with the Chicago surgeon, Frank Lydston (30), and others engaged in the notorious episode of animal organ grafting.

Testicular grafting was aimed at boosting sex hormone levels in middle-aged and old men. Brown-Sequard's theory that the signs and symptoms of ageing are secondary to gonadal hormone deficiency still had its adherents and, when testicular extracts proved ineffective, rejuvenation trials switched attention to organ grafting. This development seemed propitious at the time since the Nobel Prize had been awarded to Alexis Carrel in 1912 for transplantation surgery in animals, but it led to the most notorious blind alley in the annals of clinical endocrinology.

Lydston grafted the testes of young victims of accidents and executed prisoners to restore strength and virility to hypogonadal men. Although always controversial, the supply of human organs could not keep up with the demands for transplantation and so some of his fellow surgeons began to experiment with animal grafts in their patients. Some grafters relied heavily on farm animal species but the more sophisticated workers advocated ape and monkey gonads because of their closer genetic affinity to man. Organ slices were stitched into the scrotum beside the resident pair of organs (49,51) or injected as a mince into the abdominal rectus muscle and at other sites (45). The so-called 'monkey gland' treatment became one of the fads of the frothy society of the 1920s. Similar operations were used to restore the stud performance of prize animals and to improve wool production. Rather less attention and publicity attended attempts to reinstate ovarian function by grafting (38). Such was the attention by government agencies on Voronoff's work that an international delegation was sent to his research station in Algeria in 1927 to investigate his claims. The visitors were divided about the value of the work, though the British group was distinctly sceptical (32).

Hubris of the 1920's was followed by nemesis in the 1930's as growing evidence proved that their operations had been more-or-less worthless. The exaggerated statements of the gland grafters were not borne out by clinical histories and doubts were growing whether allografts or xenografts could survive for more than a few weeks (25). Finally, trials with synthetic sex hormones proved that hormonal rejuvenation had been a fallacy.

There is an interesting footnote to this history for, in 1978, an American urologist successfully transplanted a testis donated to an anorchic man by his genetically-identical twin brother (42). As a result of vasovasostomy and anastomosis of the epigastric and spermatic vessels the patient quickly experienced a rise in circulating testosterone and subsequent fathered children. A comparable operation could doubtless be successful in women if, by happy chance, a similar donor could be found.

GONADAL TRANSPLANTATION IN EXPERIMENTAL BIOLOGY

Organ grafting

Gonadal transplantation has been used extensively as an experimental tool in endocrine research from the beginning of this century and, although hindsight reveals serious flaws and deficiencies in some of the early studies (see Reference 54), it has nevertheless played a major role. When inbred strains of mice and subsequently other laboratory species became available the problem of graft rejection was eliminated and the full potential of grafting was realised. The fertility of hosts sometimes approached that of intact animals (28). Studies of gonadal maturation and ageing were particularly striking, as well as indicating possible clinical applications. Ovarian cyclicity in mouse strains genetically predisposed to early follicle depletion was significantly extended by ovarian grafts from young, syngeneic donors (16,27).

Although definitely effective, grafts suffer massive necrosis of oocytes for 1-3 days while they are revascularizing. Virtually all growing follicles and at least half the primordial stages die. Small follicles may be more resistant to ischaemia because of lower metabolic requirements and a peripheral location in the cortex which is reached first by invading capillary sprouts. The testis, in contrast, has a tough, fibrous capsule and simple implantation of this organ is inappropriate, although isolated Leydig cells survive and produce small quantities of testosterone (46).

Post-transplantation ischaemia can be minimized by vascular anastomosis.

Successful ovarian grafts have been achieved by this means in animals as small as rabbits and rats (6,9,53), and anastomosis is mandatory for the larger, more fibrous organs of dogs and farm animals (10,21). When microsurgical techniques were applied to intact rat testes, grafts soon recovered to full function (19).

The mouse, which has been the most popular model, is too small for the demanding art of microsurgery on a routine basis and it is fortunate that simple implantation is satisfactory. When fertility is required, grafts are placed in the evacuated ovarian capsule, which can be closed to avoid displacement. When only the endocrine function of the graft is being tested, well-vascularized heterotopic sites such as under the renal capsule are convenient and successful. Sites which are drained by the enteric portal system are normally undesirable because the greater metabolism of steroids passing directly through the liver reduces negative feedback on hypothalamo-pituitary function, and the consequent elevation of gonadotrophic hormones superstimulates the ovaries and can cause tumorigenesis (7). Graft activity at other sites can be monitored in castrated hosts by vaginal patency and cornification, which normally resume 1-2 weeks after surgery.

The long-term activity of ovarian grafts in rodents depends on the age of both host and donor. On the one hand, neuroendocrine dysfunction limits cyclical activity past mid-life (2,16,44) and, on the other, the age of the donor ovary sets an upper limit to fecundity because the number of follicles is finite and constantly declining (14). Immature ovaries are therefore expected to make better grafts than older ones, though neonatal ones may perform poorly (33). The neuroendocrine disorder of middle-aged rodents appears to be due to the self-limiting effects of oestrogenic stimulation on neuroendocrine centres because administration of large doses of oestrogen advances the onset of acyclicity whereas long-term castration increases the potential for cycle reinitiation by grafts later in life (17).

Ovarian hormones may also limit long-term capacity of the uterus to carry pregnancy. CBA mice were ovariectomized at either 5 or 10-11 months old (Long- and Acute-OVX, respectively) and implanted with young ovarian grafts under the kidney capsule at the latter age. A similar proportion in the two groups became sexually receptive and mated, but the survival of morulae/blastocysts transferred from young donors was significantly better in those deprived of ovarian activity for half their lives (Table 1). That hypogonadism

Table 1. *Effects of long-term ovariectomy (OVX) on pregnancy potential after heterotopic ovarian grafting and embryo transfer in middle-aged mice*

Group	No. mating (%)	Embryo survival (%)	Mean no. CL
Acute-OVX	7/21 (33.0)	8/78 (10.3)	6.25
Long-OVX	6/19 (31.7)	28/67 (41.8)*	4.5

*$P<0.001$.

can paradoxically benefit fertility is also indicated by the findings of Edwards et al. (13) from donor embryo transfer programmes for amenorrhoeic women.

While simple implantation of ovaries can be remarkably successful, it provides relatively little control over donor germ cells and suffers from ischaemia. The transplantation of isolated tissues and cells has, however, proved to be promising for panacreatic islets and brain cells and its advantages for gonadal tissues are now becoming clearer.

Transplantation of immature follicles

Organ grafting techniques are on the horns of a dilemma: either a sliced or whole organ is simply attached to host tissue, trusting that early revascularisation will mimimize ischaemia, or the demanding skills of microsurgery have to be applied. Transplantation of isolated cells or tissue is a compromise between these alternatives because, on the one hand, the surgery is elementary while, on the other, it encourages an early blood circulation.

Table 2. *Summary of principal benefits of isolating follicles and germ cells for grafting*

1) Cell sorting

2) Cell counting

3) Quality control

4) Potential for manipulating development

5) Banking at low temperatures

Rodent ovaries be can be disaggregated to single cells and granulosa-oocyte complexes in medium containing collagenase (40) Growing follicles are broken in the process and basement membrane constituents of others are eroded. The pregranulosa cells of primordial follicles may separate from the oocyte, although this damage is not necessarily terminal since a completely disaggregated ovary can be reaggregated to produce grafts which develop Graafian follicles. Isolated cells and follicles offer practical advantages outweighing the investment in additional steps and the costs of cell losses that inevitably occur. Individual cells and small follicles can be counted, tested for viability and sorted to eliminate moribund and unwanted cell types (e.g. passenger leucocytes). Moreover, they are potentially amenable to genetic manipulation and frozen storage.

While it may be possible in larger species to inject suspensions of germ cells or primordial follicles into host ovarian stroma or use an atretic follicle as a receptacle, this is not practicable in rodents. The problem has been overcome in mice by reaggregating cells from infant mouse ovaries in a vehicle of either clotted plasma or collagen gel. After stabilizing and contracting for 1-2 days in culture, grafts can be transferred to the ovarian capsule or a heterotopic site (22,48). In the former case, grafts have been successfully applied to a resected host ovary which had been sterilized by pelvic X-irradiation (Fig. 1) or become naturally sterile as a result of age (Fig. 2).

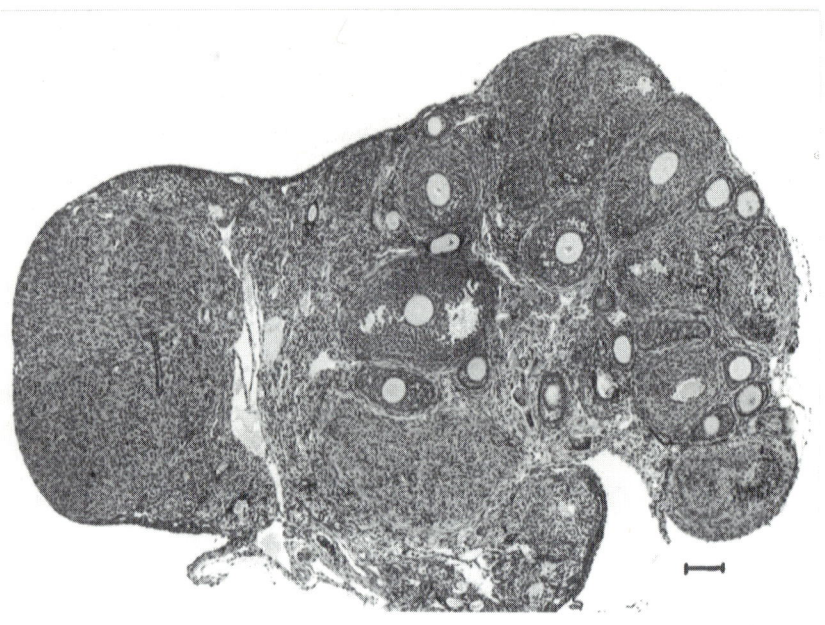

FIG. 1. Primordial follicles grafted into one side of a 3 month old X-ray-sterilized C57BL/6 mouse ovary have grown to multilaminar and antral stages within 3 weeks and eventually dominate the chimaeric organ as the sterile host tissue regresses. (H & E, bar indicates 100 μm) [Reproduced from Gosden, R.G. (1990) Mechanisms of Fertilization: Plants to Humans, edited by B. Dale, p 109. NATO ASI H45].

Grafts are rapidly invaded by sprouting blood vessels and boundaries with host ovarian tissue become blurred within a month. A host ovary is evidently not required for success because the scrambled cells in the graft have the capacity to undergo organogenesis to form histotypic associations and normal ovarian structures (22). Follicle growth rapidly resumes in the grafts and secretory Graafian stages evolve even when only small numbers survive. When several hundred or more follicles are present ovulatory cycles will occur and, provided the graft is beside a patent fallopian tube in a young host, mating can result in a viable pregnancy.

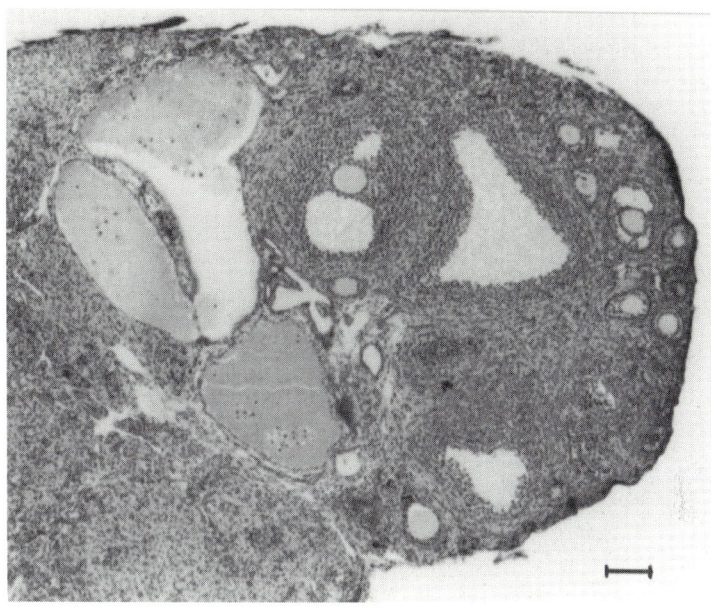

FIG. 2. As Fig. 1 except the host animal was nonirradiated and from the CBA strain that becomes spontaneously sterile at this age (15 months). (H & E, bar indicates 100 μm).

Transplantation of fetal germ cells

Cell transfer techniques which depend on recovering primordial follicles from donor organs are unlikely to be successful with the larger, fibrous ovaries of postnatal farm animals and humans because the period of incubation required for enzymatic disaggregation is too long and suitable human tissue is rarely unavailable. Fetal ovaries of these species are, however, much more delicate and contain abundant germ cells. Peak numbers of about 7 million germ cells occur in human fetuses at mid-gestation, though the majority do not survive to full-term to form primordial follicles (3).

The fetal environment is not essential for germ cells to grow, differentiate and form follicles since normal ovarian physiology, albeit with fewer follicles, can be obtained by grafting whole fetal ovaries to adult hosts (1,23). So reliable is this technique that it has been used to maintain mutant lines of mice by recovering and transplanting viable germ cells before death in utero or shortly after birth (41). Fetal germ cells at the oogonial stage and early in meiosis are easy to isolate by collagenase digestion for transplantation purposes, but cell survival is poor.

Besides fetal ovarian cells, primordial germ cells (PGC's) during their migratory phase are potential candidates for transplantation purposes. These stem cells for the germ line originate extragonadally and migrate from the yolk sac along the hindgut mesentery to the gonadal ridge where they become stationary (12). We have isolated a mixed population of mesenteric cells, including PGC's, from mice on Day 10 of pregnancy and injected them intra-peritoneally into Day 18 fetuses and neonates. Donor cells could be identified by in situ hybridisation using cDNA probes for multiple inserts of the beta-globin transgene (29), but only a few scattered somatic cells could be located in hosts 7 days later (unpublished results). It is uncertain whether PGC's can home in on the gonad when injected 'off-course', but this does not present a problem for PGC transfer in birds.

Avian PGC's migrate from their extragonadal origin to the gonad in the bloodstream from which they can be collected at an early stage of incubation and returned to by intracardiac injection. At present a small harvest of cells hampers success, though the possibility of combining this method with transfection of exogenous DNA *in vitro* could lead to a novel method for making transgenic birds (39,43,52).

Oogonia in lower vertebrates persist and generate new oocytes throughout life and there is no reason, at least in principle, why this cannot be achieved with mammals and birds by inhibiting differentiation *in vitro*. Migratory PGC's offer a better chance of success than oogonial cells, which have a more limited capacity for cell division (4,47). However, when maintained on fibroblastic feeder layers, PGC's are only able to survive for a few days before dying or differentiating and, although some cytokines can improve survival times (11,15,20), the cultivation of immortalized clones of mammalian germ cells in vitro has yet to be demonstrated.

Low temperature storage of follicles and germ cells

Frozen storage of preovulatory oocytes was first attempted in the 1950's, shortly after the successful introduction of semen banking. Ovaries were cooled in the presence of a croprotectant and cellular viability of the thawed tissue was tested by grafting (24,36). Frozen-thawed orthotopic grafts have sometimes proved to be fertile and produced live young (37), but most results have been disappointing and the field was neglected until recently.

Isolated follicles and germ cells provide significant advantages compared with larger masses of tissue for long-term cropreservation. Rapid penetration, more even cooling rates and the opportunity to test the viability of thawed cells before grafting are important benefits. Primary follicles from mouse ovaries lowered to temperatures of liquid nitrogen in dimethylsulphoxide (DMSO) remained capable of growth to Graafian size and producing fertile oocytes (8), and similar results can be obtained with primordial follicles (unpublished results). The apparent robustness of immature oocytes contrasts with problems encountered with mature oocytes. The better results may be attributable to a number of factors, including smaller size and less differentiated ooplasm, diffuse chromatin and a longer time to repair damaged organelles before the critical events of meiosis and fertilization.

APPLICATIONS OF FOLLICLE AND GERM CELL TRANSPLANTATION

Gonadal transplantation has served many aims and functions through a 200-year history, not all of them having been scientifically respectable. However, a better appreciation of the twin hazards of necrosis and transplantation immunity is enabling us to evaluate practical applications to reproductive medicine and animal breeding technology more critically than was possible in the past. The practicability of gonadal transplantation is not in doubt under the special circumstances of vascular anastomosis and a genetically identical graft and host, but the method will not be widely used if these strict criteria are mandatory. Originally, more attention was given to testicular than ovarian grafts, but it is the latter that now hold most promise.

Transplantation of fetal germ cells opens the possibility of establishing menstrual cycles and fecundity in individuals with gonadal dysgenesis and premature menopause for whom the donation of mature oocytes would provide only a partial solution based upon a limited supply of oocytes. Any forecasts must be qualified though because this manouevre would have to break new ground in both medical ethics and law and it is questionable whether otherwise healthy women should be administered potentially harmful drugs to suppress graft rejection. The pioneering transplanters were sanguine about graft tolerance, but it is now quite clear that tissues from either fetal or older gonads are not specially immunologically privileged. Marshall & Jolly working in our Department as long ago as 1908, had in fact shown that allografted rat and monkey ovaries seldom survived: "Homoplastic transplantation of ovaries is very considerably easier to perform successfully than heteroplastic transplantation, (but the latter) is apparently easier to perform successfully when... near relatives of each other" (31). We find that human and murine granulosa cells, and perhaps immature oocytes, express histocompatibility antigens (unpublished observations). An immunological problem would not exist for fetal hosts and might offer an alternative strategy for producing transgenic animals, but antenatal germ cell transfer is unlikely to assume the significance that somatic cell treatment could hold for human fetal medicine (50).

If gonadal transplantation is to have any role in reproductive medicine it is likely to be introduced first as autografting for cancer patients to avoid ovarian damage before radio- or chemotherapy. This would not pose any ethical or immunological problems and they might be able to look forward to the possibility of conceiving with their own oocytes rather than donor cells after recovering from disease. Experimental studies offer some encouragement for this strategy.

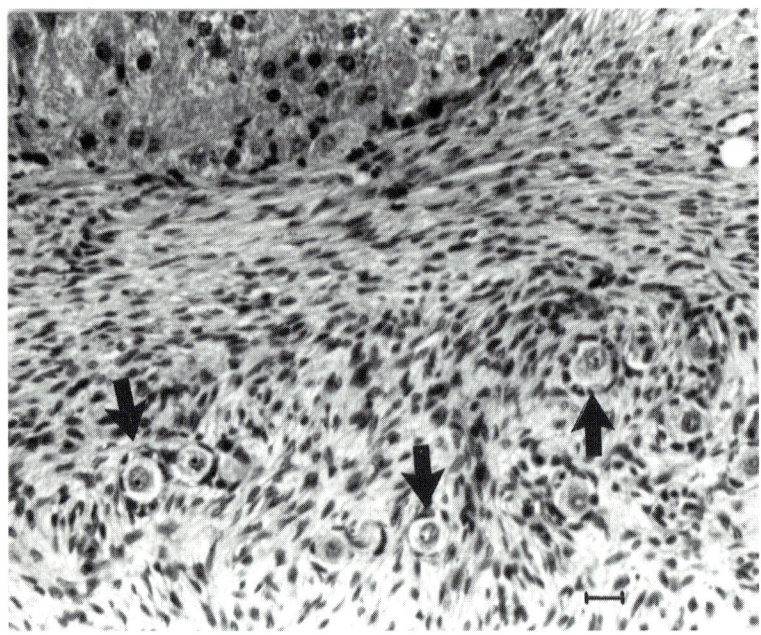

FIG. 3. Cortical slice of sheep ovary 18 days after grafting to the kidney of a scid mouse (upper left) following slow freezing to -196°C, rapid thawing and grafting. Many primordial follicles survive (arrows) (bar indicates 50 μm) (Roger Gosden & Jean Wade, unpublished results).

Sheep ovaries obtained from the abattoir were cut into thin slices, cooled in DMSO and stored for 24 hours at -196°C. The thawed tissue was grafted under the renal capsule of scid mice which lack an immune system and thus tolerate ovarian xenografting (23). Three weeks later, many primordial follicles remained in the grafts, testifying to their robustness to ischaemia and freeze-thawing (Fig. 3). A clinical application would require recovering tissue before commencing cytotoxic therapy and grafting back onto the broad ligament close to the fallopian tube after an appropriate period of low temperature storage.

In conclusion, there are distinctly promising applications for germ cell transplantation in reproductive medicine as well as in experimental science, though significant technical hurdles will have to be overcome before they can be realised.

The authors thankfully acknowledge financial support from The Wellcome Trust and The Galton Institute (London).

REFERENCES

1. Arrau, J., Roblero, L., Cury, M. and Gonzalez, R. (1983) Effect of exogenous sex steroids upon the number of germ cells and the growth of foetal ovaries grafted under the kidney capsule of adult ovariectomized hamsters. J. Embryol. Exp. Morph., 78:33-42.
2. Aschheim, P. (1965) Resultats fournis par la greffe heterochrone des ovaires dans l'etude de la regulation hypothalamo-hypophyso-ovarienne de la ratte senile. Gerontologia, 10:65-75.
3. Baker, T.G. (1963) A quantitative and cytological study of germ cells in human ovaries. Proc. Roy. Soc. B, 158:417-433.
4. Baker, T.G. and Neal, P. (1977) Action of ionizing radiations on the mammalian ovary. In: The Ovary, Volume 1, edited by Lord Zuckerman and B.J. Weir, pp 1-58. Second edition. Academic Press, London.
5. Berthold, A.A. (1849) Transplantation der Hoden. Archiv. für Anat. Physiol. Med., 16:42-46.
6. Betteridge, K.J. (1970) Homotransplantation of ovaries with vascular anastomoses in rabbits: response of transplants to human chorionic gonadotrophin. J. Endocrinol., 47:451-461.
7. Biskind, G.R., Kordan, B. and Biskind, M.S. (1950) Ovary transplanted to spleen in rats: the effect of unilateral castration, pregnancy, and subsequent castration. Cancer Res., 10:309-318.
8. Carroll, J., Whittingham, D.G., Wood, M., Telfer, E. and Gosden, R.G. (1990): Extraovarian production of mature viable mouse oocytes from frozen primary follicles. J. Reprod. Fertil., 90:321-327.
9. Cornier, E., Sibella, P. and Chatelet, F. (1985) Etudes histologiques et devenir fonctionnel des greffes de trompe et d'ovaire chez la ratte (isogreffes et allogreffes traittees par cyclosporine A). J. Gynecol. Obstet. Biol. Reprod., 14:567-573.
10. Dempster, W.J. (1954) A technique for the study of the autotransplanted kidney, adrenals and ovary of the dog. J. Physiol., 124:xv-xvi.
11. Dolci, S., Williams, D.E., Ernst, M.K., Resnick, J.L., Brannan, C.I., Lock, L.F., Lyman, S.D., Boswell, H.S. and Donovan, P.J. (1991) Requirement for mast cell growth factor for primordial germ cell survival in culture. Nature, 352:809-811.
12. Donovan, P.J., Stott, D., Cairns, L.A., Heasman, J. and Wyllie, C.C. (1986) Migratory and postmigratory mouse primordial germ cells behave differently in culture. Cell, 44:831-838.
13. Edwards, R.G., Morcos, S., Macnamee, M., Balmaceda, J.P., Walters, D.E. and Asch, R. (1991) High fecundity of amenorrhoeic women in embryo-transfer pregrammes. Lancet, 338:292-294.
14. Faddy, M.J., Gosden, R.G. and Edwards, R.G. (1983) Ovarian follicle dynamics in mice: a comparative study of three inbred strains and an F1 hybrid. J. Endocrinol., 96:23-33.
15. De Felici, M. and Dolci, S. (1991) Leukaemia inhibitory factor sustains the survival of mouse primordial germ cells cultured on TM4 feeder layers. Dev. Biol., 147:281-284.
16. Felicio, L.S., Nelson, J.F., Gosden, R.G. and Finch, C.E. (1984) Restoration of ovulatory cycles by young ovarian grafts in aging mice: potentiation by long-term ovariectomy decreases with age. Proc. Natl. Acad. Sci. USA, 80:6076-6080.
17. Finch, C.E., Felicio, L.S., Mobbs, C.V. and Nelson, J.F. (1984) Ovarian and steroidal influences on neuroendocrine aging processes in female rodents. Endocr. Rev., 5:467-497.
18. Foa, C. (1900) La greffe des ovaires en relation avec quelques questions de biologie generale. Arch. Ital. Biol., 34:43-73.
19. Gittes, R.F., Altwein, J.E., Yen, S.S.C. and Lee, S. (1972) Testicular transplantation in the rat: long-term gonadotropin and testosterone radioimmunoassays. Surgery, 72:187-192.
20. Godin, I., Deed, R., Cooke, J., Zsebo, K., Dexter, M. and Wyllie, C.C. (1991) Effects of the steel gene product on mouse primordial germ cells in culture. Nature, 352:807-809.
21. Goding, J.R., McCracken, J.A. and Baird, D.T. (1967) The study of ovarian function in the ewe by means of a vascular autotransplantation technique. J. Endocrinol., 39:37-52.
22. Gosden, R.G. (1990) Restitution of fertility in sterilized mice by transferring primordial ovarian follicles. Hum. Reprod., 5:499-504.

23. Gosden, R.G. (1992) Transplantation of ovaries and testes. In: Fetal Transplants in Medicine, edited by R.G. Edwards. Cambridge Univ. Press (in press).
24. Green, S.H., Smith, A.U. and Parkes, A.S. (1956) The numbers of oocytes in ovarian autografts after freezing and thawing. J. Endocrinol., 13:333-334.
25. Hamilton, D. (1986) The Monkey Gland Affair. Chatto & Windus, London.
26. Knauer, E. (1896) Einige Versuche uber Ovarientransplantation bei Kaninchen. Zentralblatt. für Gynakol., 20:524-528.
27. Krohn, P.L. (1962) Review Lectures on Senescence. II. Heterochronic transplantation in the study of ageing. Proc. Roy. Soc. Lond. B, 157:128-147.
28. Krohn, P.L. (1965) Transplantation of endocrine organs. With special reference to the ovary. Brit. Med. Bull., 21:157-162.
29. Lo, C.W. (1986) Localization of low abundance DNA sequences in tissue sections by in situ hybridization. J. Cell Sci., 81:143-162.
30. Lydston, G.F. (1916) Sex gland implantation. Additional cases and conclusions to date. J. Am. Med. Assoc., 66:1540-1543.
31. Marshall, F.H.A. and Jolly, W.A. (1908) On the results of heteroplastic ovarian transplantation as compared with those produced by transplantation in the same individual. Q. J. Exp. Physiol., 1:115-120.
32. Marshall, F.H.A., Crewe, F.A.E., Walton, A. and Miller, W.C. (1928) Report on Dr. Serge Voronoff's experiments on the Improvement of Livestock. Ministry of Agriculture & Fisheries and Board of Agriculture for Scotland. 24/108. HMSO, London.
33. Mayer, G. and Duluc, A.J. (1970) Reactions of the postnatal ovary after transplantation into castrated normal and sterilised rats. In: Gonadotrophins and Ovarian Development, edited by W.R. Butt, A.C. Crooke and M. Ryle, pp 332-336. Livingstone, Edinburgh and London.
34. Morris, R.T. (1895) The ovarian graft. New York Med. J., 62:436.
35. Palmer, J.F. (1837) The Works of John Hunter, F.R.S., with notes. Vol. III, p 273. Longman, Rees, Orme, Brown, Green & Longman, London.
36. Parkes, A.S. and Smith, A.U. (1953) Regeneration of rat ovarian tissue grafted after exposure to low temperatures. Proc. Roy. Soc. B, 140:455-470.
37. Parrot, D.M.V. (1960) The fertility of mice with orthotopic ovarian grafts derived from frozen tissue. J. Reprod. Fertil., 1:230-241.
38. Pettinari, V. (1928) Greffe ovarienne et action endocrine de l'ovaire. Doin, Paris.
39. Pettite, J.N., Clark, M.E. and Etches, R.J. (1991) Assessment of functional gametes in chickens after transfer of primordial germ cells. J. Reprod. Fert., 92:225-229.
40. Roy, S.K. and Greenwald, G.S. (1985) An enzymatic method for dissociation of intact follicles from the hamster ovary: histological and quantitative aspects. Biol. Reprod., 32:203-215.
41. Russell, W.L. and Gower, J.S. (1950) Offspring from transplanted ovaries of fetal mice homozygous for a lethal gene (Sp) that kills before birth. Genetics, 35:133.
42. Silber, S.J. (1978) Transplantation of a human testis for anorchia. Fertil. Steril., 30:181-187.
43. Simkiss, K. (1990) Primordial germ cells and the scope for genetic manipulation using embryos. In: Avian Incubation. Poultry Science Symposium 22, edited by S.G. Tullet, pp 125-136. Butterworth-Heinemann.
44. Sopelak, V.M. and Butcher, R.L. (1982) Contribution of the ovary versus hypothalamus-pituitary to termination of estrous cycles in aging rats using ovarian transplants. Biol. Reprod., 27:29-37.
45. Stanley, L.L. (1922) An analysis of one thousand testicular substance implantations. Endocrinology, 6:787-794.
46. Tai, J., Johnson, H.W. and Tze, W.J. (1989) Successful transplantation of Leydig cells in castrated inbred rats. Transplantation, 47:1087-1089.
47. Tam, P.P.L. and Snow, M.H.L. (1981) Proliferation and migration of primordial germ cells during compensatory growth in mouse embryos. J. Embryol. Exp. Morph., 64:133-147.
48. Telfer, E., Torrance, C. and Gosden, R.G. (1990) Morphological study of cultured preantral ovarian follicles of mice after transplantation under the kidney capsule. J. Reprod. Fertil., 89:565-571.
49. Thorek, M. (1924) Experimental investigations of the role of the Leydig, seminiferous and Sertoli cells and effects of testicular transplantation. Endocrinology, 8:61-90.
50. Touraine, J.-L. (1992) In-utero transplantation of fetal liver stem cells into human fetuses. Hum. Reprod., 7:44-48.
51. Voronoff, S. (1923) Greffes Testiculaires. Doin, Paris.

52. Wentworth, B.C., Tsai, H., Hallett, J.H., Gonzales, D.S. and Rajcic-Spasojevic, G. (1989) Manipulation of avian primordial germ cells and gonadal differentiation. Poultry Sci., 68:999-110.
53. Winston, R.M.L. and McClure Browne, J.C. (1974) Pregnancy following autograft transplantation of fallopian tube and ovary in the rabbit. Lancet, ii:494-495.
54. Woodruff, M.F.A. (1960) The Transplantation of Tissues and Organs. C.C. Thomas, Springfield, Illinois.

Management of Male Infertility

F.C.W. Wu

Department of Medicine, University of Manchester Medical School, Hope Hospital, Salford, Greater Manchester, UK

DIAGNOSIS OF MALE INFERTILITY

The accepted definition of infertility is the inability to initiate a pregnancy after 12 months of unprotected intercourse. However, it is extremely important to realise that there is a significant spontaneous pregnancy rate, albeit decreased (10-30% in 12 months), amongst the partners of those with reduced sperm counts. The conventional semen profile has proved to be an unreliable predictor of male fertility potential with a substantial overlap between normal and infertile men. Most patients are therefore subfertile rather than sterile or infertile. While more accurate diagnostic and prognostic information can be derived from tests of sperm functions, these are usually complicated biological assays which are expensive and restricted in their general availability. These considerations highlight the fundamental inadequacies in the diagnosis of male infertility; they underlie the difficulties in identifying genuine as opposed to presumptive aetiological factors, in formulating rational rather than empirical management strategies and in the critical evaluation of treatment results.

MANAGEMENT OF MALE INFERTILITY

The management of male infertility remains a difficult and somewhat frustrating experience for patients as well as doctors. The majority of patients present no recognizable or reversible aetiological factors for specific treatment (3). Advising those whose semen abnormalities seem more compatible with fertility are fraught with uncertainties due to the poor predictive powers of currently available investigations. Nevertheless, there have been a number of advances in the last few years which are beginning to make a significant impact in our therapeutic capabilities. The approach to management suggested by Baker (1) highlights the scope and limitations of currently available treatments. Accordingly, patients are allocated into three categories: 1) potentially treatable subfertility, 2) subfertility due to idiopathic hypospermatogenesis and 3) untreatable sterility.

Potentially treatable subfertility
The number of infertile patients with potentially treatable conditions are unfortunately still small (about 10% excluding varicocoele and 30% including varicocele). Nevertheless, they form a disproportionately important group for whom rational therapies of proven efficacy can be offered.

Testicular toxins
Medications such as sulphasalazine, nitrofurantoin, anabolic steroids, sex steroids and anticonvulsants and recreation drugs such as cigarettes, alcohol and cannibis should be substituted, withdrawn or avoided if possible. In view of the recent evidence of an overall decline in sperm density in the general population (2), it is important for the clinician to be alert to the possibility of testicular toxin exposure in the environment or work place of an infertile patient.

Gonadotrophin deficiency
Patients with pituitary gonadotrophin deficiency, secondary to pituitary tumours, usually respond to human chorionic gonadotrophin alone or with the addition of human menopausal gonadotrophin containing both FSH and LH. In general, 64-76% show some degree of spermatogenesis and 54-60% could be expected to achieve pregnancies (6). Chronic subcutaneous pulsatile LHRH delivered by portable pump is an effective physiological replacement in patients with congenital hypothalamic LHRH deficiency (Kallmann's syndrome); 70% of patients achieve spermatogenesis although sperm density is often below the normal adult range (15).

Sperm antibody
Immunosuppression with high dose glucocorticoid (8) has been reported to reduce antibody titres, improve sperm mucus penetration and achieve significant improvements in pregnancy rates (25-30%). However, a placebo-controlled study was unable to confirm any improvement in pregnancy rate with methylprednisolone treatment (7). Side effects are common and can be potentially life-threatening and chronically disabling.

Excurrent duct obstruction
In the last decade, microsurgical techniques of epididymo-vasostomy to bypass epididymal obstruction have achieved patency rates of 78% and pregnancy rates of 56% (11). Pregnancies have also recently been reported in patients with agenesis of the vasa when sperm aspirated from the caput epididymis were used successfully for IVF (12). These techniques are extremely expensive and available only in very few centres. Since the highest

incidence of post-infective obstructive azoospermia occur in developing countries, their outlook remains bleak.

Varicocele

The position of varicocele treatment in the management of the infertile male has continued to generate much controversy. Some studies report a favourable effect of treatment (5) but others found no difference in pregnancy outcome (13). Many published studies had unsatisfactory designs. Until a proper therapeutic trial is carried out, the significance of varicocele in male infertility must remain an open question.

Coital disorders

If semen of good quality can be obtained with masturbation, vibrators or electroejaculation from patients with various coital dysfunctions, and functional spermatozoa recovered from patients with retrograde ejaculation, AIH and/or IVF can be reasonably successful.

Idiopathic subfertility

This forms by far the largest and most difficult group of male patients in infertility clinics. They have reduced fertility as a result of poor sperm quality but pregnancies can occur without treatment. Subfertility in these men may be associated with a significant but subtle contribution from their female partners. Thus optimising the female partner's fertility by correcting any coexisting disorders is a key aspect of management.

A wide variety of essentially empirical treatments have been used in attempts to improve fertility in subfertile men. These include testosterone suppression and rebound, gonadotrophins, pulsatile LHRH, clomiphene, tamoxifen, testolactone, antibiotics, bromocriptine, pentoxiphylline, pancreatic kallikrein, vitamin C, zinc and homologous artificial insemination. However, the vast majority of these regimes have not been subjected to controlled clinical trials and most are no longer used. The few treatments that were evaluated properly were shown to be ineffective.

In the last 8 years, in vitro fertilization (IVF) has been increasingly applied to treat patients with mild to moderate impairments in sperm quality (4). It is now generally accepted that fertilization *in vitro* can be achieved by spermatozoa recovered from poor quality semen albeit at a significantly reduced rate (30-50%) compared to those obtained from normal ejaculates (60-80%). Despite the lower fertilization rate however, the overall pregnancy (10-15%) and live birth rates (8-10%) per treatment cycle were not significantly different from that expected with normal semen quality. The low fertilization rate can be overcome to some extent by maximizing the number of follicles inseminated and increasing the number of embryos transferred. There remains however a significant proportion in whom fertilization repeatedly fails completely. For these patients and those whose semen quality were considered inadequate for successful conventional IVF, various micromanipulation strategies have been developed recently to breach the zona barrier and to promote sperm-egg fusion. They involve either placing spermatozoa directly into the perivitelline space by subzonal microinjection (9) or creating a slit-like opening in the zona pellucida to facilitate sperm access to the egg - partial zona dissection (10). Although fertilization can be achieved, the pregnancy rates remain poor (3-5%). Problems of polyspermy, manipulation damage, non-selective fertilization and toxin damage to the embryo are inherent in these methods which disturb the structural integrity of the oocyte. While technically appealing, the efficacy and the safety of micromanipulation techniques in the management of male infertility remain to be established.

Untreatable sterility

Patients with azoospermia or extreme oligozoospermia (<1 million/ml), atrophic testes and elevated FSH have irreversible primary seminiferous tubular failure and are to all intents and purposes sterile. The commonest known aetiologies are Klinefelter's syndrome, cryptorchidism, cytotoxic or irradiation treatment and testicular torsion or trauma. The poor prognosis of these patients should be sensitively explained and the couple should be counselled regarding the options of continuing childlessness, adoption and donor insemination. Androgen replacement is required in those with subnormal plasma testosterone and orchidectomy considered in those with an ectopic testis.

EVALUATION OF TREATMENT

Assessment of patients who are otherwise sterile is relatively straightforward. However, determining the true efficacy of treatment in subfertile patients is difficult. This is because of the significant background treatment-independent pregnancy rate, the inherent day-to day variabilities in semen parameters and their tendency for regression towards the mean on repeat analyses, as well as the high incidence of co-existing abnormalities in the female partners. It is therefore imperative that any treatment for male subfertility must be evaluated by prospective randomised controlled trials. It is also important to include a sufficient number of patients into these trials. Since the anticipated improvement in pregnancy rates in most treatments are likely to be fairly small, it follows that the a very large number of subjects (500-800 in each group) are usually required to obtain statistically valid conclusions.

CONCLUSIONS

Despite the dramatic technological advances, it should be made clear that treatment of male infertility by various assisted conception procedures is only moderately successful at present (14). This is perhaps not surprising since the underlying abnormalities in spermatogenesis is not being corrected. The predicted live birth rates are certainly not so much higher than spontaneous pregnancy rates in some patients that treatment can be recommended unreservedly. Bearing in mind the considerable financial and emotional investments, it is prudent therefore to recommend IVF and related procedures only for couples with longstanding infertility who have virtually exhausted their spontaneous fertility potential. The wider use of sperm functional analyses and more detailed morphological assessments may, in future, improve the selection of suitable patients for assisted conception treatment. More critical appraisals of the results of treatment under controlled conditions are also much needed. Finally, in our enthusiasm for new treatments, we should not forget the basic objectives of understanding the aetiology and pathophysiology of male infertility through research. This may ultimately lead to prevention of male infertility and possibly new strategies for fertility regulation in men.

REFERENCES

1. Baker, H.W.G. (1989) Clinical evaluation and management of testicular disorders in the adult. In: The Testis. Second Edition. Eds. H Burger, D M de Kretser. Raven Press, New York, pp 419-440
2. Carlsen, E., Giwercman, A., Keiding, N. and Skakkebaek, N. (1992) Evidence for decreasing semen quality during the last half-century. Brit. Med. J., in press
3. Cates, W., Farley, T.M.M., Rowe, P.J. (1985) Worldwide patterns of infertility: is Africa different? Lancet, ii:596-598
4. Cohen, J., Fehilly, C.B., Fishel, S.B., Edwards, R.G., Hewitt, J., Rowland, G. F. and Steptoe P.C. (1984) Male infertility successfully treated by in vitro fertilization. Lancet, i:1239
5. Comhaire, F.H. (1986) In: Oxford Reviews of Reproductive Biology. Ed. J.R. Clarke, Clarenden, Press, Oxford, 8:165-213
6. Finkel, D.M., Phillips, J.L. and Snyder, P.J. (1985) Stimulation of spermatogenesis by gonadotropins in men with hypogonadotropic hypogonadism. New. Eng. J. Med., 313:651-655
7. Haas, G.G. and Manganiello, P. (1987) A double-blind placebo-controlled study of the use of methylprednisolone in infertile men with sperm-associated immuno-globulins. Fertil. Steril., 47:295-301.
8. Hendry, W.F., Treehuba, K. and Hughes, L. (1986) Cyclic prednisolone therapy for male infertility associated with autoantibodies to spermatozoa. Fertil. Steril., 45:249-254
9. Laws-King, A., Trouson, A., Sathamanthan, H. and Kola, I. (1987) Fertilization of human oocytes by micro injection of a single spermatozoa under the zona pellucida. Fertil. Steril. 48:637-642
10. Malter, H.E. and Cohen, J. (1989) Partial zona dissection of the human oocyte: a non traumatic method using micromanipulation to assist zona pellucida penetration. Fertil. Steril. 51:139-148
11. Silber, S.J. 1989 Results of microsurgical vasoepididymostomy: role of epididymis in sperm maturation. Human. Reprod., 4:298-303
12. Silber, S.J., Ord, T., Balmaceda, J., Patrizio, P. and Asch, R.H. (1990) Congenital absence of the vas deferens does not affect the fertilizing capacity of the human epididymal sperm. New. Eng. J. Med., 323:1788-92
13. Vermeulen, A. and Vandeweghe, M. (1984) Improved fertility after varicocoele correction: fact or fiction. Fertil. Steril., 42:249-256
14. Wagner, M.G. and St. Clair, P.A. (1989) Are in vitro fertilization and embryo transfer of benefit to all. Lancet., 2:1027-1029
15. Whitcombe, R.W. and Crowley, W.F. Jr. (1990) Diagnosis and treatment of isolated gonadotropin-releasing hormone deficiency in men. J. Clin. Endocrinol. Metab., 70:3-7

Treatment of Male Infertility

E. Nieschlag, H.M. Behre, C. Keck and S. Kliesch

*Institute of Reproductive Medicine of the University
Steinfurter Str. 107 Münster, Germany*

INTRODUCTION

Disturbances of male fertility have a high prevalence of about 5% and thus belong to the most common disorders of young and middle-aged men. However, disturbances of male fertility may go unrecognized for a long time and become evident only when a marriage or (in more modern terms), a relationship remains without issue despite intentionally unprotected intercourse. If, after 6 to 12 months of unprotected intercourse no pregnancy occurs, a fertility problem must be assumed. Fertility disturbances of one partner may only become evident through the other partner's problems, while optimal reproductive functions in one partner may compensate for impaired functions of the other and may thus prevent the couple from attending a fertility clinic. Thus, infertility is most often a disorder of the couple that should at best be investigated and treated as a single entity, or at least in parallel. Therefore, as a general principle, the optimization of female reproductive functions must be an essential part of any treatment regimen for male infertility.

Compared to the high prevalence of male fertility disturbances, the therapeutic possibilities are rather limited. The reasons for these shortcomings rest with the fact that the pathogenesis of many fertility disturbances has not yet been elucidated and therefore rational approaches to treatment are lacking in these cases. Careful diagnostic procedures will allow the physician to identify cases which can be treated in a rational fashion and separate them from those which cannot be treated or can only be treated on an experimental basis. Some conditions cannot be treated in their final stages when the patient consults for infertility, but could have been prevented by early intervention long before fertility was at stake.

Following from these considerations, for the purposes of this chapter, male infertility disorders will be classified according to therapeutic possibilities into those 1) requiring preventive treatment or 2) rational treatment, 3) those where treatment is still experimental or disputed and 4) those where rational treatment cannot yet be offered.

PREVENTIVE TREATMENT

Maldescended Testes

The incidence of maldescended testes among infertile patients is high. 8% of the men attending our fertility clinic have a history of maldescended testes, but of these only a few present with testes still in a dystope position. This indicates that prior treatment may have resulted in scrotal position of the testes, but did not necessarily lead to completely normal fertility. In the past it was usual to treat maldescended testes in advanced childhood or in puberty. This opinion has changed and for the past 20 years it has become accepted that the position of the testes should be corrected by the end of the second year of life. Most recently consensus was formed that treatment by hCG, GnRH or orchidopexy should be initiated even before the end of the first year of life. As most patients consulting for infertility are in their late 20s or early 30s, patients given such early treatment will only begin to turn up gradually in fertility clinics or will remain conspicuous by their absence if the concept of early treatment as a preventive measure will have proven itself.

Conventional treatment consists of intramuscular hCG injections or intranasal GnRH application. Both treatments are reported to have similar success rates and may be repeated if the testes should not reach a scrotal position after the first course of treatment. Also, switching from one regimen to the other has been recommended if one is not successful. More recently, the simultaneous combination of both GnRH and hCG has been advocated (18,28), but definite results have not yet been reported. If both treatments fail or if there are other anatomical abnormalities such as hernias, orchidopexy should be performed by a surgeon experienced in this delicate operation of the vulnerable testes.

hCG may not be effective in all cases, but it has always been considered a harmless treatment resulting only in transitory side effects such as increased aggressiveness or untimely erections due to stimulation of Leydig cells and testosterone production. In rats, however, it was shown that hCG causes an inflammation-like reaction in the testes with increased vascular permeability and leucocyte infiltration (6). While this was first considered a reaction specific to the rat, Hjertkvist et al. (21) recently demonstrated that such infiltrations are also observed in boys following hCG treatment. Although these alterations had largely disappeared 6-12 months after hCG therapy, the question may be raised whether hCG treatment is as harmless as it is thought to be and whether hCG treatment may in fact be harmful rather than beneficial for fertility. Since prospective studies addressing this question will be difficult to perform due to the long time spans of 2 to 3 decades involved, retrospective analysis of patients treated with different modalities will help to clarify this question.

In the adult infertile patient with a history of maldescended testes there is no possibility of improving seminal parameters. Whether chances of fertilization and pregnancy may be increased by techniques of assisted reproduction, is the object of ongoing investigations. Since maldescended testes show a higher incidence of malignancy, they should be investigated regularly (e.g. at annual intervals) by palpation and ultrasonography. In addition, the patient should learn to palpate the testes himself and seek medical advice as soon as he has any suspicious findings.

Infections

Another area where prevention of infertility plays an almost more important role than later treatment, are infections of the reproductive organs. Before antibiotics were introduced into clinical medicine, occlusion of the excurrent ducts as a sequelae of veneral disease, in particular, gonorrhea was the most common reason for male infertility (as a relic of that era, in Germany male infertility is still part of training in dermatology and venereology). While occlusion as a major cause of infertility still prevails in some areas of Africa, it became a minor problem in countries where early antibiotic treatment is practiced. Today, reconstructive microsurgery offers such patients good chances for refertilization which may, however, be impeded by sperm antibodies.

The best known cause of orchitis is the mumps virus. In addition, other viruses such as ECHO virus, Marburg virus, Chorionmeningitis virus and Arbo virus B as well as bacteria may cause orchitis. In the acute phase, usually glucocorticoids are administered. Whether they may help to prevent the permanent destruction of the seminiferous tubules is not known. If this occurs, the tubules are devoid of sperm cells and only Sertoli cells remain. When all tubules are afflicted, hypergonadotropic azoospermia occurs. In other cases, sperm may still be produced, however, their reduced quantity and quality cannot be improved. Thus, prevention of such a condition is the only useful therapy, but can only be effected by vaccination in the case of mumps.

In the course of assisted reproduction it became clear that subclinical infections also impair fertility. For this reason, infections, as evidenced by elevated seminal leucocytes, are now generally treated by antibiotics even if no specific pathogenic microorganisms can be identified.

Cryopreservation of Sperm

As chances of surviving malignant diseases have significantly increased in recent years due to modern chemo- and radiotherapy, patients (and their doctors) are becoming more concerned about the quality of life after therapy. Since these therapies may result in destruction of the seminal epithelium and in infertility, patients may be offered the possibility of cryopreservation of their semen. Unfortunately, testicular tumours and other malignant diseases may be associated with impaired seminal parameters even before therapy (7,13,44). As even under the best technical condition cryopreservation leads to a further decrease in sperm quality, it may be not worthwhile cryopreserving sperm of some of these patients.

This is illustrated by our own experience. Of 118 patients with testicular tumours (38%), hematologic (40%) or other (22%) neoplasias who consulted our clinic in the last 4 years for this purpose, semen samples went into long-term cryo-storage in only 51 cases. In the others, semen parameters were already too poor before cryopreservation or following a thawing trial. In cases where sperm are cryopreserved, however, chances of inducing pregnancy by insemination or in vitro fertilization are quite good, as published figures indicate (11,48,59).

Since dividing cells are more sensitive to cytotoxic effects than cells at rest, it had been suggested that suppression of spermatogenesis may protect patients undergoing chemotherapy from ensuing infertility (24). The GnRH-agonists, when given in high enough doses, desensitize the pituitary and lead to suppression of spermatogenesis. Exploiting this effect in trials for male contraception proved disappointing when given together with testosterone, as is necessary in hormonal male contraception (for review see Reference 39). Similarly, GnRH-agonists did not lead to the desired protection of spermatogenesis in patients undergoing chemotherapy (22). Now it is expected that GnRH-antagonists may be better suited for this purpose. It could, however, also be that this concept is incorrect and that spermatogenesis should not be suppressed but rather stimulated by gonadotropins, as van Alphen *et al.* (60) could demonstrate in monkeys exposed to X-ray irradiation. Future studies may provide therapeutic modalities to protect men undergoing cancer therapy from infertility, but for the time being, cryopreservation of sperm is an option that can be offered.

RATIONAL TREATMENT

Hypogonadism due to Hypothalamic or Pituitary Failure

The endocrine regulation of testicular function is the best elucidated aspect of male reproductive function. Therefore, endocrinology is often considered the backbone of andrology. The well-known feedback mechanisms between hypothalamus, pituitary and testes and their disturbances result in rational diagnostic and therapeutic measures in the case of secondary hypogonadism due to hypothalamic or pituitary failure.

In monkeys serving as a model for the human, testosterone in pharmacologic doses or FSH alone were sufficient to induce or maintain qualitatively normal spermatogenesis (for review see Reference 66). If such high doses of the hormones could be used in humans, similar effects would probably be achieved. However, for qualitatively and quantitatively normal spermatogenesis the interplay of both hormones, FSH and testosterone is required. Therefore, secondary hypogonadism has to be treated with a combination of hCG (LH, which stimulates testosterone production) and hMG (FSH) to induce spermatogenesis or alternatively, in the case of idiopathic hypogonadotropic hypogonadism (IHH) caused by hypothalamic dysfunction, GnRH must be administered in pulsatile fashion. Unless other confounding factors are encountered, such as maldescended testes, these therapies are effective in inducing spermatogenesis and pregnancies.

The current schemes of hCG/hMG and GnRH application may not entirely reflect the physiological situation since normal testes sizes and sperm counts are not achieved in most cases (29,47,52,67). This may, for example, be due to insufficient administration of FSH as current therapeutic schemes appear to provide FSH at too long intervals (23). Perhaps, in the course of introducing biosynthetic FSH (31) pharmacokinetic studies may be performed and result in improved therapeutic schemes.

Despite the need of further optimization of these treatment modalities, even the subnormal numbers of sperm produced by the current regimen are sufficient to induce pregnancies, since these are probably healthy sperm. Of the 18 patients with secondary hypogonadism whom we recently treated with hCG/hMG or pulsatile GnRH, all nine who intended to father a child, achieved pregnancies. These occurred after treatment periods of 12 months on average (ranging from 4-27 months) and with sperm counts in 8/9 patients well below the normal limit of 20 million/ml, as measured in the semen samples closest to the time of impregnation. Only in one of the remaining nine cases with a history of bilateral cryptorchidism and orchidopexy could spermatogenesis not be induced. The data illustrate the effectiveness of the current therapeutic regimens.

If the goal of pregnancy has been reached, GnRH or gonadotropic treatment can be terminated and therapy continued with testosterone substitution. The conventional substitution therapy consists of intramuscular injection of testosterone enanthate, subcutaneous implantation of cristalline testosterone or oral application of testosterone undecanoate (for review see Reference 36). Currently new forms of substitution therapy are under development, such as transdermal testosterone (4) or the long-acting testosterone buciclate (5) which may provide serum testosterone levels closer to physiology, thus providing the patient with improved well-being and long-term effects.

If another pregnancy should be desired, testosterone substitution is discontinued and stimulation by GnRH or hCG/hMG again implemented. Intermittent testosterone therapy does not reduce the chances that spermatogenesis can again be stimulated.

Obstruction of the Efferent Ducts

If antibiotic treatment is not used, or not used in time, acute inflammations of the epididymis, deferent ducts and other accessory organs may lead to obstruction of the efferent ducts, so that despite regular spermatogenesis, azoospermia may result. As mentioned above, reconstructive microsurgery may be applied in these cases, often resulting in regained fertility. The same microsurgical techniques can be applied for reanastomosis of the defective ducts after vasectomy, if fertility is requested again. In cases where surgery has failed or is not possible due to extensive obstruction, the insertion of alloplastic spermatoceles had been attempted. However, to 79 couples in whom 2-37 (!) inseminations with aspirated sperm were attempted, no child was born (63). The failure of pregnancy induction prevented wider use of this technique. More recently, pregnancies were reported following in vitro fertilization with sperm aspirated from the epididymis proximal of the occlusion (32). With improving IVF techniques, this approach may provide an alternative if surgery is not possible or failed to achieve reanastomosis.

Aspiration of sperm from the epididymis followed by IVF and pregnancy has also been reported in cases with congenital absence of the ductus deferentes (54). Since a high proportion of these patients carry gene mutations for cystic fibrosis (1,15), sperm aspiration and IVF must be preceded by genetic screening of the patient and his wife and proper counselling of the couple if the risk of cystic fibrosis in the offspring should be high.

Treatment of Basal Diseases and Elmination of Toxins

Male hypogonadism and infertility may occur in severe acute or systemic disorders such as liver diseases, diabetes mellitus, renal failure, hemochromatosis and neoplasia (30,55). One of the most extensively studied effects of chronic disease on reproductive function is the impairment of spermatogenesis and testicular steroidogenesis by chronic renal failure. These dysfunctions are not correctable by hemodialysis, but can be reversed by renal transplantation which is thus the best treatment for the associated infertility (for review see Reference 19). About half of the patients with full-blown AIDS present with hypogonadotropic or hypergonadotropic hypogonadism (10,12).

Occupational and environmental chemicals, such as carbon disulfide, dibromochloropropane and lead, are well known to have adverse effects on male reproductive function (for review see Reference 53). Of major clinical importance are the negative effects of radiation and chemotherapy on testicular function. In addition, a large number of different drugs has been identified as having negative effects on male fertility (for review see Reference 14). GnRH analogs (for review see Reference 39) and steroid hormones including anabolic steroids (26) suppress gonadotropin secretion and lead to suppression of spermatogenesis. Morphine analogs interfere with endogenous opiate metabolism and suppress LH secretion via changes in central neurotransmitter metabolism. Psychotropic drugs, antihypertensives such as alphamethyldopa or reserpine, dopamine antagonists such as metoclopramide, and H2-receptor antagonists such as cimetidine or ranitidine interfere with hypothalamic dopamine metabolism leading to an increase in prolactin and suppression of GnRH and gonadotropin secretion, or may interfere with ejaculation. Among others, antibiotics including salicylazosulfapyridine, and psychotropic drugs may have direct effects on spermatogenesis and/or sperm function (14,16,51). Rational treatment would be withdrawal of these drugs or replacement by drugs with no adverse effects on male fertility.

NO TREATMENT AVAILABLE

In primary hypogonadism both spermatogenesis and testosterone production are impaired or absent. One of the most frequent syndromes encountered in this category is the Klinefelter syndrome, characterized by azoospermia and various degrees of testosterone deficiency, caused by a numerical chromosomal abnormality. In the XX-male caused by translocation of the Y-chromosome, in gonadal dysgenesis and the male Turner syndrome azoospermia and testosterone deficiency are also found. Of course, in bilateral anorchia, congenital or acquired, both testosterone and sperm production are lacking. In other cases, defects in spermiogenesis may render the patient infertile. For example, defects in the axonemata structure of the sperm flagellum may cause immotility of the sperm (35) and the failure of acrosome development may lead to globozoospermia where the sperm cannot interact with the zona pellucida and infertility results. With the advancement of techniques of molecular genetics, more and more genetically caused defects in spermatogenesis may be identified. For example, identification of the azoospermia factor on the long arm of the Y-chromosome may explain why an otherwise normal patient may be azoospermic (62).

For the time being, however, these diagnoses will not lead to therapeutic possibilities of treating infertility. Nevertheless, a firm diagnosis, though disappointing, dispels uncertainty and it puts an end to false hopes. While the infertility cannot be abolished, it is important to emphasize that any accompanying endocrine insufficiency in these patients can and must be treated by testosterone substitution according to the principles outlined above (36). Testosterone substitution must be performed as a lifelong therapy.

DISPUTED AND EXPERIMENTAL TREATMENT

Varicocele

Varicoceles have a high incidence in the general male population above the age of puberty; conservative estimates assume about 5%. Among infertile men the incidence may be 3 to 6 times higher. The different incidence of varicocele in fertile and infertile men suggests that there is a causal relationship between this condition and infertility. However, this infertility is not absolute and may be compensated by optimal female reproductive functions, while they may become evident when the female partner's functions are also impaired. It is established that varicoceles are associated with impaired seminal and hormonal parameters even in fertile men (34) and may progressively deteriorate with time (8).

While the relationship between varicocele and impaired fertility is established, the influence of therapy is much less certain. Although surgical ligation of the vena spermatica, and more recently, angiographic methods for the occlusion of the spermatic vein are generally considered integral parts of male infertility treatment, not all investigators are convinced that this therapy really improves the chances for fertility. Uncontrolled studies usually report satisfactory results. A review of 50 publications comprising 5471 patients treated by surgical ligation found an average pregnancy rate of 36% with indications for surgery, surgical techniques, observation periods and other criteria varying considerably (33). The only studies comparing surgical treatment with no treatment concluded that ligation does not increase the chances for pregnancy in the treated patients (42,46,61). However, two of these studies were criticized since real randomization of the patients was not carried out and over all, these studies did not exert much influence on the therapeutic approach to varicocele. It appears that larger controlled studies fulfilling strict criteria are required to resolve the question whether, and under which conditions, varicoceles should be treated or not.

Meanwhile, we have recently concluded a study addressing the question whether surgical ligation or angiographic occlusion by tissue adhesive may result in better seminal parameters and higher pregnancy rates. The results showed that pregnancy rates among the 71 couples in the 12 months follow-up treatment were similar in both groups (29% in the surgical and 33% in the angiographic group) so that the two techniques can be considered equivalent (40). The advantage of the angiographic procedure is that it can be performed on an outpatient basis without general anaesthesia. The shorter time requested from the otherwise healthy patient is generally considered to be of advantage.

Immunological Infertility

Antibodies to sperm can lead to a decrease in sperm motility, to agglutinations and to fertility disturbances. Antibodies may arise from autoimmune processes initiated by infection, traumas, obstruction of the epididymis and deferent ducts, as well as other events. Insofar as possible, therapy should include the correction of anatomic anomalies and obstructions (20). In addition, immunosuppressive therapy with corticosteroids, often administered in high doses, was recommended for many years. More recent double-blind, placebo-controlled studies were able to show that this therapy which is not free of side effects, could not induce higher pregnancy rates (2,17). In our study, 20 selected couples were enrolled and husbands were treated in a randomized cross-over fashion with either placebo or prednisolone (40 mg on day 1-10 and 5 mg on day 11-12 of the wife's cycle for 3 cycles each). No pregnancy occured under either treatment (2). While some authors continue to recommend this treatment (e.g., see Reference 20), the lack of effectiveness should direct the therapist to alternative modalities.

As discussed in the following chapter by Brindson (page 273), such new modalities are offered by techniques of assisted fertilization. It ist not yet clear whether intrauterine insemination using prepared sperm in stimulated and carefully monitored cycles or *in vitro* fertilization, more complex and time-consuming, achieves better results. In addition, sperm preparations may be further improved by adding proteolytic enzymes which will dissolve sperm agglutinations (43).

Idiopathic Infertility

The largest group of patients with disturbed fertility suffer from idiopathic infertility. These patients show impaired spermatogenesis and subnormal semen parameters with or without elevated FSH, but the pathologic course of this disturbance remains unclear. This diagnosis probably harbours a multitude of different pathologies and represent a constant challenge to andrologic research. New insights are expected from molecular biology, paracrinology and gamete biology (for reviews see References 38 and 45). However, since the patients require treatment now, there is a constant temptation to use a variety of drugs and procedures without final proof of effectiveness.

Since GnRH, gonadotropins and testosterone are required for normal testicular function and are also effective in the treatment of hypogonadism, it was and is tempting to try their application in idiopathic infertility as well, although endocrine defects could not be demonstrated as the pathogenetic causes of this type of infertility. Ever since gonadotropins became available for clinical use in the early 60s, they were also applied in this condition. Surprisingly, they were used without their effectiveness being properly assessesd. A review summarizing 39 studies, all uncontrolled and reporting pregnancy rates on average of 8 or 14% depending on sperm concentrations below or above 10 million/ml respectively, concluded that controlled double-blind studies were urgently needed (49). At last, such a study was performed by us in patients with normogonadotropic oligoasthenoteratozoospermia and we could demonstrate that, in comparison to the placebo group, no improvement of seminal parameters (Fig. 1) or increase in pregnancy rates could be produced (25).

In a preliminary observation Wagner and Warsch (64) suggested that oligoasthenoteratozoospermia in patients with elevated FSH levels may be

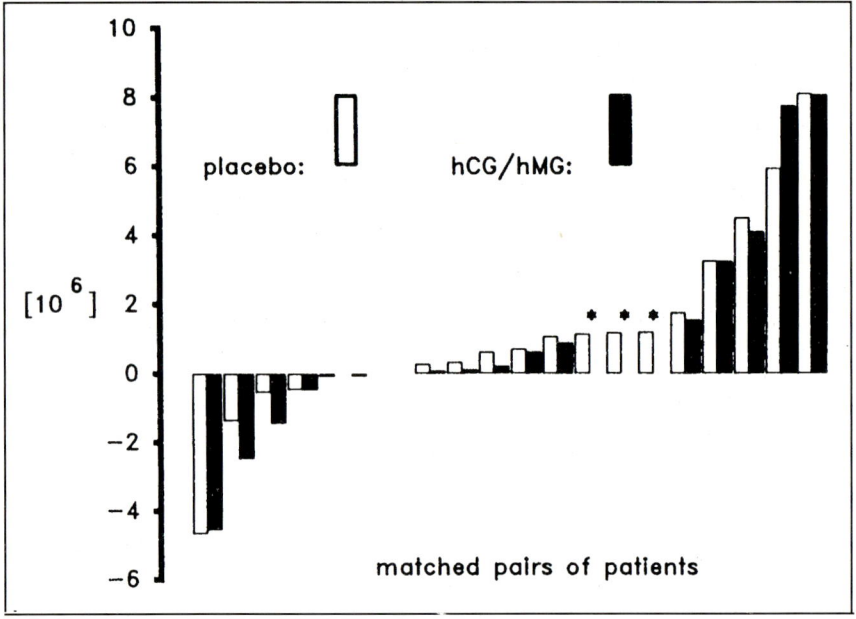

FIG. 1. Results of a placebo-controlled, double-blind, randomized trial of hCG/hMG treatment for normogonadotropic oligoasthenoteratozoospermia. The differences in the means of the total number of normally formed, motile sperm are shown. Individual values of patients (placebo, n = 20, hCG/hMG, n = 17) are matched between groups according to the magnitude of the differences. Asterisks indicate lack of appropriate counterpart (25).

caused by too infrequent GnRH pulses and claimed improved seminal parameters by pulsatile GnRH therapy delivered at a physiologic frequency. We tried to confirm these findings and treated seven patients with oligoasthenoteratozoospermia and elevated FSH levels with 5 µg GnRH pulses every 120 minutes for 12 weeks and nine such further patients with pulses every 90 minutes over 24 weeks. Despite a significant reduction of FSH levels (Fig. 2) no improvement in seminal parameters as analyzed according to WHO guidelines could be observed (3). Due to the lack of positive effects on seminal parameters a further and controlled study appeared superfluous.

The requirement of testosterone for normal spermatogenesis under physiologic conditions lead to the use of androgens in idiopathic male infertility, although abnormalities in serum or intratesticular testosterone could not be demonstrated in this condition (41). Even without a clear pathophysiologic concept, mesterolone was used over many years in idiopathic infertility. Finally, WHO (68) performed a randomized, controlled double-

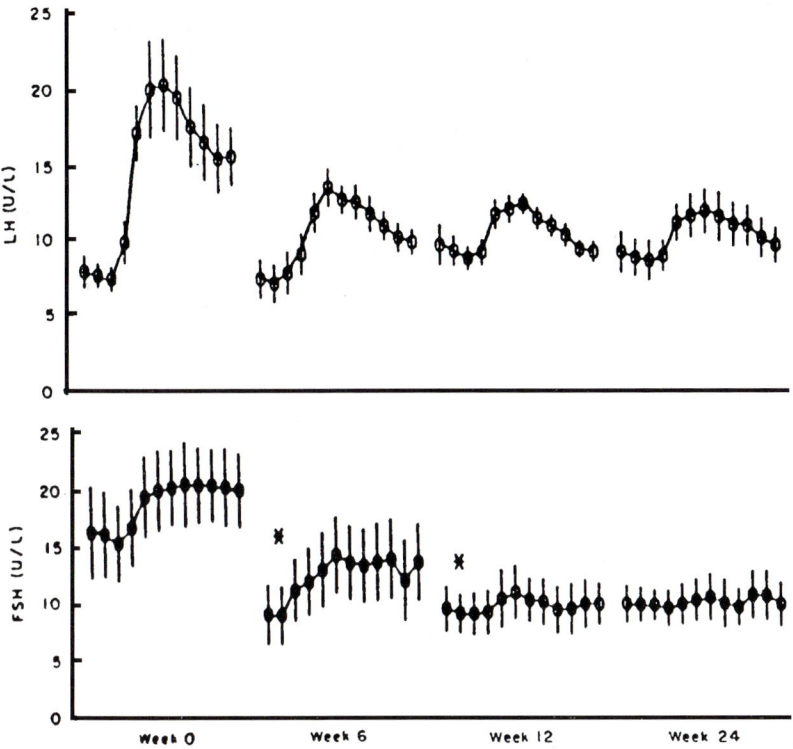

FIG. 2. Basal and GnRH (5 μg) stimulated LH and FSH serum levels in seven patients with idiopathic infertility and elevated FSH treated by pulsatile GnRH at 90 min. intervals for 24 weeks (means ± SEM). Asterisks indicate $P < 0.05$ compared with preceding basal values (3).

blind study involving 256 couples. Compared to placebo, no significant increase in pregnancy rates could be demonstrated. More recently, the oral effect of testosterone undecanoate has been advocated for the treatment of male infertility, but again, convincing results have not yet been produced. Earlier, testosterone rebound therapy was used in order to prove fertility (for review see Reference 37); however, the resulting semen parameters and pregnancy rates were obviously so unconvincing that this modality became unpopular even without properly designed controlled studies.

Currently, antiestrogens (in particular tamoxifen) have taken over from mesterolone. Antiestrogens block estrogen action in the pituitary and thereby increase gonadotropins in serum. Assuming that an increase in LH and FSH may improve sperm production, antiestrogens are used in idiopathic infertility. The studies carried out so far have produced negative or conflicting results (27,56,58,65). Larger double-blind placebo-controlled studies would be required to establish their effectiveness. In addition, Tamoxifen has recently been reported in association with the development of lethal liver damage (9) so that it should not be used indiscriminantly.

Although there is no clear therapeutic concept supporting the use of kallikrein, it has been in use for many years as a treatment of idiopathic infertility, especially to improve sperm motility. Results concerning the improvement of seminal parameters and induction of pregnancy are contradictory. Today, the effectiveness of kallikrein cannot be considered proven and further results of large-scale studies presently being conducted must be awaited (50).

In addition to insemination techniques, of which intrauterine application of prepared sperm in stimulated and well-monitored cycles are currently favoured, other techniques of assisted reproduction have been introduced to male infertility treatment. As a recent worldwide survey revealed, of 47,192 IVF cycles and of 4,647 GIFT cycles, 15 and 23%, respectively, were performed for 'male factor only' (57), indicating the order of magnitude of this kind of treatment. While these techniques will be discussed in detail in the following chapters by Brindson (page 273) and by Fishell (page 293), it should be emphasized here that techniques of assisted reproduction have to be subjected to the same strict evaluation criteria as any other method in order to establish their effectiveness and their proper rank in the treatment of male infertility. In particular, comparisons between these techniques and natural, yet timed intercourse in stimulated cycles appear to be mandatory.

CONCLUSIONS

Although not based on strict pathogenetic criteria, the classification of male infertility into disorders which can be prevented, which can be treated on a rational basis, which cannot be treated and where experimental treatment may be performed, proved useful when discussing the therapeutic possibilities of increasing the chances of an infertile male to induce a pregnancy. All treatments should be evaluated in properly designed trials. The requirements in the design of such studies may be least stringent in the case of substitution therapy where, e.g., the application of gonadotropins leads from azoospermia to the presence of sperm sufficient for fertilization. If modifications to an established regimen or new gonadotropins (e.g. produced by recombinant synthesis) are introduced, they should be evaluated in comparison to the existing treatments. Treatments for other conditions require strictly controlled, prospective studies. A genuine therapeutic effect can only be considered to have taken place when changes in seminal parameters differ significantly from those of a placebo-treated, control group and only when pregnancies accumulated over time are significantly more numerous in the treated group than in the control group. Such studies are, however, extremely complex. Not only must the patients in the verum and in the control group be alike in order to be randomized, but thorough examination of the partners must also exclude any disturbances of female reproductive function. As any anticipated changes in seminal parameters and pregnancy rates will occur in a narrow range, reasonably large groups are required to produce convincing results. The standards demanded by such a study often exceed the capacities of a single center and multicenter studies, while fulfilling these criteria, presuppose a high level of organization.

As in any other field of medicine, only therapies with definitely proven effectiveness should be used in the treatment of male infertility. Any therapeutic procedures whose effectiveness has not been verified by control studies should be applied only in the context of clinical studies until their effectiveness has been proven.

REFERENCES

1. Anguiano, A., Cates, R.D., Amos, J.A, Dean, M., Gerrard, B., Stewart, C., Maner, T.A., White, M.B., and Milunsky, A. (1992) Congenital bilateral absence of the vas deferens. A primarily genital form of cystic fibrosis. JAMA, 267:1794-1797.
2. Bals-Pratsch, M., Dîren, M., Karbowski, B., 1. Schneider, H.P.G. and Nieschlag, E. (1992) Cyclic corticosteroid immunosuppression is unsuccessful in the treatment of sperm antibody-related male infertility: a controlled study. Hum. Reprod., 7:99-104.
3. Bals-Pratsch, M., Knuth, U.A., Hinigl, W., Klein, H.M., Bergmann, M. and Nieschlag, E. (1989) Pulsatile GnRH-therapy in oligozoospermic men does not improve smeinal parameters despite decreased FSH levels. Clin. Endocrinol. (Oxf)., 30:549-560.
4. Bals-Pratsch, M., Knuth, U.A., Yoon, Y.D. and Nieschlag, E. (1986) Transdermal testosterone substitution therapy for male hypogonadism. Lancet, ii:943-946.
5. Behre, H.M. and Nieschlag, E. (1992) Testosterone buciclate (20-Aet-1) in hypogonadal men: Pharmacokinetics and pharmacodynamics of the new long-acting testosterone ester. J. Clin. Endocrinol. Metab. (in press).
6. Bergh, A., Rooth, P., Widmark, A., and Damber, J.E. (1987) Treatment of rats with hCG induces inflammation-like changes in the testicular microcirculation. J. Reprod. Fertil, 79:135-143.
7. Carson, S.A., Gentry, W.L., Smith, A.L and Buster, J.E. (1991) Feasibility of semen collection and cryopreservation during chemotherapy. Hum. Reprod., 6:992-994.
8. Chehval, M.J. and Purcell, R.N. (1992) Deterioration of semen parameters over time in men with untreated varicocele: evidence of progressive testicular damage. Fertil. Steril., 57:174-177.
9. Ching, C.K., Smith, P.G. and Long, R.G. (1992) Tamoxifen-associated hepatocellular damage and agranulocytosis. Lancet, 339:940.
10. Croxson, T.S., Chapman, W.E., Miller, L.K., Levit, C.D., Senie, R., Zumoff, B. (1989) Changes in the hypothalamic-pituitary-gonadal axis in human immunodeficiency virus-infected homosexual men. J. Clin. Endocrinol. Metab., 68:317-321.
11. Davis, O.K., Bedford, J.M., Berkeley, A.S., Graf, M.J. and Rosenwaks, Z. (1990) Pregnancy achieved through in vitro fertilization with cryopreserved semen from a man with Hodgkin's lymphoma. Fertil. Steril., 53:377-378.
12. Dluhy, R.G. (1990) The growing spectrum of HIV-related endocrine abnormalities. J. Clin. Endocrinol. Metab., 70:563-565.
13. Drasga, R.E., Einhorn, L.H., Williams, S.D., Patel, D.N. and Stevens, E.E. (1983) Fertility after chemotherapy for testicular cancer. J. Clin. Oncol., 1:179-184.
14. Drife, J.O. (1987) The effects of drugs on sperm. Drugs, 33:610-622.
15. Dumur, V., Gervais, R. Rigot, J.M., Lafitte, J.J., Manouvrier, S., Biserte, J., Mazemann, E. and Roussel, P. (1990) Abnormal distribution of CF delta F 508 allele in azoospermic men with congenital aplasia of epididymis and vas deferens. Lancet, 336:512.
16. Giwercman, A. and Skakkebaek, N.E. (1986) The effect of salicylazosulphapyridine (sulphasalazine) on male fertility: A review. Int. J. Androl., 9:38-52.

17. Haas, G.G., and Manganiello, P. (1987) A double-blind, placebo-controlled study of the use of methylprednisolone in infertile men with sperm-associated immunoglobulins. Fertil. Steril., 47:295-301.
18. Hagberg, S. and Westphal, O. (1987) Results of combined hormonal and surgical treatment for undescended testis in boys under 3 years of age. A randomized study. Eur. J. Pediat. 146: Suppl., 2:38-39.
19. Handelsman, D.J. (1985) Hypothalamic-pituitary gonadal dysfunction in renal failure, dialysis and renal transplantation. Endocr. Rev., 6:151-182.
20. Hendry, W.F. (1992) The significance of antisperm antibodies: measurements and management. Clin. Endocrinol. (Oxf)., 36:219-221.
21. Hjertkvist, M., Läckgren, G., Plöen, L. and Bergh, A. (1992) Does hCG-treatment induce inflammation-like changes in undescended testes in boys? J. Pediat. Surg. (in press).
22. Höffken, K. (1988) LHRH agonists in oncology. Springer. Verlag, Heidelberg.
23. Jockenhîvel, F., Fingscheidt, U., Khan, S.A., Behre, H.M. and Nieschlag, E. (1990) Bio- and immuno-activity of FSH in serum after intramuscular injection of highly purified urinary human FSH in normal men. Clin. Endocrinol. (Oxf)., 33:573-584.
24. Johnson, D.H., Linde, R., Hainworth, J.D., Vale, W, Rivier, J., Stein, R., Flexner, J., Van Welch, R. and Greco, A. (1985) Effect of a luteinizing hormone releasing hormone agonist given during combination chemotherapy on posttherapy fertility in male patients with lymphoma: preliminary observations. Blood, 65:832-836.
25. Knuth, U.A., Hönigl, W., Bals-Pratsch, M., Schleicher, G. and Nieschlag, E. (1987) Treatment of severe oligozoospermia with hCG/hMG. A placebo-controlled double-blind trial. J. Clin. Endocrinol. Metab., 65:1081-1087.
26. Knuth, U.A., Maniera, H. and Nieschlag, E. (1989) Anabolic steroids and semen parameters in bodybuilders. Fertil. Steril., 52:1041-1047.
27. Krause, W., Holland-Moritz, H. and Schramm, P (1992) Treatment of idiopathic oligozoospermia with tamoxifen - a randomized controlled study. Int. J. Androl., 15:14-18.
28. Lala, R., Canavese, F., Matarazzo, P., Chiabotto, P., and De Sanctis, C. (1991) Trattamento medico del criptorchidismo nella prima infanzia. Pediat. Med. Chir., 13(1):73-75.
29. Liu, L., Banks, S.M., Barnes, K.M. and Sherins R.J. (1988) Two-year comparison of testicular responses to pulsatile gonadotropin-releasing hormone and exogenous gonadotropins from the inception of therapy in men with isolated hypogonadotropic hypogonadism. J. Clin. Endocrinol. Metab., 67:1140-1145.
30. Luppa, P., Munker, R., Nagel, D., Weber, M. and Engelhardt, D. (1991) Serum androgens in intensive-care patients: correlations with clinical findings. Clin. Endocrinol. (Oxf)., 34:305-310.
31. Mannaerts, B., De Leeuw, R., Geelen, J. and Van Ravestein, A. (1991) Comparative *in vitro* and *in vivo* studies on the biological characteristics of recombinant human follicle stimulating hormone. Endocrinology, 129:2623-2630.
32. Mathieu, C., Guérin, J.-F., Cognat, M., Lejeune, H., Pinatel, M.-C. and Lornage, J. (1992) Motility and fertilizing capacity of epididymal human spermatozoa in normal and pathological cases. Fertil. Steril., 57:871.
33. Mordel, N., Mor-Yosef, S., Margalioth, E.J., Simon, Menashe, A.M., Berger, M. and Schenker, J. (1990) Spermatic vein ligation as treatment for male infertility. J. Reprod. Med., 35:123-127.
34. Nagao, R.R, Plymate, S.R., Berger, R.E., Perin, E.B. and Paulsen, C.A. (1986) Comparison of gonadal function between fertile and infertile men with varicoceles. Fertil. Steril., 46:930-933.
35. Neugebauer, D.-Ch., Neuwinger, J., Jockenhîvel, F. and Nieschlag, E. (1990) "9+0" axoneme in spermatozoa and some nasal cilia of a patient with totally immotile spermatozoa associated with thickened sheath and short midpiece. Hum. Reprod., 5:981-986.
36. Nieschlag, E. and Behre, H.M. (1990) Pharmacology and clinical use of testosterone. In: Testosterone: Action, Deficiency, Substitution, edited by Nieschlag, E. and Behre H.M., pp 92-114. Springer Verlag, Heidelberg.
37. Nieschlag, E. and Freischem, C.W. (1982) Androgen therapy in hypogonadism and infertility. In: Treatment of male infertility, edited by Bain, J., Schwarzstein, A. and Schill, W.-B., pp. 103-113. Springer Verlag, Heidelberg.
38. Nieschlag, E. and Habenicht, U.F. (eds.) (1992) Spermatogenesis - fertilization - contraception: Molecular, Cellular and Endocrine Events in Male Reproduction. Schering Foundation Workshop 4, Springer, Heidelberg.
39. Nieschlag, E., Behre, H.M and Weinbauer, G.F. (1992) Hormonal male contraception: A

real chance? In: Spermatogenesis - fertilization - contraception: Molecular, Cellular and Endocrine Events in Male Reproduction, edited by Nieschlag, E. and Habenicht, U.F., pp 477-502. Schering Foundation Workshop 4, Springer, Heidelberg.
40. Nieschlag, E., Behre, H.M., Schlingheider, A., Nashan, D., Pohl, J. and Fischedick, A.R. (1992) Surgical ligation versus angiographic embolisation of the vena spermatica: A prospective randomized study for the treatment of varicocele-related infertility. (Submitted).
41. Nieschlag, E., Wickings, E.J. and Mauss, J. (1979) Endocrine testicular function in vivo and in vitro in infertile men. Acta Endocrinol. (Copenh)., 90:544-551.
42. Nilsson, S., Edvinsson, A. and Nilsson, B. (1979) Improvement of semen and pregnancy rate after ligation and division of the internal spermatic vein: fact or fiction? Br. J. Urol., 51:591-596.
43. Pattinson, H.A., Mortimer, D. and Taylor, P.J. (1990) treatment of sperm agglutination with proteolytic enzymes. II. sperm function after enzymatic disagglutination. Hum. Reprod., 5:174-178.
44. Ragni, G. Bestetti, O., Santoro, A., Viviani, S., Di Pietro, R. and De Lauretis, L. (1985) Evaluation of semen and pituitary gonadotropin function in men with untreated Hodgkin's disease. Fertil. Steril., 43:927-930.
45. Robaire, B. (ed.) (1991) The male germ cell: spermatogonium to fertilization. Ann. NY Acad. Sci., 637. New York.
46. Rodriguez-Rigau, L., Smith, K. and Steinberger, E. (1978) Relationship of varicocele to sperm output and fertility of male partners in infertile couples. J. Urol., 120:691-694.
47. Saal, W., Happ, J. Cordes, U., Baum, R.P., and Schmidt, M. (1991) Subcutaneous gonadotropin therapy in male patients with hypogonadotropic hypogonadism. Fertil. Steril., 56:319-324.
48. Scammel, G.D., White, N., Stedronska, J., Hendry, W.F., Edmonds, D.K. and Jeffcoate, S.L. (1985) Cryopreservation of semen in men with testicular tumour or Hodgkin's disease results of artificial insemination of their partners. Lancet, 2:31-32.
49. Schill, B.-W. (1986) Medical treatment of male infertility. In: Infertility: Male and female, edited by Insler, V. and Lunenfeld, B., pp 533-573. Churchill Livingstone, Edinburgh.
50. Schill, B.-W., Miska, W. (1992) Possible effects of the kallikrein-kinin system on male reproductive functions. Andrologia, 24: 69-75.
51. Schlegel, P.N., Chang, T.S.K., Marshall F.F. (1991) Antibiotics: potential hazards to male fertility. Fertil. Steril., 55: 235-242.
52. Schopohl, J., Mehltretter, G., von Zumbusch R., Eversman, T. and von Werder, K. (1991) Comparison of gonadotropin-releasing hormone and gonadotropin therapy in male patients with idiopathic hypothalamic hypogonadism. Fertil. Steril., 56:1143-1150.
53. Schrag, S.D. and Dixon, R.L. (1985) Occupational exposures associated with male reproductive dysfunction. Annu. Rev. Pharmacol. Toxicol, 25:567-592.
54. Silber, S., Ord, T., Balmaceda, J., Patrizio, P. and Asch, R. (1990). Congenital absence of the vas deferens. The fertilizing capacity of human epididymal sperm. N. Engl. J. Med., 323:1788-1792.
55. Sobel, R.J., Liel, Y., Glick, S.M. (1986) Medical conditions leading to infertility. In: Infertility: male and female, edited by Insler, V. and Lunenfeld, B. pp. 673-696. Churchill Livingstone, Edinburgh.
56. Sokol, R., Steiner, B., Bustillo, M., Petersen, G. and Swerdloff, R. (1988) A controlled comparison of the efficacy of clomiphene citrate in male infertility. Fertil. Steril., 49:865-870.
57. Testart, J., Plachot, M., Mandelbaum, J., Salat-Baroux, J., Frydman, R. and Cohen, J. (1992) World collaborative report on IVF-ET and GIFT: 1989 results. Hum. Reprod., 7:362-369.
58. Török, L. (1984) Treatment of oligozoospermia with tamoxifen (open and controlled studies). Andrologia, 17:497-501.
59. Tournaye, H., Wisanto, A., Camus, M. van Steirteghem, A.C., Bollen, N. and Devroey, P. (1991) In vitro fertilization techniques with frozen-thawed sperm: a method for preserving the progenitive potential of Hodgkin patients. Fertil. Steril., 55:443-445.
60. van Alphen, M.M.A, van de Kant, H.J.G. and de Rooij, D.G. (1989) Protection from radiation-induced damage of spermatogenesis in the rhesus monkey (macaca mulatta) by FSH. Cancer. Res., 49:533-536.
61. Vermeulen, A., Vandeweghe, M. and Deslypere, J.P. (1986) Prognosis of subfertility in men with corrected or uncorrected varicocele. J. Androl., 7:147-155.
62. Vogt, P. (1992) Y-chromosome function in spermatogenesis. In: Spermatogenesis - ferti-

lization - contraception: Molecular, Cellular and Endocrine Events in Male Reproduction, edited by Nieschlag E. and Habenicht U.F., pp 225-266. Springer, Heidelberg.
63. Wagenknecht, L.V. (1991) Aktueller Erfahrungsstand zur alloplastischen Spermatozele. Fertilität, 7:185-189
64. Wagner, R.O.F. and Warsch, F. (1984) Pulsatile LHRH therapy of "slow pulsing oligospermia": indirect evidence for a hypothalamic origin of the disorder. Acta Endocrinol. (Copenh)., 105: suppl. 264:142-145.
65. Wang, C., Chan, C.W, Wong, K.K. and Yeung, K.K. (1983) Comparison of the effectiveness of placebo, clomiphen citrate, mesterolone, pentoxifylline, and testosterone rebound therapy for the treatment of idiopathic oligospermia. Fertil. Steril., 40:358-365.
66. Weinbauer, G.F. and Nieschlag, E. (1991) Peptide and steroid regulation of spermatogenesis in primates. In: The germ cell: spermatogonium to fertilization, edited by Robaire, B., Ann. N.Y. Acad. Sci., 637:107-121.
67. Whitcomb, R.W. and Crowley, W.F. (1990) Clinical review 4: diagnosis and treatment of isolated gonadotropin-releasing hormone deficiency in men. J. Clin. Endocrinol. Metab., 70:3-7.
68. WHO Task Force on the Diagnosis and Treatment of Infertility (1989) Mesterolone and idiopathic male infertility: a double-blind study. Int. J. Androl., 12:254-264.

Assisted Reproductive Technology in the Treatment of Male Infertility

P.R. Brinsden and S. Avery

Bourn Hall Clinic, The Bourn-Halam Group, Bourn, Cambridge, CB3 7TR, UK

INTRODUCTION

Following the development of in vitro fertilisation (IVF) for the treatment of tubal and idiopathic infertility, it became apparent by the mid-1980's that good pregnancy rates were achievable for couples whose principal cause of infertility was sperm dysfunction. As the success of this treatment became more evident, so it became obvious that much more detailed studies of actual sperm function rather than the existing crude categorisations were required. With increasing experience of IVF for male infertility, it also became apparent that, while the conventional World Health Organisation (WHO) (71) classification of male fertility might apply to natural fertility, it bore no relationship to fertility using assisted fertilisation techniques which had evolved out of IVF.

Because the treatment of male infertility by conventional means remains so unsuccessful, and because of the high incidence of the problem, very great efforts are being made in units practising assisted reproductive technology (ART), both on the scientific and medical sides, to solve some of the problems of male infertility and to achieve better pregnancy success rates. The different ART techniques which have evolved for the treatment of male infertility are reviewed in this chapter. Discussion and emphasis is placed on the vital importance of adequate assessment of sperm function prior to entering treatment and will be considered before discussion of the clinical aspects of treatment.

THE DIAGNOSIS OF DISORDERS OF SPERM FUNCTION

The cause of failure to fertilise oocytes, either *in vivo* or *in vitro* in the presence of male factor infertility is, in general, seldom adequately diagnosed because the basic cause of the sperm dysfunction of infertile men is poorly understood. This makes diagnosis difficult and therefore also makes rational treatment of the problem often impossible.

SPERM FUNCTION TESTING

Matson *et al.* (47), in examining the outcome of IVF with low numbers of motile sperm, showed that, following exclusion of those cases where fertilization failed completely, fertilization rates were comparable with those of normospermic men. This led to the suggestion that there were two types of oligospermic patient, those whose problem was simply one of sperm numbers, and those who also had a problem of sperm dysfunction, and were likely to fail completely at IVF. Equally there are many cases where semen parameters are normal, but fertilization persistently fails to occur. This illustrates the weakness of using the WHO standard for semen analysis (71) as the only assessment of male fertility. Over recent years, a number of tests has been developed enabling more detailed assessment of sperm function.

Tests can be divided into two main groups; motility/transport and zona/oocyte binding and penetration. Sperm motility can be assessed quantitatively by routine methods, but there are specifics of sperm motion that are critical for fertility *in vivo* and *in vitro*. Penetration of cervical mucus is dependent on lateral displacement of the sperm head being >4.5 μm and less than 10 μm (2). In addition, sperm velocity below 25 μm/sec may also impair mucus penetration. This aspect of sperm function can be assessed by the use of mucus penetration tests using a flat capillary tube containing cervical mucus and assessing the degree of penetration achieved in terms of numbers and distance. Bovine mucus may also be used, or artifical mucus columns such as those consisting of hyaluronic acid. While values outside these limits do not preclude fertility, they represent a significant disadvantage. As sperm undergo the process of capacitation, the pattern of motion alters considerably, with the development of hyperactivated or whiplash motility. The amplitude of the flagellar wave increases, and the path of sperm movement becomes erratic, rather than straight. This type of activity is thought to play a major role in penetration of the zona pellucida by setting up shearing forces once the sperm is tightly bound to the zona surface. Sperm motion can be analysed using a number of techniques, by time lapse photography, using a stroboscope, or frame by frame analysis of film/video tape. However the only practial method for routine use involves the use of computerised motion analysis. There are a number of commercially available machines which allow the operater to set his own parameters, and which can give rapid assessment of all the relevant parameters, including the percentage of sperm that have undergone hyperactivation. This is likely to be the most significant aspect of sperm motility as far as IVF is concerned, and is important, not only for assessing the proportion of sperm capable of undergoing capacitation, but also for assessng the response of sperm to stimulants that might enhance fertilizing capacity.

In terms of sperm oocyte interraction, the acrosome reaction is a convenient process to measure since it has a definite end point. Much attention has been focussed on methods of testing acrosomal function using various markers and dedicated commercial products are now available. Spontaneous acrosome reactions give no useful information about fertilizing capacity and therefore assays need to be based on the acrosomal response to suitable stimuli. Increasing levels of intracellular calcium play an important role in triggering the acrosome reaction and the calcium ionophore A23187 has been used to bring about this increase. Cummins *et al.* (23) used a score based on the difference between stimulated and unstimulated rates of acrosome reaction to successfully predict fertilizing capacity. This group used the lectin *Pisum sativum* linked to fluoroscein isothyacyanate as a marker for the presence of the acrosome, and considered this test to be an accurate predictor of IVF outcome, although the predictive value varied according to the cut off score used. Aitken *et al.* (2) had already proposed the used of calcium ionophore in sperm function testing, in this case in relation to the zona free hamster egg penetration test. While this addition clearly increased the predictive value of this test, such tests are always likely to produce false positives, since they do not test all aspects of sperm function in particular zona binding and penetration. The hemizona assay, which involves the use of unfertilized human oocytes, is not possible in many units, due to the non availability of suitable oocytes. This is unfortunate, since this test has a pivotal role in the diagnosis of fertilisation ability (2). Failure at the level of zona binding is likely to negate subsequent functional assays.

There are more generalised assays of sperm physiology such as the hypoosmotic sperm swelling test, and 24 hour sperm survival rates. Opinions differ as to the predictive accuracy of these assays. Some authors have found hypoosmotic swelling to be highly predictive of fertilizing capacity (37), while other have found it to be of little value (7). Thus, sperm function testing still presents a number of problems, particularly of accuracy, and availability. IVF itself remains the best test of sperm function, although a single failed cycle is not considered to be sufficient evidence of lack of fertilizing capacity (47). However, sperm function testing will yield conclusive results in some patients, and may prevent them from undergoing traumatic and expensive treatments in cases where sperm function is totally impaired.

SPERM PREPARATION FOR ART PROCEDURES

In vitro fertilization (IVF) originally evolved as a treatment for female infertility due to blocked Fallopian tubes (60,61). It was soon realised however that it was also useful in the treatment of other infertility problems, including male infertility (18).

In assessing the relationship between sperm parameters and the outcome of assisted conception, it should be remembered that the truly relevant statistics are those relating to the sperm preparation, rather than those of the semen. Preparation of sperm considerably distorts these characteristics by mainly selecting the normal motile sperm.

The most frequently used method of sperm preparation is the standard 'swim up' technique, sperm being allowed to swim up from a centrifuged pellet following separation from the seminal plasma and washing in culture medium (25). Aitken (2) has demonstrated that centrifugation of sperm results in a burst of reactive oxygen species production, which may result in peroxidative damage to the sperm membrane. Human sperm membranes contain high proportions of unsaturated fatty acids, and are therefore susceptible to peroxidation, resulting in a loss of membrane fluidity (38). Damage caused to sperm by centrifugation prior to selection may be a cause of fertilization failure (51). We believe there is no reason to continue to use this technique, since a direct swim-up from liquified semen followed by a centrifugation washing step is as simple to carry out, and has been shown to result in significantly lower levels of reactive oxygen species (2). The results reported by Cohen *et al.* (18), which have been reported as optimistic (47), were achieved using the direct swim up method as well as sedimentation under paraffin oil (54), which was used in extreme cases. The success rates reported by Cohen *et al.* (18) have been maintained using the original preparation methods, with the addition of a two-step Percoll gradient (8), a method which has also been shown to have little damaging effect in terms of reactive oxygen species (2).

Percoll, a suspension of silica beads, is used to form a buoyant density gradient, which not only represents an atraumatic method of sperm preparation, but has also been shown to be efficient at removing lymphocytes and other contaminants (30). It is a highly adaptable technique. Ord *et al.* (53) have developed a 'mini Percoll' technique using small volumes of Percoll (0.3 ml) for each layer in a three step gradient, which was shown to be highly efficient in the preparation of severely oligoasthenospermic samples, with encouraging IVF results.

Success at IVF with low sperm numbers will depend on retrieving maximum numbers of normal motile sperm and therefore selection of the appropriate preparation technique is critical. While it is essential that efficient and appropriate sperm preparation techniques are employed in cases of defective sperm, it is also possible to adapt culture conditions to optimize the chances of fertilization.

Other alternative culture methods include the removal of cumulus cells in order to improve access of sperm to the zona pellucida (45). Cumulus disperses rapidly in IVF conditions, and this technique may only be applicable in cases of severely defective sperm motility.

ANTISPERM ANTIBODIES

Five to 9% of men attending infertility clinics are likely to have antisperm antibodies in their semen and their serum, or occasionally in their serum alone. Fertilization *in vitro* in the presence of antisperm antibodies has been shown to be impaired (16,39), although the mechanisms of this effect are not entirely clear.

It has been shown that the presence of sperm antibodies may be detrimental to fertilization in vitro if the majority of the sperm are antibody coated (15). IgA class antibodies have been shown to inhibit fertilization to a greater extent than those of the IgG class (20), These effects on in vitro fertilization were subsequently confirmed by Junk *et al.* (39) and Clark *et al.* (15), both studies suggesting a synergistic action of the two classes in inhibiting fertilization.

A simple method of preparation in the presence of antisperm antibodies was proposed by Fishel and Edwards (28), and the effect on IVF outcome was shown by Elder *et al.* (26). Semen samples were collected in to culture medium, supplemented with 50% maternal serum, and immediately centrifuged to remove the seminal plasma. Although there was no detailed immunological data to assess the effects of this method on the depletion of antibodies, there was a significantly higher pregnancy rate, compared to antibody positive patients whose semen was treated in the normal way. In 59 patients who underwent cycles with and without collection into 50% serum, fertilization was improved in every case. The rate of failure to fertilise oocytes was reduced from 37.2% in the controls to 9.2% in the treated group and the pregnancy rate improved from 5.1% to 24.1%. It is thought that the presence of serum in this high concentration inhibits the binding of antibodies to the sperm surface (26). Thus, by relatively simple methods a measure of success may be obtained in this group of patients, although those cases with both IgG and IgA antibodies remain a problem.

SPERM STIMULATION

A variety of methods have been used in an attempt to stimulate sperm activity where this is defective. Since follicular fluid is present in the environment where the sperm makes contact with the oocyte, a number of authors have investigated its possible effect on sperm function. Mbizvo *et al.* (48) assessed the stimulating capacity of follicular fluid before and after removal of the steroid content, and found no effect in the absence of steroids, but a considerable improvement in fertilization rates in their presence. This suggests that some steriod component is responsible for the stimulatory effect.

Phosphodiesterase inhibitors, such as caffeine or pentoxifylline may improve sperm function by correcting defective energy metabolism. Human sperm obtain the bulk of their ATP from glycolysis, and both caffeine and pentoxifylline raise the rate of glycolysis (56). Pentoxifylline has also been shown to increase the swimming velocity of sperm (56). As a phosphodiesterase inhibitor, pentoxifylline will raise the intracellular concentration of cyclic AMP (cAMP), by preventing its breakdown. cAMP has a role in both capacitation and the acrosome reaction, and thus pentoxifylline may also have a role in stimulating these events (77).

The clinical significance of the effects of pentoxifylline has been shown by Yovich et al. (77) in a group of patients undergoing IVF. Oocytes inseminated with pentoxifylline incubated sperm had a significantly higher fertilization rate than those inseminated with control sperm. The successful results obtained with patients who had failed fertilization in a previous cycle without pentoxifylline, have led this group to suggest that pentoxifylline should be used routinely in cases with previous fertilization failure (77).

2-deoxyadenosine has also been shown to enhance sperm motility. This compound also increases intracellular levels of cAMP, by stimulating production. Imoedemhe et al. (34) showed a significant improvement in sperm motility and fertilisation rates with IVF following incubation of sperm with 2-deoxyadenosine.

Without any exposure to inducing agents, only some 5 to 10% of the motile population of spermatozoa undergo capacitation and complete the acrosome reaction. Even in response to powerful stimuli such as the calcium ionophore A 23187, as few as twenty percent of motile sperm will acrosome react. However, the toxicity of calcium ionophore restricts its use to sperm function testing. In an effort to synchronise the acrosome reaction so that a maximum number of reacting cells are available, particularly for sub-zonal insertion, Mortimer (50) suggested the substitution of strontium ions for calcium ions. The presence of strontium stalls those cells that were about to undergo the acrosome reaction so that when the sperm are transferred to calcium containing medium, a larger number will undergo the acrosome reaction simultaneously.

Pentoxifylline is thought to have some potential for increasing the rate of acrosome reaction (23). Observations from our own laboratory suggest that, rather than stimulating the reaction directly, it may increase the potential for acrosome reaction in response to stimuli.

Tomkins and Houghton (64) induced the acrosome reaction in sperm to be used in the zona free hamster oocyte penetration test by subjecting them to short pulses of voltages ranging from 750 to 1500 V/cm^{-1} electroporation. This gave rise to membrane fusion, as a result of depolarisation, similar to the processes associated with exocytosis. Van Steirteghem (68) used this method in conjunction with subzonal insertion, but, while a high rate of acrosome reaction was induced, fertilization rates were no higher than those achieved by sperm that had been incubated with follicular fluid.

There is considerable room for further refinement of methods used for sperm stimulation, and with improved sperm function tests it may be possible to apply them more appropriately. It does, however seem logical to adopt this type of approach, i.e. that of attempting to correct defects in sperm function by the use of stimulants, rather than trying to circumvent them by more invasive procedures such as microinsemination.

THE CLINICAL TREATMENT OF MALE INFERTILITY

The clinical treatment of male infertility may be divided into the following main categories:

- Conventional treatment

- Treatment by insemination procedures

- Treatment of men with antisperm antibodies

- Treatment by chemical enhancement of sperm function

- Assisted fertilization procedures
  - by in vitro fertilization (IVF)
  - by Gamete Intrafallopian Transfer (GIFT)
  - by Zygote Intrafallopian Transfer (ZIFT)
  - by micromanipulation of oocytes
  - by microinsemination procedures

- Other procedures such as
  - Microepidydimal sperm aspiration (MESA)
  - Treatment of ejaculatory dysfunction

CONVENTIONAL TREATMENT

Conventional methods of treatment are considered in detail elsewhere in this volume (see page 257) and only techniques involving ART for the treatment of male infertility will be considered here.

INSEMINATION PROCEDURES

In general, insemination procedures not involving superovulation, the preparation of sperm and intra-uterine insemination (IUI) with that preparation are not successful in the treatment of severe degrees of oligospermia and/or asthenoteratospermia. The technology involved with the preparation of sperm for IVF over the years has meant the development of techniques such as 'wash and swim up' (73) and Percoll preparations, wherebye only clean samples of the most actively motile spermatozoa are isolated from the ejaculate. Table 1 shows the pregnancy rates that can be achieved by intrauterine insemination of prepared sperm and show some of the earliest results that were obtained for different categories of male infertilty.

Table 1. *Pregnancy rates achieved with IUI of prepared husband sperm with superovulation for male infertility*

Factor	No. Couples	Pregnancy rate % Per couple	Per cycle
Negative PCT	88	30.7	15.8
Male antisperm antibodies	14	35.7	18.5
Oligozoospermia	42	21.4	10.3
Asthenozoospermia	13	0	0
Unexplained infertilty	68	17.7	9.0

(Yovich & Matson, 1988) (76).

In a more recent review of the efficacy of IUI in the treatment of male infertility, Tarlatzis *et al.* (62) achieved pregnancy rates of between 3.9 and 16.6% for intrauterine insemination, depending on whether treatment was in a natural cycle or using ovulation induction.

Table 2. *Pregnancy rates in spontaneous and induced cycles among male infertile patients undergoing IUI with husbands sperm*

	Male only infertility	Cervical factor and male
Spontaneous cycles	4/48 (8.3%)	1/4 (25%)
Induced cycles (all)	4/63 (6.3%)	2/6 (33.3%)
- Clomiphene only	2/51 (3.9%)	0/1 (0%)
- hMG	2/12 (16.6%)	2/5 (40%)

(Tarlatzis *et al.* 1991) (62).

Although no significant difference was found in this series between spontaneous cycles and the combined ovulation induction group, there was a significant difference between the increased pregnancy rate in the group treated with Human Menopausal Gonadotrophins (hMG) when considered alone. This study also confirmed that the large majority of pregnancies in superovulated IUI cycles occur in the first two or three cycles of treatment. 92% of pregnancies occurred in the first two cycles in this series. This is confirmed by the findings of Confino *et al.* (19) and Allen *et al.* (4) who agreed that the maximum number of 3 IUI cycles should be attempted before abandoning it as worthwhile treatment. In both of these papers, pregnancies were reported with severe degrees of oligospermia and teratospermia but, as has been found in IVF (17,18) and natural conception (3), it is the sperm motility which is the parameter that is the most sensitive indicator of sperm function and therefore success in ACT. The benefits of adding hMG stimulation are evident in the series of Tarlatzis et al. (62). Serhal et al. (57) have also reported the beneficial effects of adding hMG to IUI cycles in a series on idiopathic infertility.

The results of treatment of male factor infertility using the WHO standards (71) at The Hallam Medical Centre over a four year period are shown in Table 3.

Table 3. Results of treatment by IUI for male factor infertility* only at The Hallam Medical Centre (November 1987 - December 1991)

Total no. cycles	167
Abandoned	6
Hyperstimulated/abandoned	13
Inseminations	148
Pregnancies	22
Pregnancy rate/cycle	14.9%

(Bekir et al - unpublished data). (*Definition: <WHO standard).

In conclusion, we believe that IUI is a useful treatment option that may be used with benefit on couples with male infertility for up to three cycles of treatment, provided that it is combined with superovulation. This may be carried out before proceeding to IVF or while on a waiting list for IVF, provided that the female patient's tubal function is normal. In general, however, it is not considered to be useful for treatment of male infertility due to severe oligospermia or asthenospermia.

IN VITRO FERTILIZATION (IVF) IN THE MANAGEMENT OF MALE INFERTILITY

The technique of IVF has changed little since the earliest descriptions (60,61,66,67). During the early years of IVF, it became apparent that insemination with very high concentrations of sperm was unnecessary. Indeed, better results were achieved in IVF with low concentrations of 0.5-1 million motile spermatozoa (60,66). The concentration of spermatozoa for insemination was further reduced and optimum results were then found with concentrations of between 50,000 and 100,000 (70). The minimum sperm parameters that were considered necessary for successful IVF by a number of different authors is shown in Table 4.

Table 4. *Minimum sperm parameters required to achieve successful IVF as suggested by previous Authors*

	Sperm Density*	Motile Sperm Density*	% Sperm Motility
Mahadevan and Trounson (1984)	—	—	>20%
Van Uem et al. (1985)	—	>1.5 million	—
Cittadini et al. (1988)	—	>1.5 million	—
Riedel et al. (1989)	>5 million	—	—
Hinting et al. (1989)	—	>0.4 million	—
Barlow et al. (1990)	>2 million	—	—

*per ml

Whereas men with severe degrees of oligospermia, asthenospermia or teratospermia were initially excluded from treatment in IVF programmes, it was found that, provided actively motile sperm concentrations of 50,000 - 100,000 were able to be achieved in the final preparations of sperm for insemination of oocytes, good fertilization rates and pregnancies could be achieved (17,18). The successful pregnancies reported by Cohen et al. (17) were all achieved from sperm specimens with less than 10 million per ml, asthenospermia of <20% and teratospermia of >80%. Pregnancies are reported from sperm samples of <0.5 million spermatozoa/ml and even one from a sample of < 100,000/ml weakly active spermatozoa in the best fraction of a split ejaculate. The only earlier report on the treatment of male infertility by IVF was by Mahadevan et al. (44). They reported three pregnancies in 30 couples in whom the male partner had sperm counts of <10 million/ml or asthenospermia of <50%.

From these early reports on the treatment of male factor infertility has evolved a number of different treatments involving assisted fertilization, but IVF remains the cornerstone of treatment. To take a number of mature pre-ovulatory oocytes and a preparation of sperm and place them together in culture in vitro and observe the outcome provides the maximum of information about an individual couples ability to fertilize and gives them an optimum chance of conception following the transfer of any resulting embryos.

The importance of the proper preparation of sperm for IVF cannot be overstated and has already been discussed. It is because of the improved methods of sperm preparation that better pregnancy rates are constantly being achieved for the partners of infertile men. Yovich and Stanger (72) reported pregnancies and deliveries in couples in whom the male partner had severe oligospermia, defined as motile sperm counts of <5 million/ml. The problem with the data from these series and many others since is that they have shown IVF to be successful in the treatment of oligospermia and asthenoteratospermia but, in actually treating these men, they have only been treating those for whom they have been able to achieve adequate sperm numbers in the insemination preparation of sperm. They are thus treating those men who may be defined as having normal sperm function, since sperm function was good enough to be able to achieve a preparation at all. Hull (33) thus maintains that in treating oligospermic men who can achieve good sperm preparations, we are not treating men with true sperm dysfunction and that we should therefore abandon traditional semen analysis, and that much of the past literature on the treatment of male infertility by ART should be completely re-interpreted.

Avery et al. (8) made a retrospective analysis of the data of 300 couples with known oligospermia of less than 8 million spermatazoa per ml. in the original ejaculate. They studied the mean sperm characteristics of three groups: those who failed fertilisation, fertilised oocytes normally and who achieved a pregnancy. Analysis of the sperm parameters of the three groups revealed no significant difference in the sperm characteristics. One couple achieved fertilisation with a sperm density of <10,000/ml. and a pregnancy was achieved with a sperm density of 220,000/ml. in the ejaculate.

The recent study of Tournaye et al. (65) comparing the outcome of IVF for couples with pure tubal infertility and male infertility showed that, although the pregnancy rate in the male infertility group was significantly lower per cycle than the tubal groups, per transfer the results were the same. Thus, as expected, the fallout with infertile males is at the fertilization stage. In this series, only 23% of the male factor group fertilized oocytes compared with 67.9% ($P < 0.001$) of the tubal group. Other studies (18,27) have in fact shown higher implantation rates in cases of sperm defect. Thus, with male infertility treated by IVF, if the critical fertilization process can be achieved, then pregnancy, ongoing pregnancy and delivery rates will be normal (65).

It is possible that the newer techniques of microinjection of oocytes with sperm (29,42), which are dealt with in detail elsewhere in this volume (see page 293), and possibly the chemical enhancement of sperm motility by agents such as pentoxifylline (75,77) will do much to increase the chances of fertilization occurring; but this will still need to be combined with IVF for couples to achieve their best chance of successful pregnancy.

Oehninger et al. (52) studied in detail 58 cases of failure to fertilise (FTF) following attempted IVF in 583 patients who had undergone 1,067 IVF attempts. In the original evaulation of the cause of the FTF, sperm factors were thought to be responsible in 40.3% of cases. However, when the sperm morphology was re-examined by newer, stricter criteria (40,41), this figure was revised to 74.9% sperm factors being responsible for the FTF, thus confirming the importance of assessing sperm function rather than absolute numbers when assessing male infertility.

GAMETE INTRA-FALLOPIAN TRANSFER (GIFT)

The argument for placing oocytes and sperm into the physiological environment of the distal Fallopian tube would seem to be strong, and yet the majority of workers in ART support our view that, at least in the initial treatment cycle, IVF remains the treatment of choice. GIFT was proposed as a treatment for infertile couples in whom the female partner had at least one normal Fallopian tube, primarily those with idiopathic infertility (5,6). In the report of their first series of GIFT cases, Asch and his colleagues (6) report that three of the couples had male infertility and one of these became pregnant. Since then, there have been a number of reports of good results from GIFT for male infertility (46,75,31,21). Yovich et al. (75) indeed recommend that all non tubal infertility, including male factor, should be offered tubal transfer of gametes (GIFT) or zygote intra-fallopian transfer (ZIFT) or pronuclear intra-Fallopian transfer (PROST) rather than IVF. Most workers now agree that, at least on the first attempt at treatment, IVF should be performed, with subsequent uterine or tubal transfers of the embryos. Thus the maximum information on the fertilizing ability and sperm function can be obtained from that cycle.

At Bourn Hall Clinic, we have found no difference in the pregnancy rates between IVF/ET and GIFT and have therefore largely abandoned GIFT, especially since GIFT requires the more traumatic procedure of laparoscopy - at least for the present, until trans-cervical Fallopian tube transfers can be improved. This philosophy is shared by Leeton and colleagues (43), who found no difference in success rates between IVF and GIFT.

The question of whether the fate of supernumerary oocytes from GIFT is helpful or provides useful information on the likely outcome of the GIFT procedure, has produced conflicting results. Abdulla et al. (1) showed that when fertilization of supernumerary oocytes failed to occur in vitro, the chances of pregnancy was significantly reduced to 9.1% and when fertilisation did occur, the pregnancy rate was 57.1%. This report was on small numbers of patients but Critchlow et al. (22) reported on a larger series of 130 treatment cycles. Failure of supernumerary oocytes to fertilize was associated with the 13% GIFT pregnancy rate compared with 37% when fertilization occurred. They felt that this confirmed that IVF with GIFT was of particular diagnostic value. Other studies have shown the limited value of IVF of supernumerary oocytes at GIFT as regards prognosis for the outcome, but found it useful if the GIFT failed, as confirmation at least that fertilization was possible (46,49).

In order to combine the improved benefits generally achieved with tubal transfer with the diagnostic benefits of IVF, the tubal embryo transfer procedures PROST and ZIFT were developed.

TUBAL EMBRYO TRANSFER PROCEDURES

Yovich et al. (75) showed a significant benefit of tubal over uterine transfer procedures with pregnancy rates of: IVF 14/112 (12.5%), GIFT 66/184 (35.9%), PROST 30/81 (37.0%) and ZIFT 3/3 (all donor oocytes).

They postulated that the improved rates achieved in tubal transfer procedures may be due to the tubal milieu being more favourable than the culture dish; the possible presence of a 'tubal factor' which improves embryo quality; and the possible hostility of the early postovulatory uterine environment. One of the major concerns of many Clinics against using PROST and ZIFT more frequently is that patients require two operative procedures within 48 hours - vaginal ultrasound oocyte recovery, followed by laparoscopy to replace the embryos. This problem may soon be resolved following work done by Jansen and Anderson who pioneered the technique of transferring sperm initially (35) and later embryos (36) to the Fallopian tubes by the trans-cervical route. More recently, Diedrich et al. (24) reported a series of 95 trans-cervical tubal embryo transfers for couples with male infertility; 29 (31%) became pregnant. As other units start to achieve comparable results for trans-cervical transfers, so we believe that tubal embryo transfer will became more widely used as a treatment option, especially in male infertility.

THE TREATMENT OF OTHER SPECIAL MALE INFERTILITY PROBLEMS

Following on the technological advances in sperm preparation that have arisen out of IVF and the realisation that fertilization can be achieved *in vitro*, sometimes with as few as 2,000 - 3,000 motile spermatozoa per oocyte (65), it was realised that it may be possible to extend treatment to men hitherto considered untreatable - of whom there are two main groups:

1. Men with irreversible obstruction of the vasa with functioning testes, who may benefit from micro-epididymal sperm aspiration (MESA)

2. Spinal cord injured (SCI) men and men with other disorders of erection and ejaculation

1. MICRO-EPIDYDIMAL SPERM ASPIRATION (MESA)

MESA involves the aspiration of multiple minute samples of sperm from different levels of the epidydimis by microsurgical methods. Silber, in collaboration with Asch, (58, 59) first successfully described this procedure in association with ZIFT for two men with congenital absence of the vasa. In spite of the fact that some 20 million sperm were retrieved, only 5% were motile with 20% normal forms.

The technique has also achieved success for men with failed vasectomy reversal (63) and post inflammatory vasal obstruction. A recent survey of the literature by Bladou et al. (10) showed that in 130 attempts of MESA combined with IVF by 7 groups, the overall fertilization rate per oocyte varied between 25 and 35% with pregnancy rates ranging between 0 and 50% per IVF attempt. In their own series of 58 sperm aspirations on 23 men, only 14 patients achieved the stage of attempted IVF, of whom 5 had a mean of 2.1 embryos transferred, 2 pregnancies were achieved, both of which aborted. This shows that this is still a relatively unsuccessful treatment but there is no doubt that improvements will be achieved with better results as our experience grows.

In our own experience at the Hallam Medical Centre and Bourn Hall Clinic with MESA, results have been encouraging. One pregnancy was reported in our first series of four patients and this patient has now delivered twins. Results since then have been less successful, although sperm has been retrieved from 93% of the cases done so far and fertilization achieved in 46% of couples, including one with aspiration from the vas. Two of 26 couples have ongoing pregnancies or have delivered, a pregnancy rate of 7.5% per cycle started and 16.6% per embryo transfer (Bourn-Hallam unpublished data).

2. TREATMENT OF MEN WHOSE INFERTILITY IS DUE TO SEXUAL DYSFUNCTION.

There are five main groups of men with varying degrees of sexual dysfunction who may be helped to achieve a pregnancy for their partners by the stimulation of ejaculation, combined with IVF:

1. Spinal cord injured (SCI) men
2. Impotence due to diabetes
3. Impotence due to multiple sclerosis
4. Pharmacologically induced impotence
5. Men with psychosexual problems

These men may be helped to produce semen by various techniques including:

1. Pharmacological means using intra-cavernous papaverine (69).
2. Surgical methods using semen capsules (14).
3. Hypogastric plexus stimulator inserted at laparotomy (13).
4. Microepidydimal sperm aspiration as described above
5. The use of a vibrator applied to the penis (12).
6. The use of electroejaculation techniques (11, 9).

This last technique has been used in humans since 1948 and extensive experience has also been gained worldwide from its use in endangered species of animals (11,9).

At Bourn Hall over the past two years we have gained extensive experience from the use of the electroejaculation technique, primarily in spinal cord injured (SCI) men. We have used the Seagar model 12 electroejaculation unit to achieve the sperm samples, followed by IVF. The details of the procedure are reviewed by Rainsbury (55). In his analysis of the first 12 couples treated, with 17 IUI and 17 IVF cycles, 8 have achieved pregnancies, of which 7 were ongoing or delivered at the time of writing. The quality of the sperm from these men is very poor indeed. The first pregnancy was achieved from an ejaculate containing no spermatozoa in the antegrade part, but with 200 million spermatozoa in the retrograde catheter specimen, with less than 1% motility. This was spun down, washed, treated by the Percoll method and layered under paraffin, achieving a stock of only 7,500 motile spermatozoa in a volume of 0.25 ml. Four oocytes were inseminated with this stock, all in one droplet of medium. Two embryos (2-cell and 4-cell) were transferred and a baby subsequently delivered. These details give a very good indication of how adequate sperm preparations for successful IVF can be achieved from very poor semen samples.

We have also used the rectal electroejaculation (REE) technique for the other groups of men listed above with success. REE, when combined with IVF would appear to be a useful additional treatment option to help a number of men who are infertile because of ejaculatory dysfunction, most of whom also have disorders of sperm function.

MICROMANIPULATION TECHNIQUES TO ASSIST FERTILISATION

We have limited experience using the methods of partial zona dissection (PZD) sperm microinjection (MI) and sub-zonal insertion (SUZI) and in common with other workers have found very limited success. Fischel *et al.* (29) have recently reported a very large series of SUZI, the details of which are presented in the next chapter.

CONCLUSIONS

In this brief review of the usefulness of ART procedures in the treatment of male infertility we have attempted to show the importance of adequate assessment of sperm function before starting treatment, as well as the very great effect that improved methods of sperm preparation have made on the outcome of ART. A number of sophisticated preparation techniques now exist, with the selection being decided by the type of sperm disorder and the ART procedure proposed. The management of couples with antisperm antibodies has become more effective by the simple expedient of ejaculating into medium containing protein. The use of pentoxifylline has added yet another dimension to improving sperm function *in vitro*.

We believe that there is a place for IUI when combined with limited superovulation in the treatment of less severe degrees of male infertility. For the more severe forms, then IVF remains the mainstay of treatment, with GIFT and ZIFT showing certain advantages in selected cases. It is now possible to achieve pregnancies by azoospermic men from whom we can retrieve sperm capable of fertilising oocytes *in vitro* from the epididymis. Finally, we have shown that by combining rectal electro-ejaculation techniques combined with IVF, it is possible to achieve pregnancies for couples where the husband is unable to ejaculate.

With the introduction of micromanipulation methods it has become possible to achieve success for couples with severe degrees of sperm dysfunction; indeed, it may eventually be possible to achieve fertilisation and pregnancies when only one non-motile sperm can be found and injected into the ooplasm.

REFERENCES

1. Abdalla, H.I., Ahuja, K.K., Leonard, T. and Morriss, N.N. (1988) The value of IVF-ET in patients undergoing treatment by the GIFT procedure. Hum. Reprod., 3:944-947.
2. Aitken, R.J. (1988) Assessment of sperm function for IVF. Hum. Reprod., 3:89-95.
3. Aitken, R.J., Best, F.S.M., Richardson, D.W., Djahanbakhch, O., Templeton, A. and Lees, M.M. (1982) An analysis of semen quality and sperm function in cases of oligozoospermia. Fertil. Steril., 38:705-711.
4 Allen, N.C., Herbert, C.M., Maxson, W.S., Rogers, B.J., Diamond, M.P. and Wentz, A.C. (1985) Intra uterine insemination: a critical review. Fertil. Steril., 44:569-580.
5. Asch, R.H., Elsworth, L.R., Balmaceda, J.P. and Wong, P.C. (1984) Pregnancy after trans laparoscopic gamete intra fallopian transfer. Lancet, 2:1034.
6. Asch, R.H., Balmaceda, J.P., Elsworth, L.R. and Wong, P.C. (1986) Preliminary experience with GIFT (Gamete Intra Fallopian Transfer). Fertil. Steril., 45:366-371.
7. Avery, S., Bolton, V. and Mason B.A. (1990) An evaluation of the hypo-osmotic sperm swelling test as a predictor of fertilizing capacity in-vitro. Int. J. Androl., 13:93-99.
8. Avery, S., Elder, K. and Edwards, R.G. (1990) IVF as a treatment for oligospermia - experiences of 300 cases. abstract of the Second Joint Meeting of the European Society of Human Reproduction and Embryology and the European Sterility Congress Organisation. Hum. Reprod., abstract 70, p. 22.
9. Bennett, C.J., Seager, S.W. and McGuire, E.J. (1987) Electroejaculation for recovery of semen after retroperitoneal lymph node dissection: Case report. J. Urol., 137:513.
10. Bladou, F., Grillo, J.M., Rossi, D., Noizet, A. Gamerre, M., Erny, R., Luciani, J.M. and Serment, G. (1991) Epidydimal sperm aspiration in conjunction with in vitro fertilization and embryo transfer in cases of obstructive azoospermia. Hum. Reprod., 6:1284-1287.
11. Brindley, G.S. (1981) Electroejaculation: its technique, neurological implications and uses. J. Neurol. Neurosurg. Psychiatr., 44:9-18.
12. Brindley, G.S. (1984) The fertility of men with spinal cord injuries. Paraplegia, 22:337-348.
13. Vindley, G.S., Sauerwein, D. and Hendry, W.F. (1986) Hypogastric plexus stimulators for obtainaing sperm from paraplegic men. Br. J. Urol., 64:72-77.
14. Brindley, G.S., Scott, G.I. and Hendry, W.F. (1986) Vas cannulation with implanted sperm reservoirs for obstructive azoospermia or ejaculatory failure. Br. J. Urol., 58:721-723.
15. Clarke, G.N., Lopata, A., McBain, J.C., Baker, H.W. and Johnston, W.I. (1985) Effect of antisperm antibodies in males on in vitro fertilisation. Am. J. Reprod. Immunol. Microbiol., 8:62-66.
16. Clarke, G.N., Hyne, R.V., du Plessis, Y. and Johnston, W.I. (1988) Fertil. Steril., 49:1018-1025.
17. Cohen, J., Fehilly, C., Fishel, S.B., Edwards, R.G., Hewitt, J., Roland, G.F. and Steptoe, P.C. (1984) Male infertility successfully treated by in vitro fertilization. Lancet, 1:1239.
18. Cohen, J., Edwards, J.G., Fehilly, C., Fishel, S.B., Hewitt, J. Purdy, J., Roland, G., Steptoe, P.C. and Webster, J. (1985) In vitro fertilization: a treatment for male infertility. Fertil. Steril., 43:422-432.
19. Confino, E. and Friberg, J. (1986) Intra uterine insemination with washed human spermatozoa. Fertil. Steril., 46:55-60.
20. Coombs, R.R.A., Rumke, P. and Edwards, R.G. (1973) Immunoghlubulin classes reactive with spermatazoa in the serum and seminal plasma of vasectomised and infertile men. In: Immunology of Reproduction, edited by Bratanov, K., Edwards, R.G., Vulchanov, V.H., Dikov, V. and Somlev, B. p 354. Bulgarian Academy of Science Press, Sofia.

21. Craft, I. and Brinsden, P. (1989) Alternatives to IVF: the outcome of 1071 first GIFT procedures. Hum. Reprod., 4:29-36.
22. Critchlow, J.B., Matson, P.L., Troop, S.A., Ibrahim, Z.H.Z., Burslem, R.W., Buck, P. and Lieberman, B.A. (1990) Fertilization in vitro from supernumery oocytes following gamete intra fallopian transfer (GIFT). Hum. Reprod., 5:853-856.
23. Cummins, J.M., Pember, S.M., Jequier, A.M., Yovich, J.L. and Hartmann, P.E. (1991)A test of the human sperm acrosome reaction following ionophore challenge - relationships to fertility and other seminal parameters. Int. J. Androl., 12:98-103.
24. Diedrich, H., Bauer, O., Werner, A., van der Ven, H., Al-Hasani, S. and Krebs, D. (1991) Transvaginal intra-tubal embryo transfer: a new treatment of male infertility. Hum. Reprod., 6:672-675.
25. Drevius, L.O. (1971) The sperm rise test. J. Reprod. Fertil., 24:427-429.
26. Elder, K.T., Wick and K.L., Edwards, R.G. (1990) Seminal plasma antisperm antibodies and IVF: the effect of semen sample collection into 50% serum. Hum. Reprod., 5:179-184.
27. Englert, Y., Vekemans, M., Lejeune, B., Van Rysselberge, M., Puissant, F., Degueldre, M. and Leroy, F. (1987) Higher pregnancy rates after in vitro fertilization and embryo transfer in cases with sperm defects. Fertil. Steril., 48:254-257.
28. Fishel, S.B. and Edwards, R.G. (1982) The essentials of fertilisation. In: Human Conception in Vitro, edited by Edwards, R.G. and Purdy, J.M. p 157. Academic Press, London.
29. Fishel, S., Timson, J., Faratian, B. and Symonds, E.M. (1992) Sub-zonal insemination. Lancet, 1:932-933.
30. Gorus, R.K. and Pipeleers, D.G. (1981) A rapid method for the fractionation of human spermatozoa according to their progressive motility. Fertil. Steril., 35:662-665.
31. Hinting, A., Comhaire, F., Vermeulen, L., Dhont, M., Vermeulen, A. and Vandekerckhove, D. (1990) Possibilities and limitations of techniques of assisted reproduction for the treatment of male infertility. Hum. Reprod., 5:544-548.
32. Hull, M.G.R., Glazener, C.M.A. and Kelly, N.J. (1985) Population study of causes, treatment, and income of infertility. Br. Med. J., 291:1693-1697.
33. Hull, M.G.R. (1990) Indications for assisted conception. In: Assisted Human Conception, edited by Edwards, R.G., pp 580-595. Churchill Livingstone, London.
34. Imoedemhe, D.A.G., Sigue, A.B., Pacpaco, E.A. and Olazo, A.B. (1992) Successful use of the sperm motility enhancer 2-deoxyadenosine in previously failed human in Vitro fertilisation. J. Assist. Reprod. Genetics, 9:53-56.
35. Jansen, R.P.S., Anderson, J.C., Radonic, I., Smit, T. and Sutherland,P.D. (1988) Pregnancies after ultrasound-guided fallopian insemination with cryostored donor semen. Fertil. Steril., 49:920-922.
36. Jansen, R.P.S., Anderson, J.C. and Sutherland,P.D. (1988) Nonoperative embryo transfer to the fallopian tube. N. Engl. J. Med., 319:288-291.
37. Jeyendran, R.S., van der Ven, H.H., Perez-Palez, M., Crabo, B.G. and Zaneveld, L.J.D. (1984) Development of an assay to assess the functional integrity of the human sperm membrane and its relationship to other semen characteristics. J. Reprod. Fertil., 70:219-228.
38. Jones, R., Mann, T. and Sherins, R. (1979) Peroxidative breakdown of phospholipids by spermatozoa spermicidal properties of fatty acid peroxides and protactive action of seminal plasma. Fertil. Steril., 31:531-537.
39. Junk, S.M., Matson, P.L., Yovich, J.M., Bootsma, B. and Yovich, J.L. (1986) The fertilisation of human oocytes by spermatazoa from men with antispermatazoal antibodies in semen. J. in Vitro. Fert. Embryo Transf., 3:350-352.
40. Kruger, T.M., Menkveld, R., Stasnder, F.S.H, Lomkbard, C.J., Van der Merwe, J.P., van Zyl, J.A. and Smith, K. (1986) Sperm morphologic features as a prognostic factor in in vitro fertilisation. Fertil. Steril., 46:1118-1123.
41. Kruger, T., Acosta, A.A., Simmons, K.F., Swanson, R.J., Matta, J.F., Veek, L., Morshedi, M. and Brugo, S. (1987) A new method of evaluating sperm morphology with predictive value for human in vitro fertilisation. Urology, 30:248-251.
42. Laws-King, A., Trounson, A., Sathanthan, H. and Kola, I. (1987) Fertilisation of human oocytes by microinjection of a single spermatazoon under the zona pellucida. Fertil. Steril., 48:637-642.
43. Leeton, J., Healey, D., Rogers, P., Yates, C. and Caro, C. (1987) A controlled study between the use of gamete intrafallopian transfer (GIFT) and in vitro fertilisation and embryo transfer in the management of idiopathic and male infertility. Fertil. Steril., 48:605-607.
44. Mahadevan, M.M., Trounson, A.O. and Leeton, J.F. (1983) The relationship of tubal blockage, infertility of unknown cause, suspected male infertility and endometriosis to success of in-vitro fertilisation and embryo transfer. Fertil. Steril., 40:755-762.

45. Mahadevan, M.M. and Trounson, A.O. (1984) The influence of seminal characteristics on the success rate of human in vitro fertilisation. Fertil. Steril., 42:400-405.
46. Matson, P.L., Blackledge, D.G., Richardson, P.A., Turner, S.R., Yovich, J.M. and Jovich, J.L. (1987) The role of gamete intrafallopian transfer (GIFT) in the treatment of oligospermic infertility. Fertil. Steril., 48:608-612.
47. Matson, P.L., Troup, S.A., Lowe, B., Ibrahim, Z.H.Z., Burslem, R.W. and Lieberman, B.A. (1989) Fertilisation of human oocytes in vitro by spermatazoa from oligospermic and normospermic men. Int. J. Androl., 12:117-123.
48. Mbizvo, M.T., Burkman, L.J. and Alexander, N.J. (1990) Human follicular fluid stimulates hyperactivated motility in human sperm. Fertil. Steril., 54:708-711.
49. McKenna, K.M., McBain, J.C., Speirs, A.L., Jones, G., Du Plessis, Y. and Johnston, W.I.H. (1988) The fate of supernumerary oocytes in a gamete intrafallopian transfer (GIFT) program is not predictive of a poor outcome: The effect of oocyte selection. J. in Vitro Fert. Embryo Transf., 5:261-264.
50. Mortimer, D., Chorney, M.J., Curtis, E.F. and Trounson, A.O. (1988) Calcium dependence on human sperm fertilizing ability. J. Exp. Zool., 246:194-201.
51. Mortimer, D. (1991) Sperm preparation and iatrogenic failures of in vitro fertilisation. Hum. Reprod., 6:173-176.
52. Oehninger, S., Acosta, A.A., Kruger,T., Veeck, L.L., Flood, J. and Jones, H.W. (1988) Failure of fertilisation in in vitro fertilisation: The «occult» male factor. J. in Vitro Fert. Embryo Transf., 5:181-187.
53. Ord, T., Patrizio, P., Marello, E., Balmaceda, J.P. and Asch, R.H. (1990) Mini-Percoll: a new method of semen preparation for IVF in severe male factor infertility. Hum. Reprod., 5:987-989.
54. Purdy, J.M. (1985) Methods for fertilisation and embryo culture in vitro. In: Human Conception in Vitro. Academic Press: 135-148.
55. Rainsbury, P.A. (1992) The treatment of male fasctor infertility due to sexual dysfunction. In: A Textbook of in Vitro Fertilisation and Assisted Conception, edited by Brinsden, P.R. and Rainsbury, P.A., pp 345-359. Parthenon, Carnforth, UK.
56. Rees, J.M., Ford, W.C.L. and Hull, M.G.R. (1992) Effect of caffeine and of pentoxifylline on the motility and metabolism of human spermatazoa. J. Reprod. Fertil., 90:147-156.
57. Serhal, P.F., Katz, M., Little, V. and Woronowsji, H. (1988) Unexplained infertility - the value of Pergonal superovulation combined with intrauterine insemination. Fertil. Steril., 49:602-606.
58. Silber, S., Ord, T., Borrero, C., Balmaceda, J. and Asch, R. (1987) New treatment for infertility due to congenital absence of the vas deferens. Lancet, 2:850-851.
59. Silber, S.J., Balmaceda, J., Borrero, C., Ord, T. and Asch, R. (1988) Preganacy with sperm aspiration from the proximal head of the epididymis: A new treatment for congenital absence of the vas deferens. Fertil. Steril., 50:525-528.
60. Steptoe, P.C. and Edwards, R.G. (1976) Reimplantation of a human embryo with subsequent tubal pregnancy. Lancet, 1:880-882.
61. Steptoe, P.C., Edwards, R.G. and Purdy, J. (1980) Clinical aspects of pregnancies established with cleaving embryos grown in vitro. Br. J. Obstet. Gynaecol., 87:757-768.
62. Tarlatzis, B.C., Bontis, J., Kolibianakis, E.M., Sanopoulou, T., Papadimas, J., Lagos, S. and Mantanakis, S. (1991) Evaluation of intrauterine insemination with washed spermatazoa from the husband in the treatment of infertility. Hum. Reprod., 6:1241-1246.
63. Temple-Smith, P.D., Southwick, G.J., Yates, C.A., Trounson, A.O. and De Kretser, D.M. (1985) Human pregnancy by in vitro fertilisation (IVF) using sperm aspirated from the epididymis. J. in Vitro Fert. Embryo Transf., 2:119-122.
64. Tomkins, P.T. and Houghton, J.A. (1988) The rapid induction of the acrosome reaction of human spermatazoa by electropermeabilization. Fertil. Steril., 50:329-366.
65. Tournaye, H., Devroey, P., Camus, M., Staessen, C., Bollen, N., Smitz, J. and Van Steirteghem, A. (1992) Comparison of in vitro fertilisation in male and tubal infertility: A 3 year survey. Hum. Reprod., 7:218-222.
66. Trounson, A.O., Leeton, J.F., Wood, E.C., Webb, J. and Kovacs, G. (1980) The investigation of idiopathic infertility by in vitro fertilisation. Fertil. Steril., 34:431-438.
67. Trounson, A.O., Leeton, J.F., Wood, E.C., Webb, J. and Wood, J. (1981) Successful human pregnancies by in vitro fertilisation and embryo transfer in a controlled ovulatory cycle. Science, 212:681-682.
68. Van Steirtegham, A.C. (1991) Assessment of procedures enhancing recovery, capacitation and acrosome reaction in human spermatazoa. Hum. Reprod., 6, Suppl., 1:157.

69. Virag, R., Frydman, D. and Legman, M. (1984) Intracavernous injection of papaverine as a diagnostic and therapeutic method in erectile failure. Angiology, 35:79-87.
70. Wolf, D.P., Byrd, W., Dandekar, P. and Quigley, M.M. (1984) Sperm concentration and the fertilisation of human eggs in vitro. Biol. Reprod., 31:837-848.
71. World Health Organisation. (1987) Laboratory Manual for the Examination of Semen and Semen-cervical Mucus Interactions. Cambridge University Press, Cambridge.
72. Yovich, J.L. and Stanger, J.D. (1984) The limitations of in Vitro Fertilisation from males with severe oligospermia and abnormal sperm morphology. J. In Vitro Fert. Embryo Transf., 1:172-179.
73. Yovich, J.L., Matson, P.L., Blackledge, D.G., Turner, S.R., Richardson, P.A. and Draper, R. (1987) Pregnancies following pronuclear stage tubal transfer. Fertil. Steril., 48:851-857.
74. Yovich, J.L., Yovich, J.M. and Edirisinghe, W.R. (1988) The relative chance of pregnancy following tubal or uterine transfer procedures. Fertil. Steril., 48:858-864.
75. Jovich, J.M., Edirisinghe, W.R., Cummins, J.M. and Jovich, J.L. (1988) Preliminary results using pentoxifylline in a pronuclear stage tubal transfer (PROST) program for severe male factor infertility. Fertil. Steril., 50:179-181.
76. Yovich, J.L., Matson, P.L. (1988) The treatment of infertility by the high intrauterine insemination of husband's washed spermatazoa. Hum. Reprod., 3:938-943.
77. Yovich, J.M., Edirisinghe, W.R., Cummins, J.M. and Yovich, J.L. (1990) Influence of pentoxifylline in severe male factor infertility. Fertil. Steril., 53:715-722.

Subzonal Insemination

S. Fishel and J. Timson

NURTURE (Nottingham University Research and Treatment Unit in Reproduction)
Department of Obstetrics & Gynaecology, Floor 'B', East Block University Hospital
Queen's Medical Centre, Nottingham NG7 2UH, UK

INTRODUCTION

The essential developments in micro-assisted fertilisation for infertility must be set against the backdrop of research in animals. The manipulation of animal gametes has occurred over the last four decades, and it has been a natural progression for embryologists to utilise these techniques for conception in our own species.

The early investigations into the injection of sperm into eggs, which began in earnest in the mid-1960's, were primarily to investigate the initial events of fertilisation: viz, membrane fusion between homologous and heterologous gametes, activation of the ooplasm and formation of the pronuclei. (10,16,17,29).

Experiments of this kind made an enormous contribution to our understanding of the biological mechanisms of fertilisation. Apart from the increase in fundamental knowledge of the processes of capacitation and acrosome reaction, surface membrane fusion between the gametes, activation of the oocyte and cytoplasmic control of the formation of pro-nuclei, this work led to the appliance of techniques for animal production. It was eventually perceived that sperm micro-injection could be used effectively for the preservation of genetically valuable material in certain domestic and wild animal species where biological defects prevent conception. Methods of micro-manipulating gametes during the 1980's resulted in enormous advances in techniques for increasing the incidence of fertilisation and cleavage, with the eventual birth of live offspring of domestic and livestock animals (28,25,19,11,12).

However, most of this work involved the direct injection of spermatozoa into the ooplasm, and it was clear that this approach compromised the developmental rate of transferred embryos. In 1986 Gordon and Talansky (9) reported on a method by which a portion of the zona pellucida could be digested, using an acidified culture medium gently released from a micropipette pressing up against the zona pellucida. This was the first in the series of experiments for creating a breach in the zona pellucida. Although using an acidified medium was successful in animal studies, it was soon apparent that this particular technique was flawed for use in human conception. However, using micro-needles to cause a mechanical breach in the zona pellucida was soon to prove successful in procuring fertilisation with human gametes and, in 1988, the first human pregnancy by this method was reported by Cohen *et al.* (2).

The clinical application of micro-insemination techniques was first reported in 1985 by Metka *et al.* (20). In 1987, Laws-King and co-workers (15) reported on the insertion of a single spermatozoon into the perivitelline space with subsequent fertilisation. Thus, by the end of the 1980's, there were two major approaches to overcoming the problem of failure to achieve fertilisation with human gametes; one which required creating a mechanical breach in the zona pellucida (which has been called Partial Zona Dissection - PZD; Zona Cutting - ZC; Zona Tearing - ZT, or, by some, is still referred to as Zona Drilling - ZD), and the approach of subzonal insemination (SUZI). Much of the early work with SUZI, in a clinical context, was performed by the group in Singapore and ourselves. In 1988 there was the first report of a human pregnancy after subzonal sperm injection (22) by Ng and co-workers, shortly followed by the first published birth by Fishel *et al.* (5).

Although these techniques have now resulted in the birth of more than 100 babies, there still remains enormous difficulties in evaluating the efficacy, efficiency and safety of these procedures.

To keep within the scope of this chapter we will deal mainly with subzonal insemination, and our experiences with this technique.

PATIENTS AND METHODS

Patients

The criteria for inclusion into the subzonal insemination programme were an overt severe male factor problem which had precluded these patients from being admitted to an *in vitro* fertilisation (IVF) programme, or patients with either no discernible male factor problem or only moderately severe problems who had previously attempted IVF but failed to achieve fertilisation on at least one attempt. If patients had only failed to achieve fertilisation on a single attempt previously, and there were more than 4 or 5 oocytes recovered in the current study, it was advised that subzonal insemination and routine IVF should be performed in individual oocytes from the same cohort. Each couple was given an extensive consultation to explain the practicalities of the procedure involved and was informed about the lack of knowledge concerning this technique in human beings. Women were between 22 and 45 years of age. No female factors which could have affected outcome were obvious.

Follicular Stimulation

Each patient was administered a GnRH agonist (Suprefact: Hoeschst, Hounslow, UK) as a nasal spray to desensitise the pituitary gonadotropes. The dosage was 2 sprays per nostril every 8 hours commencing on day 21 of the cycle before treatment. The start of menses was designated day one of the treatment cycle. Patients who were not synchronised with the proposed starting date of treatment were maintained on Suprefact.

Follicular stimulation was initiated with 150 IU of follicle stimulating hormone (FSH; Metrodin; Serono, Rome, Italy), administered either on days one and two, or days one, two and three, i.e. a dose of four or six ampoules of Metrodin in total. On day three of follicular stimulation, patients were administered either two, three or four ampoules of human menopausal gonadotrophin (hMG; Pergonal; Serono, Rome, Italy), according to their age, weight and previous response, until the administration of 10,000 IU human chorionic gonadotrophin (hCG; Profasi; Serono, Rome, Italy) to induce ovulation. Throughout follicular stimulation, patients continued with daily doses of Suprefact to maintain pituitary desensitization. Evaluation of data according to variations in stimulation regimes showed no statistical differences.

Oocyte Recovery and Stimulation

Oocytes were recoved by the sonographic transvaginal technique. The procedures for culturing oocytes, embryology and replacement of embryos have been described previously (4). The oocyte cumulus complexes were subject to digestion by hyaluronidase (0.15% w/v). For comparing SUZI, PZD and IVF in sibling oocytes, it was important to evaluate the maturity of the oocytes, and to compare only those at metaphase II. Patients had their oocyte cumulus complexes subjected to hyaluronidase as an additional step in the IVF procedure, generally because of a very low sperm count, to isolate the individual oocytes for insemination in a single microdrop containing the spermatozoa concentrated from the whole ejaculate (microdrop IVF).

Preparation of Spermatozoa

The majority of seminal plasma samples were prepared utilising Percoll (Sigma, Poole, UK) with two discontinuous gradients of 45% and 90%.

Centrifugation was at 350-400 g for 10 minutes, followed by a second wash and centrifugation at 250 g for 5 minutes before final resuspension in culture medium.

Evaluation of the Morphology of Spermatozoa

All semen samples were obtained after a split ejaculate. Both portions were assessed independently, and the data combined for the total morphology for the purposes of this analysis. Slides were thoroughly washed with 70% ethyl alcohol before use. Staining was by the Diff Quik Staining Kit methodology (Baxter Dade Diagnostics AG, Dubinger, Switzerland). After the fixing and staining protocol, slides were air dried and cover slips were applied using XAM neutral medium (Searle, Hopkin & Williams, UK). The morphology of spermatozoa was assessed according to the parameters in Table 1. For each assessment 200 spermatozoa were counted.

Preparation of the Oocyte and the Micro-insemination Procedures

The procedures used for SUZI have been detailed elsewhere (6,7).

Control Studies

The great difficulty that practitioners face in this work is to strike a balance between offering what is perceived to be the 'best' treatment for the patient to establish a pregnancy, against the necessity to validate the data with matched controls. Where possible in a group of patients, sibling oocytes from the same cohort were divided into a group undergoing in-vitro insemination and micro-assisted fertilisation (MAF). All oocytes were subject to hyaluronidase to ensure that the oocytes used for both IVF and MAF were at metaphase II. Conditions which prevented the use of control studies in some patients included: inhibited progressive motility or too few spermatozoa to reasonably attempt IVF, too few oocytes, and those patients who had previous failures of IVF who expressly wished their oocytes to be used for SUZI only.

Statistics

Statistical evaluation between groups was assessed using the χ^2 (2) test. The Student's t-test was used where appropriate.

Table 1. *Sperm morphology evaluation*

Type
Normal Forms
Amorphous
Megalo
Small
Elongated
Duplicated
Immature
Loose
Midpiece Abnormality
Cytoplasmic Droplets
Coiled Tails
Multiple Tails

RESULTS

Overall Data for SUZI - Patients and Oocytes

Of the 307 patients undergoing oocyte recovery, 147 (47.9%) achieved fertilisation with 43.6% (134) having embryo transfer. Thirty-one pregnancies were established, representing an overall incidence of pregnancy of 23.1% per transfer and 10.1% of all oocyte recoveries. Approximately 54% of patients had one embryo transferred compared with 28% and 17% having two and three embryos transferred, respectively (Fig. 1). There was no difference in the mean age of patients who became pregnant ($\bar{x}$ 34.6±5.01

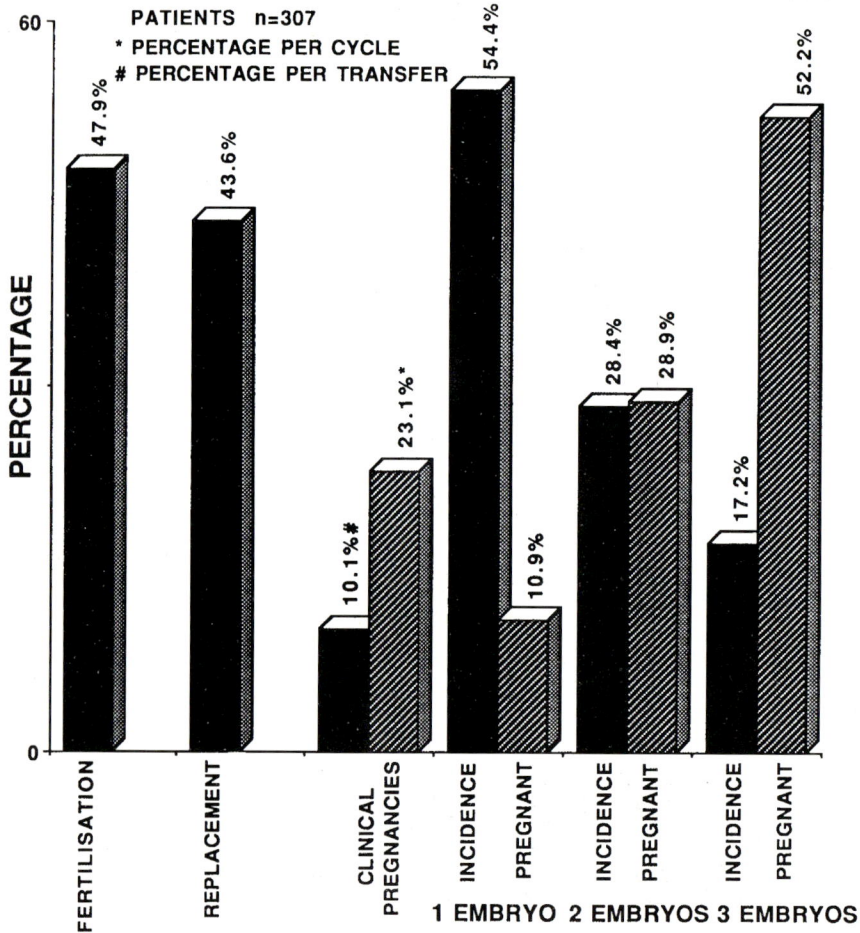

FIG. 1. Overall data from those patients having SUZI transfer only.

SD), whose embryos did not cleave (x̄ 34.8±4.78 SD), and in those patients where fertilisation failed to occur (x̄ 32.9±4.17 SD). Overall, the mean age of patients was 34.9±5.87 SD. Of all the recovered oocytes that appeared to have a mature oocyte-cumulus complex before digestion with hyaluronidase (2,476), 82% were observed in metaphase II compared with 14.6% in metaphase I. Three per cent still had a germinal vesicle and 8 (0.32%) appeared to have been parthenogenetically activated *in vitro*, as a single pronucleus was present after the removal of the cumulus cells. The number of oocytes available for SUZI was 1,384. Of all the oocytes undergoing SUZI, 21% were fertilised; 92.4% cleaved and 77.3% fertilised oocytes were replaced (16.3% of the total number of oocytes undergoing SUZI). The highest order of multiple pronucleate eggs observed was five pronuclei which arose in 1% of oocytes. Overall, 9% of fertilised oocytes were multi-pronucleate. The incidence of parthenogenetic activation by SUZI was observed at 0.58% (Fig. 2).

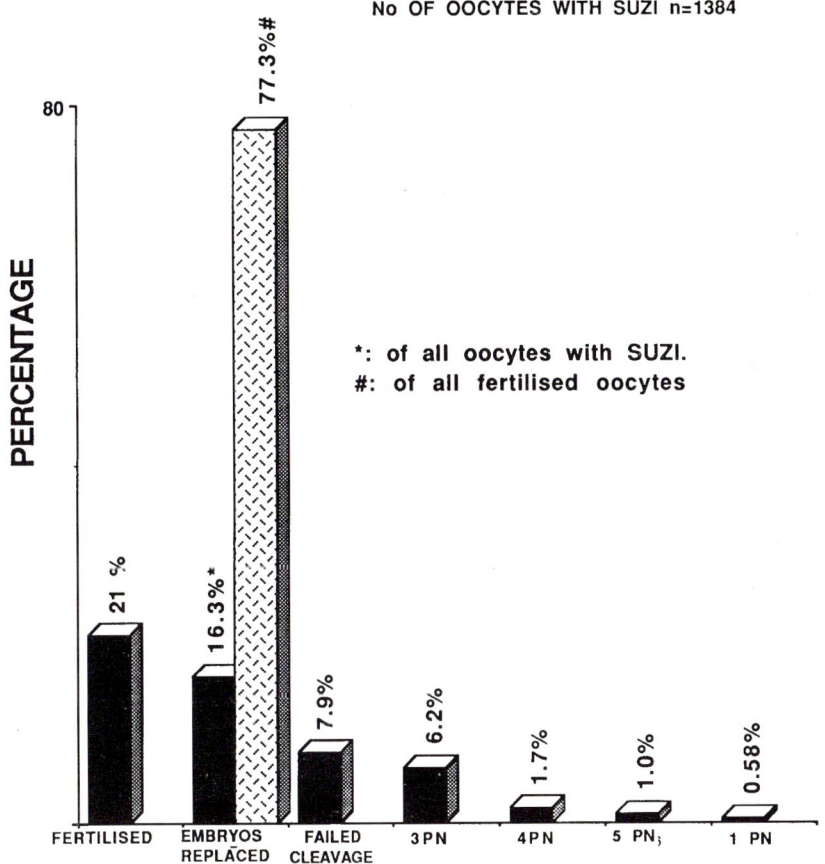

FIG. 2. Outcome of oocytes with SUZI.

The mean number of spermatozoa injected for all oocytes was 5.13±1.06 (SEM). The mean number of spermatozoa injected into oocytes that were not fertilised, or that achieved fertilisation with two or three pronuclei was 4.07±0.14, 4.91±0.28, and 7.11±0.97 (SEM), respectively. The difference in the mean number of spermatozoa injected in the fertilised oocytes was significantly greater than those injected into the oocytes that were not fertilised ($P<0.001$), and similarly for the oocytes that had three pronuclei compared to those with two pronuclei ($P<0.002$).

SUZI vs IVF with Sibling Oocytes

Table 2 shows the outcome of fertilisation in those patients for whom it was possible to compare IVF with SUZI in the same cohort of oocytes. Significantly ($P<0.0001$) more patients (44%) achieved fertilisation with SUZI compared to those who achieved fertilisation with both SUZI and IVF (8.4%). Only 1.6% of patients achieved fertilisation with IVF only.

Table 2. *Comparison between SUZI and IVF sibling oocytes*

Total number of patients with both SUZI and IVF	191	
Number with fertilisation with SUZI and IVF	16	(8.4%)
Number of patients with fertilisation with SUZI only	84	(44.%)
Number of patients with fertilisation with IVF only	3	(1.6%)
Total number of EGGS with SUZI	821	
Number fertilised	220	(26.8%)
Total number of EGGS with IVF	571	
Number fertilised	25	(4.4%)

($P<0.0001$)

In this group of patients the incidence of fertilisation per egg with subzonal insemination was significantly higher (26.8%) than with IVF (4.4%).

Assessment and Classification of Semen Parameters

Six parameters were used to assess the semen: volume (ml), total count (TC x 10^6), total motility (TM percentage), total count x 10^6/ml (TC/ml), total motile count x 10^6 (TMC) and progression (P on a scale 0-4). The arithmetic mean and the standard error of the mean for volume, TC, TM, TC/ml and P were 3.64±0.09, 33.87±3.90, 18.20±1.10, 10.68±1.34, 7.62±1.31 and 1.62±0.05, respectively (8). In earlier studies assessing the semen parameters according to four groups of patients: (those in whom fertilisation did not occur, where fertilisation occurred but without cleavage, where there was fertilisation with cleavage but not pregnancy, and where pregnancy occurred) it was found that only the total motile count and progression showed a significant difference. There was a higher total motile count (TMC) ($P<0.005$) in the group of patients which achieved fertilisation compared with those which failed to achieve fertilisation, and similarly for a rating of progression of spermatozoa ($P< 0.0001$) for the same two groups. However, the latter is a subjective score and as such is not considered as a prognosticator.

The incidence of fertilisation was assessed according to two classifications of seminal parameters. Classification of seminal parameters into the standard World Health Organisation (WHO) characteristics (Classification 1) was difficult as these parameters do not consider the various degrees of severity of asthenozoospermia and oligozoospermia and the various combinations. For example the classification according to asthenozoospermia and oligozoospermia resulted in 16 groups (A-P) ranging from the 'normal' to the very severe oligozoospermia/very severe asthenozoospermia samples. The division into 16 groups resulted in some groups having very few patients, thus presenting a difficulty for valid analysis (8).

According to the fertilisation data, the incidence of fertilisation was significantly affected when the total motile count (TMC) was taken into consideration. The calculation of TMC x 10^6 takes into account the volume of semen and the density and motility of spermatozoa; providing information on the total number of motile spermatozoa available. A second classification (Classification 2) was therefore devised expressing five groups of patients according to the TMC, Groups 1-5 (8) which correspond to <1, 1-5, 6-10, 11-20 and >20 TMC. The incidence of fertilisation with SUZI according to the new classification is shown in Tables 3 and 4. The majority of patients (68%) were in Groups 1 and 2. The incidence of fertilisation per patient was approximately 40%, or per oocyte approximately 21%. On a patient basis, there was a trend to decreasing fertilisation with increasing total motile count (Table 3). In Group 1, none of the 72 patients had fertilisation with IVF.

Table 3. *SUZI vs IVF and Sperm Classification 2*

	1. Patients			
Classification	Total number	Incidence	Fertilisation SUZI only	Fertilisation SUZI and IVF
Group 1	72	0.40	28 (38.9%)	0
Group 2	49	0.28	26 (53.1%)	4 (8.2%)
Group 3	16	0.09	57 (43.8%)	2 (12.5%)
Group 4	16	0.09	3 (18.8%)	3 (18.8%)
Group 5	25	0.14	7 (28.0)	2 (8.0%)

Evaluating the data on a per egg basis, all groups excepting Group 4 had a significant increase in the incidence of fertilisation with SUZI compared with IVF (Table 4).

Table 4. *SUZI vs IVF and Sperm Classification 2*

Classification	2. Eggs				
	SUZI		IVF		
	Total number	Number fertilised (%)	Total number	Number fertilised (%)	
Group 1	424	89	(21.0)^a	252	0^a	
Group 2	49	66	(23.5)^b	172	11	(6.4)^b
Group 3	16	15	(19.0)^c	59	6	(10.2)^c
Group 4	16	12	(16.0)^d	70	5	(7.1)^d
Group 5	25	22	(17.1)^e	98	5	(5.1)^e

a) $\chi^2_2 = 59.059$, $P<0.0001$.
b) $\chi^2_2 = 20.898$, $P<0.0001$.
c) $\chi^2_2 = 65.014$, $P<0.0001$.
d) N.S.
e) $\chi^2_2 = 6.494$, $P<0.0001$.

Sperm Morphology v SUZI

Using Classification 2, the incidence of fertilisation, cleavage and fragmentation after SUZI was evaluated (Fig. 3). Patients with the severest morphology (>95% abnormal forms) tended to a reduced incidence of fertilisation between groups and within each group. The lowest incidence of fertilisation occurring in patients with a TMC <1 and >95% abnormal forms. In TMC Group 1, a high incidence of patients had a sperm morphology of >95% abnormal forms (36%). The incidence of pronuclei stage arrest and, possibly, the level of cytoplasmic fragments, appeared to be related more to the degree of abnormal forms than the actual TMC (Fig. 4). Overall, there was a significant reduction in the incidence of fertilisation, multi-pronucleate oocytes and cleavage, and a significant increase and cytoplasmic fragments in patients with >95% abnormal forms.

DISCUSSION

A number of reports in recent years have confirmed that SUZI can achieve fertilisation and cleavage even with the most severe seminal defects associated with the density, motility and morphology of spermatozoa (6,8,15,21,23). This study demonstrates that SUZI significantly increased the number of oocytes fertilised and the number of patients whom achieved fertilisation compared with standard IVF, and, in addition, this can be

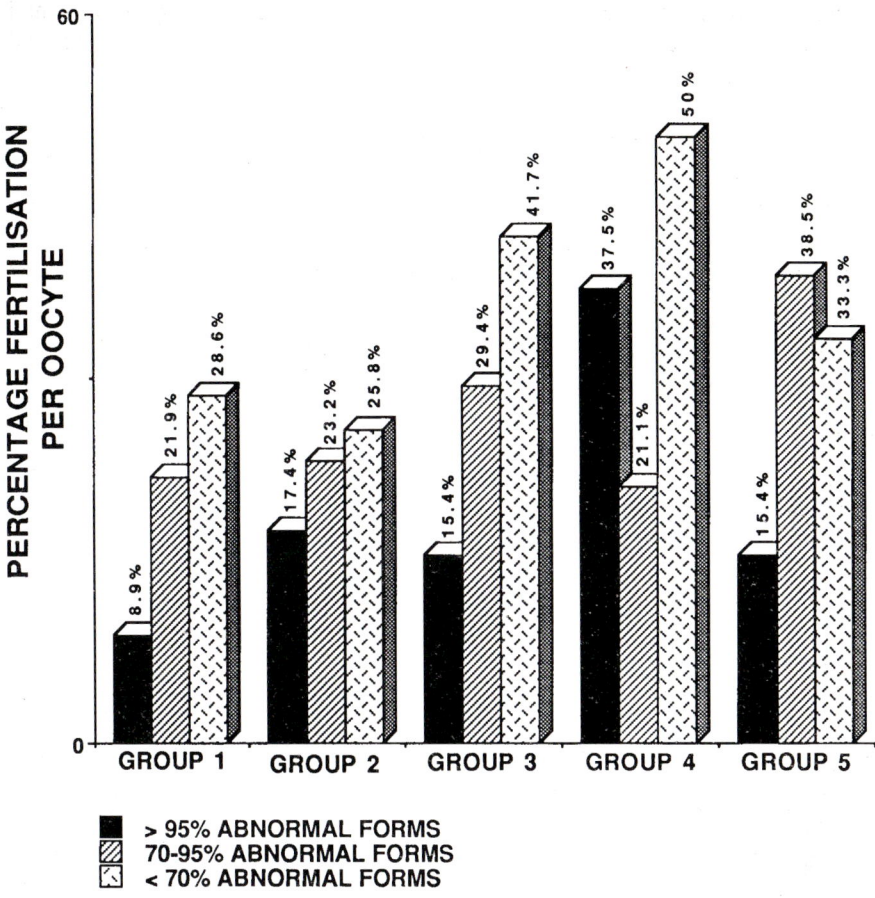

FIG. 3. SUZI in relation to sperm morphology and Classification 2.

achieved in those patients where fertilisation with IVF has never occurred. Studies using sibling oocytes to assess SUZI versus IVF for the same population of spermatozoa resulted in only 6% of eggs fertilised with IVF compared with 20.8% with SUZI.

The relevance of sperm morphology to SUZI needs to be clarified. A relationship of sperm function to particular morphological abnormalities remains unclear. Sperm morphology has consistently been shown to be of value as a prognosticator of spermatozoa function with the zona free hamster egg assay and human oocyte fertilising ability after IVF. However, the particular relevance of sperm morphology in relation to SUZI is unclear. One third of spermatozoa located in the perivitelline space after SUZI from men with severe oligozoopermia were found to be abnormal; defects of the nucleus, acrosome, midpiece and axoneme have been observed (27).

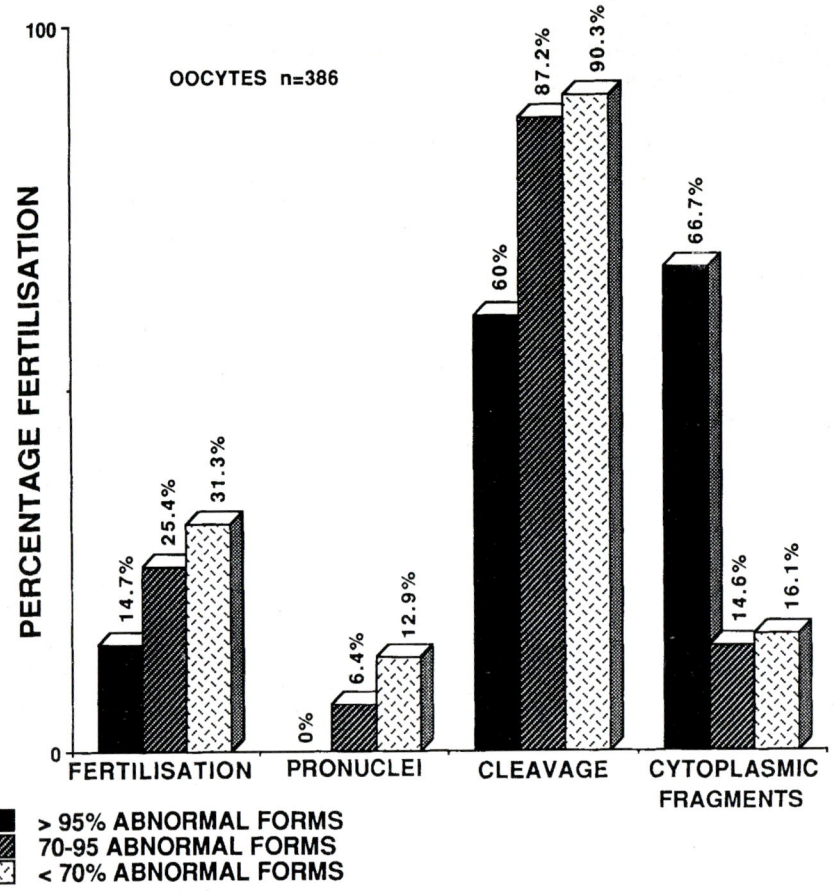

FIG. 4. SUZI and sperm morphology vs fertilisation, pronuclei, cleavage and cytoplasmic fragments.

In this study, a critical assessment of sperm morphology revealed that 26% of patients had >95% abnormal forms. The incidence of fertilisation was clearly affected by the severity of both the TMC and the morphology of spermatozoa. By distinguising the groups of patients before SUZI it is necessary to evaluate the need to modulate the numbers of sperm used for SUZI in each particular group. For example, with TMC Group 1 and morphology of >95% abnormal forms, i.e. the group with the lowest incidence of fertilisation, it might be advantageous to inject more sperm into the perivitelline space. The low incidence of polyspermia in this group might reduce our concern for the production of multi-pronucleate oocytes. However, the apparent high incidence of cleavage arrest in this group might be a cause for concern. For example, whether it is the fertilisation of the egg by abnormally-formed sperm or simply the presence of increased numbers of spermatozoa that might have a deleterious effect on cleavage is unknown. Previous studies (1) have suggested that the viability of embryos produced by SUZI is not significantly different from embryos produced after IVF. The data in the present series do not confirm this. Cohen *et al.* (1) reported that embryos produced from men with severe teratozoospermia had a much better prognosis than after embryos produced as a result of PZD or IVF, and also from those embryos produced by SUZI from men with moderate teratozoospermia. Arguments propounded include the method of insemination or the selection of normal spermatozoa during the SUZI procedure. As Cohen and co-workers acknowledge, this latter argument is most unlikely, and the former argument relates to the presence of many immotile cells and possible contamination with particulate matter which may result in the release of toxic elements such as reactive oxygen species. However the data remains an apparent paradox especially as it is not consistent with our experience.

Different results have been published, and this may be the reflection of different patient populations. Palermo *et al.* (26) demonstrated that in 43 couples who had previous failure of fertilisation, 30.9% of oocytes fertilised with a 3% polyspermia rate. Thirty-four patients had embryo transfer and 7 pregnancies resulted. However, the classification of sperm as abnormal in their lowest group demonstrated a mean density of $<5 \times 10^6$/ml with 35% motility and 17% normal forms. Although these were mean values, fertilisation can be achieved, especially with microdrop IVF, with considerably lower values even in patients that have previously failed to achieve fertilisation, as demonstrated using sibling oocytes in this study. Sibling oocytes were not used as controls in the study of Palermo *et al.* (25)

The recent publication by Ng *et al.* (23) using SUZI for men with severe oligoasthenoteratozoospermia demonstrated an incidence of monospermic fertilisation of 16.6% (2.3% for polyspermy) from 771 oocytes. Five pregnancies (one biochemical) resulted after 58 transfers from 131 patients with only one of the pregnancies resulting in a delivery. Further observation from this study using concomitant IVF with sibling oocytes showed the incidence of fertilisation with IVF (approximately 17%) not significantly different in all patients with a sperm concentration $>5 \times 10^6$/ml. The authors put this down to the few oocytes in each group. However, in the group with a sperm concentration $<5 \times 10^6$/ml 7 eggs undergoing IVF did not fertilise compared with 12.7% which fertilised after SUZI. One of the major differences between this study 23 and our data is the enormous centrifugal force applied to the spermatozoa. The method of sperm preparation, which included the use of Ficoll compared to our use of Percoll, was the centrifugation of sperm at 3,352 g for 20 minutes compared with our 350-400 g for 10 minutes. As the authors commented there may well be damage to the spermatozoa at this force including membrane leakage of adenosine 5-triphosphate.

In the present study there was a higher incidence, and a higher order of polyspermic oocytes than were published previously (26). This is a reflection of increasing the numbers of spermatozoa deposited in the perivitelline space. Techniques causing a breach in the zona pellucida prior to insemination with motile sperm have been reported to result in much higher levels of polyspermy than SUZI (1,2,18). Conflicting levels of polyspermy rate have also resulted after SUZI which is probably a reflection of patient selection and technique (8,23,6,26). Methods to increase the incidence of acrosome-reacted spermatozoa might be utilised in order that fewer spermatozoa would be injected into the perivitelline space. This approach would possibly increase the incidence of monospermic fertilisation and reduce the probability of polyspermy. Palermo *et al.* (26) utilised 50% follicular fluid and also electroporation in conjunction with pentoxifylline. Also using 2-dexoyadenosine in conjunction with follicular fluid and prolonged incubation of the sperm they achieve the same aim. A discussion on the existence of slow and fast blocks to polyspermy and the respective roles of the oolemma and zona pellucida in human oocytes has been discussed extensively elsewhere (6,27,24).

For clinical use it is imperative that we try to establish guidelines for the use of these procedures on particular groups of patients. In this study a modified version of the WHO classification and the classification using TMC appeared to demonstrate an increase in the incidence of oocytes fertilised after SUZI compared with IVF. However, an attempt to delineate a significant difference between different categories of male infertility for each level of severity proved non-viable on the basis of the WHO classification. In an earlier study, there was a significant demarcation in the incidence of fertilisation using the TMC classification which occurred between Group 1 and the other Groups. However, in the present study, by increasing the numbers of sperm used for SUZI in TMC Group 1 the incidence of fertilisation was increased. This resulted in no clear distinction in the incidence of fertilisation between groups. An association of TMC, morphology and other parameters needs to be assessed for a formula which may be used as a prognosticator of fertilisation.

In conclusion, this early developmental period for the clinical use of SUZI has demonstrated that these techniques can achieve fertilisation, pregnancy and birth in couples unable to conceive by other methods. The underlying concern that the incidence of abnormal embryos may increase after SUZI, or, that by bypassing the selection criteria for spermatozoa at the level of the zona pellucida, there may be an increase in the demise of embryos cannot emphatically be dismissed. Despite the study of Kola *et al.* (13) on a small number of embryos demonstrating no increase in the incidence of chromosomal abnormalities after SUZI in cases of oligoasthenoteratozoospermia, a healthy caution and strict observation is necessary before we can be assured of the overall safety of this procedure. However, the numbers of normal, ongoing pregnancies and births to date have alleviated many of the initial concerns. The different experiences and success rates of various groups obviously reflect the different populations of patients and clearly demonstrate the need to standardise patient selection and to build in the necessary control studies wherever possible during routine treatment.

Subzonal insemination is now providing a viable option for certain causes of infertility, but to increase the efficiency, improve the efficacy and to be confident of the safety much continued research is required in association with the treatment of patients.

ACKNOWLEDGEMENTS

The sincerest gratitude goes to Mrs. Barbara Gallimore, without whose help this manuscript would have been incomplete.

REFERENCES

1. Cohen, J., Alikani, M., Malter, H.E., Adler, A., Talansky, B.E. and Rosenwaks, Z. (1991) Partial zona dissection or subzonal sperm insertion: microsurgical fertilization alternatives based on evaluation of sperm and embryo morphology. Fertil. Steril., 56:696-706.
2. Cohen, J., Malter, M., Fehilly, C., Wright, G., Elsner, C., Kort, H. and Massey, J. (1988) Implantation of embryos after partial opening of oocyte zona pellucida to facilitate sperm penetration, Lancet, 2:162.
3. Cohen, J., Malter, H., Wright, G., Kort, H., Massey, J. and Metchell, D. (1989) Partial zona dissection of human oocytes when failure of zona pellucida penetration is anticipated. Hum. Reprod., 4:435-42.
4. Fishel, S. and Symonds, E.M. (1986) In-vitro fertilisation - past, present and future. IRL Press, Oxford.
5. Fishel, S.B., Antinori, S., Jackson, P., Johnson, J., Lisi, F., Chiariello, F. and Versaci, C. (1990) Twin birth after subzonal insemination. Lancet, 2:722.
6. Fishel, S.B., Jackson, P., Antinori, S., Johnson, J., Lisi, F., Cliariello, F., Versaci, C. and Lisi, R. (1990) Sub-zonal insemination (SUZI) for the alleviation of infertility. Fertil. Steril., 54:828-35.
7. Fishel, S., Antinori, S., Jackson, P., Johnson, J. and Rinaldi, L. (1991) Presentation of six pregnancies established by sub-zonal insemination (SUZI). Hum. Reprod., 6:124-30.
8. Fishel, S., Timson, J., Lisi, F. and Rinaldi, L. (1992) Evaluation of 225 patients undergoing subzonal insemination for the procurement of fertilisation *in vitro*. Fertil. Steril., 57:840-49.
9. Gordon, J.W. and Talansky, B.E. (1986) Assisted fertilization by zona drilling: A mouse model for correction of oligospermia. J. Exp. Zool., 238:347-54.
10. Hiramoto, Y. (1962) Microinjection of the live spermatozoa into sea urchin eggs. Experimental Cell Res., 27:416-426.
11. Iritani, A. and Hosoi, Y. (1989) Microfertilization by various methods in mammalian species. In: Development of preimplantation embryos and their environment, edited by Yoshinaga, K., Mori, T., pp 145-9. Allan R. Liss Incorporated, New York.
12. Keefer, C.L., Younis, A.I. and Brackett, B.G. (1990) Cleavage development of bovine oocytes fertilized by sperm injection. Mol. Reprod. Dev., 25:281-5.
13. Kola, I., Lacham, O., Jansen, R.P.S., Turner, M. and Trounson, A. (1990) Chromosomal analysis of human oocytes fertilised by micro-injection of spermatozoa into the perivitelline space. Hum. Reprod., 5:575-7.
14. Kopak, M.J. (1961) Exploring living cells by microsurgery. Transactions of the New York Academy of Sciences, II, 21:200-214.
15. Laws-King, A., Trounson, A., Sathananthan, H., Kola, I. (1987) Fertilization of human oocytes by microinjection of a single spermatozoon under the zona pellucida. Fertil. Steril., 49:835-42.
16. Lin, T.P. (1966) Microinjection of mouse eggs. Science, 151:33-37.

17. Lin, T.P. (1967) Micropipetting cytoplasm from the mouse eggs. Nature, 216:162-163.
18. Malter, H., Talansky, B., Gordon, J. and Cohen, J. (1989) Monospermy and polyspermy after partial zona dissection of reinseminated human oocytes. Gam. Res., 23: 377-86.
19. Markert, C.L. (1983) Fertilization of mammalian eggs by sperm injection. J. Exp. Zool., 228:195-201.
20. Metka, M., Haromy, T., Huber, J. and Schurz, B. (1985) Artificial insemination using a micromanipulator. Fertilität, 1:41-7.
21. Ng, S-C., Sathananthan, A.H., Edirisinghe, W.R., Kum Chue, J.H., Wong, P.C., Ratnam, S.S. and Sarla, G. (1987) Fertilization of a human egg with sperm from a patient with immotile cilia syndrome: case report. In: Advances in Fertility and Sterility, edited by Ratnam, S.S., Teoh, E.S., Anandakumar, C. 4:71-76, Parthenon Publishing, Lancaster, UK.
22. Ng, S-C., Bongso, T.A., Ratnam, S.S., Sathananthan, A.H., Chan, C.L.K., Wong, P.C., Hagglund, L., Anandakumar, C., Wong, Y.C. and Goh, V.H.H. (1988) Pregnancy after transfer of multiple sperm under the zona. Lancet, 2:790.
23. Ng, S-C., Bongso, A. and Ratnam, S.S. (1991) Microinjection of human oocytes: a technique for severe oligoasthenotenatozoospermia. Fertil. Steril., 56:1117-25.
24. Ng, S-C., Bongso, T.A., Sathananthan, H. and Ratnam, S.S. (1990) Micromanipulation: its relevant to human in vitro fertilisation. Fertil. Steril., 53:203-19.
25 Ohsumi, K., Katagiri, C. and Yanagimachi, R. (1986) Development of pronuclei from human spermatozoa injected microsurgically into Xenopus eggs. J. Exp. Zool., 237:319-325.
26. Palermo, G., Joris, H., Devroey, P. and Van Steirteghem, A.C. (1992) Induction of acrosome reaction in human spermatozoa used for subzonal insemination. Hum. Reprod., 7:248-54.
27. Sathananthan, A.H. and Chen, C. (1986) Sperm-oocyte membrane fusion in the human during monospermic fertilisation. Gamete Res., 15:177-8.
28 Thandani, V.M. (1980) A study of hetero-specific sperm-egg interactions in the rat, mouse and deer mouse using *in vitro* fertilization and sperm injection. J. Exp. Zool., 212:435-453.
29 Uehara, T. and Yanagimachi, R. (1976) Microsurgical injection of spermatozoa into hamster eggs with subsequent transformation of sperm nuclei into male pronuclei. Biol. Reprod., 15:467-470.

Subject Index

A
AA-8, 127
Abdominal aorta, 119
Acidic epididymal glycoprotein, 41
Acromegaly, 195
Acrosomal vesicle, 95
Acrosome, 41,257
Acrosome reaction, 75,273,293
ACTH, 119,207
Activin-A, 217
Activin-AB, 217
Activin-B, 217
Activin receptors, 44
Adenyl cyclase, 149,195
Adhesion molecules, 119
Adrenal glands, 195
β-Adrenergic agents, 119
Agarose gel electrophoresis, 157
AID (Artificial Insemination, Donor), 251
AIH (Artificial Insemination, Husband), 251
Albumin, 41
Allograft reaction, 237
Amphibian oocyte, 85
AMH, 1,5,17,31,45,195
Anabolic steroids, 251,257
Androgen, 49,63,119,127,139,157,179,251
Androgen Binding-Protein, 41
Androgen receptor, 49,119
Androgen-regulated genes, 127
Androgen-regulated mRNAs, 127
Andrology, 257
Angiogenesis, 167
Antiandrogens, 127
Anti-Müllerian Hormone (see also AMH,MIS), 1,5,17,31,49,195
Anti-phosphotyrosine antibodies, 99
Antibiotics, 215
Anticonvulsants, 251
Antiestrogens, 257
Antihypertensives, 257
Antisense oligonucleotides, 85
Antisperm antibodies, 273
Antral follicle, 151,159,167
Apoptosis, 159
Apoptotic bodies, 159
Arginine-vasopressin, 119
Aromatase, 145,149,179
Aromatase activity, 149,157
Aromatase Inhibitors, 1
Aromatisation, 157
ARP-1, 127
ARP-2, 127

ARP-5, 127
ARP-6, 127
ARP-7, 127
Artificial insemination, 189,251
Assisted reproduction, 273,293,225
Assisted Reproductive Technology (ART), 273
Asthenoteratospermia, 273
ATP, 273
Atresia, 157
Atrial Naturetic Factor, 119
Autocrine regulation, 1
Autoimmune orchitis, 119
Avascular cartilage, 167
Avian, 157
AVP, 119
Azoospermia, 251,257

B
Basal lamina, 157
Benzylidene malononitrile, 99
Blastocyst, 107
Blood, 119
Blood cells, 119
Blood vessels, 119
Blood-testis barrier, 119
Boys, 257
Bradykinin, 119
Branched-chain amino acid transferase, 63
Bromocriptine, 251
Bryostatin, 151
Buserilin, 207

C
Caffeine, 273
Calcium, 159,273
Calcium ionophore, 273
Calcium/magnesium-dependent endonuclease activity, 159
cAMP (see also cyclic AMP), 41,73,85, 99,107,149,195,273
cAMP-dependent protein kinase, 73,85,149
cAMP response element, 49
cAMP regulatory element, 149
cAMP response element binding-protein, 195
cAMP-dependent regulation, 149
cAMP-independent regulation, 149
α-Antitrypsin, 189
Capacitation, 75,293
Caput epididymis, 251
Carbonic anhydrase, 63
Carnitine, 41

Catecholamines, 119
Cats, 107
Cattle, 107,195
cDNA, 127,145,149,167,207
CEF-147,149
Cell, 1
Cell-cycle, 85,99
Cell death, 157
Cell growth, 145
Cell injury, 157
Cervical, 273
Chicken, 149,237
Chimeras, 1
Chimeric animals, 17
Chinese Hamster Ovary, 145
Chloramphenicol aceltyltransferase (CAT), 207
Cholesterol side chain cleavage enzyme (P450scc), 179
Chromatin, 85,237
Chromosome, 5
Chromosome mosaics, 17
Clomiphene, 251
Clomiphene citrate, 227
Cloning, 189
Collagenase, 167
Collagenase gene, 167
Collagenase IV, 167
Connective tissue remodeling, 167
Contraception, 75
Corpus luteum, 145,167,179
Corticotrophin-Releasing Factor, 119
Countercurrent transfer, 119
Cow, 85
Cropreservation, 237
Cryopreservation, 189,257
Cryptorchidism, 119,251
Cumulus oophorus, 75
Cumulus-oocyte complex, 85
Cyclic AMP (see also cAMP), 41,73,85,99,107,149,195,273
Cyclin-A, 85
Cyclin-B, 85
Cycloheximide, 85
Cysteine, 167
Cystic fibrosis, 257
Cytochrome P450, 5,31,145,149
Cytochrome P450c, 17,149
Cytochrome P450arom, 5,31,149
Cytochrome P450scc, 149,179
Cytomegalovirus expression vector, 217

D
daf-1, 49
2-Dexoyadenosine, 293
Dephosphorylation, 99
Diabetes mellitus, 257
Diacylglycerol (DAG), 149
Differentiation, 139,145
Digoxygenin-labelled riboprobe, 127
Diptheria toxin, 195,207
DNA, 17,99,167,195,207,217

DNA-binding proteins, 127
Dominant negative mutant, 217
Donor insemination, 251
Dopamine antagonists, 257
5α-Dihydrotestosterone (DHT), 157

E
EGF (see also Epidermal Growth Factor), 99,151
Egg (see also Oocyte, Ovum), 1,17,41,73, 85,99,107,167,189,207,225,227,237,251, 273,293
Egg collection (see also Oocyte collection), 227
Eicosanoid (see also Prostagandin, Leukotriene), 167
Ejaculation, 251,257,273
Electroejaculation, 251,273
Embryo, 73,107,189,217,227,237,251,293
Embryo development, 107
Embryo transfer, 189,225,227,237
Embryogenesis, 107,217
Embryonic development, 73
Embryonic epiblast, 73
Embryonic stem cells, 189
Endocrine stimulation, 145
β-Endorphin, 119
Endothelial cells, 119,179
Endothelium, 119
Epidermal Growth Factor (see also EGF), 99,151
Epididymis, 41,63,119,251,31
Epididymo-vasotomy, 251
Erythroid differentiation, 217
Erythroleukemia cells, 217
Estradiol (see also oestradiol), 207,227
Estrogen (see also oestrogen), 1,145,157, 167,207,227,237
Ethane Dimethane Sulphonate (EDS), 127
Ethidium bromide staining, 159
Eukaryotic, 99
Extracellular matrix, 167

F
Fallopian tube, 237,273
Fertilisation, 73,75,107,225,237,257,273
Fertility, 207,237,257
Fetal development, 134
Fetal ovary, 31
Fetal testis, 5,31
FGF (see also Fibroblast Growth Factor), Fibroblast Growth Factor (see also FGF), 139,167
Fibroblasts, 167
Fission yeast, 99
Flagellum, 41
Follicle cells, 1
Follicle-Stimulating Hormone (see also FSH), 41,49,75,119,139,145,149,157, 167,179,207,217,225,227,257
Follicles, 107,145,157,227
Follicular antrum, 107

Follicular development, 107,225,227
Follicular fluid, 157,273
Follicular maturation, 227
Folliculogenesis, 73,227
Forward-Motility Protein, 41
Forskolin, 149
Fragmentation, 157
Freemartins, 17
FSH (see also Follicle-Stimulating Hormone), 41,49,75,119,139,145,149 157,167,179,207,217,225,227,257
FSH receptors, 145
FSH-β subunit mRNA, 207

G

G-proteins, 75
Galactosyl transferase, 75
Gamete, 75,189
Gametogenesis, 49
Gene 'knock out', 217
Gene expression, 107,149,207
Gene therapy, 189
Genistein, 85
Genital ridge, 1,17,73
Genome, 107,195
Genome,
Germ cells, 1,5,31,73,99,119,139,195,237
Germinal cell, 139
Germinal vesicle, 99,107
GH (see also Growth Hormone), 195,207, 217,227
GH deficiency, 195
GIFT, 257
Gigantism, 195
β-Globin protein, 217
β-Globin transgene, 237
Glucocorticoid, 157,251,257
Glutathione, 49
Glycolysis, 41,273
GnRH (see also LHRH), 119,149,189, 195,207,227,251,257,293
GnRH analogue, 179,189,207,227,257, 293
GnRH receptor, 189
GnRH-agonists, 257
GnRH-like peptide, 151
Goat, 195
Gonad, 17,189,237
Gonadal dysgenesis, 257
Gonadal ridge, 17
Gonadotropes, 207
Gonadotrophin (see also FSH, HCG, HMG, LH, PMSG),107,139,145,149, 157,167,179,225,229, 251
Graafian follicle (see also Preovulatory follicle), 107,145,149,167,179,207,237
Granulosa, 139,145,149,157,167,174
Granulosa cell differentiation, 149
Granulosa cells, 167
Granulosa-luteal cell, 179
Growth factors, 49,99,119,149,139,159, 167,217,227

Growth Hormone (see also GH), 195,207, 217,227
Growth Hormone Releasing Factor (GRF), 195
G-proteins, 7,195
Guinea-pig, 63

H

Hamster, 63,273
Hamster egg penetration test, 273
HCG (see also Human Chorionic gonadotrophin), 119,225,227, 251,257, 293
Hematopoietic stem cell, 159
Hemizona asay, 273
Hemochromatosis, 257
Hermaphrodites, 17
Hernias, 257
Herpes simplex, 207
Herpes simplex virus type 1 (HSV1tk), 195
Histamine, 119
Histone H1 kinase, 85
HMG (see also Human Menopausal Gonadotrophin), 225,227,257,273,293
Human beings, 1,5,17,31,157,167,179,217, 225,227,237,251,257,273,293
Human Chorionic Gonadotrophin (see also HCG), 119,225,227,251,257,293
Human Menopausal Gonadotrophin (see also HMG)), 225,227,257,273,293
Hyaluronic acid, 75
Hyaluronidase, 75,293
Hybridisation, 167,189,237
17-Hydroxylase/C17-20 lyase, 145,159
Hydroxymethyl Glutaryl CoA Reductase (HMGCR), 195
3β-Hydroxysteroidehydrogenase/Δ^{5-4} isomerase (3β-HSD), 179
Hypogonadal mouse, 189
Hypogonadism, 237
Hypoosmotic sperm swelling test, 273
Hypophysectomy, 127
Hypothalamus, 195,207,257
Hypoxanthine, 73
Hystricomorphs, 63

I

Idiopathic Hypogonadotropic Hypogonadism, 257
IGF-1 (see also Insulin-like Growth Factor-I), 227
IL-1, 119
Immune response, 119
Immunocompetent cells, 119
Immunosupressive substances, 119
Implantation, 227
In Vitro Fertilisation (see also IVF), 225,227,251,257,273,293
Infertility, 41,195,225,227,237,251,257, 273,293
Inhibin, 41,49,119,179,207,217
Insemination, 107,273

Insulin receptor, 99
Insulin-like Growth Factor-I (see also IGF-1), 227
Intercourse, 251
Interleukins, 119
Interstitial tissue, 1
Interstitial fluid, 119
Interstitial space, 119
Interstitium, 139
Intra-Uterine Insemination (IUI), 273
Isobutlymethylxanthine (IBMX), 99
IVF (see also In Vitro Fertilisation), 225,227,251,257,273,293

K
Kallikrein, 251,257
Kallmann's syndrome, 251
Kartagener's syndrome, 195
α-Ketoisocaproate, 49
Kidney, 195
Klinefelter syndrome, 257

L
Lactate dehydrogenase, 49
Leucine, 49
Leukotriene, 119
Leydig cell, 17,41,49,119,127,139,195, 237,257
LH (see also Luteinising Hormone), 41,49,99,107,119,139,145,149,157,167, 179,207,225,227
LH receptors, 16,17,20
LH-β mRNA, 23
LH-β subunit, 23
LHRH (see also GnRH), 119,149,179, 189,195,207,227,251,257,293
Liver diseases, 257
Locus, 195
Luteal cell, 179,227
Luteal function, 179
Luteal phase, 179
Luteinising Hormone (see also LH), 41,49,99,107,119,139,145,149,157,167, 179,207,225,227
Luteinisation, 149,167,179
Luteolysis, 179
Lymph, 119
Lymphocytes, 63

M
α$_2$-Macroglobulin, 149
Male infertility, 251,257,273,293
Mammary gland, 157
Marsupials, 63
Mast cell growth factor, 49
Maturation Promoting Factor (see also MPF), 85,99
Mediastinal venous plexus, 127
Meiosis, 73,85,99,107,151,189,237
α-Melanocyte Stimulating Hormone (see also MSH), 119
Menopause, 237

Menses, 179
Menstrual cycle, 145,179,227
Menstruation, 179
Mesenchymal cell, 1,139
Mesoderm, 17
Mesodermal differentiation, 217
Mesterolone, 257
Metallothionein II (MT) gene, 195
Metaloproteinase inhibitor, 167
Metatheria, 75
Methylprednisolone, 251
Micro-assisted fertilisation, 293
Microcirculation, 119
Microsurgery, 257
Midpiece, 41
MIS (Müllerian Inhibiting Substance; see also AMH), 1,17,195
Mitochondria, 179
Mitosis, 41,85
Monoclonal antibodies, 189
Monosomies, 225
Morula, 107
Mouse, 1,17,107,167,207,237
MPF (see also Maturation Promoting Factor), 85,99
MPF kinase, 99
mRNA, 127,145,157,167,179,207
MSH (see also α-Melanocyte Stimulating Hormone), 119
Mumps, 257
Muscle, 189
Mutagenesis, 217
Mutation, 189
Myocrisin, 75

N
Necrosis, 157
Neoplasia, 257
Nerve Growth Factor, 119
Neuroblastoma cells, 217
Neurological development, 217
Neuronal cell survival, 157
Nitrofurantoin, 251
Non-aromatizable androgens, 157
Nuclear condensation, 157
Nuclear DNA, 127

O
Oestradiol (see also estradiol), 207,227
Oestrogen (see also estrogen), 1,145,157, 167,207,227,237
Oligoasthenoteratozoospermia, 257
Oligoasthenoteratozoospermia, 293
Oligonucleotides, 107
Oligospermia, 273
Oligozoospermia, 251
Oncogenes, 189,195
Oocyte (see also Egg, Ovum), 1,17,41,73, 85,99,107,167,189,207,225,227,237,251, 273,293
Oocyte collection (see also Egg collection), 227

Oocyte culture, 107
Oocyte cumulus complexes, 293
Oocyte donors, 107
Oocyte maturation, 107
Oogenesis, 73,85,99,107
Oogonia, 237
Oolemma, 63
Ooplasm, 273
Orchidopexy, 257
Orchitis, 257
Orthotopic grafts, 237
Osmotic pressure, 119
Osteoblasts, 167
Ovarian follicle, 49,145
Ovarian graft, 237
Ovarian mRNA, 145,167
Ovarian Stimulation, 225,227
Ovary, 1,5,17,31,73,75,85,99,107,145,149, 157,167,179,225,227,237
Ovotestis, 17
Ovulation, 145,149,157,167,225,227, 237,293
Ovulation induction, 273
Ovum (see also Egg, Oocyte), 1,17,41,73, 85,99,107,167,189,207,225,227,237,251, 273,293
Oxytocin, 119

P
P-aminobenzamidine, 85
P-Mod-S, 127
p34 cdc2, 85,99
p34cdc2 kinase, 85
Pampiniform plexus, 119,127
Pancreatic kallikrein, 251
Paracrine regulation, 1,139,145,157
Parenchyma, 145
PCR, 127
Pentoxifylline, 251,273,293
Percoll, 293
Peritubular cells, 1,49,127,139
Peritubular myoid cells, 1,49
Perivitelline space, 293
Peroxidation, 273
Phorbol esters, 151
Phorbol myristate acid (PMA), 149
Phosphodiesterase inhibitors, 99,273
Phosphoenolpyruvate carboxykinase, 195
Phospholipase, 151
Phosphorylation, 85,99
Pig, 85,159
Pituitary gland, 207,217,251
Pituitary cell line, 189
Pituitary gland, 179
Pituitary gonadotrope, 293
Plasmin, 167
Plasminogen, 149,167
Plasminogen activator, 41,167
Plasminogen activator inhibitor, 167
PMSG see also (Pregnant Mare Serum Gonadotrophin), 107,145,167
Point mutations, 189

Polycystic ovary syndrome, 227
Polymorphonuclear leukocytes, 119
Polyspermy, 75,251,293
Porcine follicles, 157
pp60 v-src, 151
Pre-embryo, 189
Pregnancy, 179,225,227,251,273,293
Pregnant Mare Serum Gonadotrophin (see also PMSG), 107,145,167
Premature ovarian failure, 157
Preovulatory follicle (see also Graafian follicle), 107,145,149,167,179,207,237
Primary hypogonadism, 257
Primordial follicle, 73,179,237
Primordial germ cells, 17,49,237
Pro-activin A, 217
Procollagenase, 167
Progesterone, 85,149,157,179
Progesterone receptor, 149
Progesterone secretion, 179
Programmed cell death, 157
Prolactin, 195,207
Pronuclei, 189
Prospermatogonia, 1
PROST, 273
Prostaglandin endoperoxide synthase (PGS-2), 151
Prostaglandin, 119,167,189
Prostate, 119
Protein, 157
Protein kinase, 159
Protein kinase A signalling, 73,85
Protein kinase C signalling, 149
Protein synthesis, 167
Proteinases, 167
Proteolysis, 85
Protyeolytic enzymes, 167
Psychotropic drugs, 257
Pubertal development, 139
Puberty, 119,257
Pulse-field gel electrophoresis, 195
Purkinje cell, 195
Pyknotic nuclei, 159

R
Rabbit, 63,167,195,237
RASK antibody, 85
Rat, 49,99,107,119,127,145,149,157,167
Reactive oxygen species, 273
Receptors, 49,195
Recombinant GH, 227
Recombinant FSH, 145
Renal failure, 257
Renin-angiotensin system, 119
Rete testis, 119
Retinoic acid, 49,217
Retinoic acid receptors, 49
Retroviral vectors, 189
RIIβ, 149
Round spermatid, 41
Rous sarcoma virus, 149

S

SDS-PAGE, 127
Secondary interstitial cells, 157
Secondary sexual characteristics, 1
Semen, 251,293
Semen analysis, 273,293
Seminiferous epithelium, 41
Seminiferous tubules, 5,31,41,119,127,139,257
Serine, 49,99
Serotonin, 119
Sertoli cell, 1,5,17,31,41,49,119,127,139,195,257
Sertoli cell differentiation, 139
Sex determination, 17
Sex differentiation, 5,31
Sex reversal, 17
Sex steroids, 251
Sheep, 85,107,157,189,195,207
Sister chromatids, 189
Site-directed muragenesis, 85
Smooth endoplasmic reticulum, 179
Somatotropes, 195
Sperm anitibodies, 257
Sperm biology, 41
Sperm development, 49
Sperm dysfunction, 257,273,293
Sperm micro-injection, 293
Sperm morphology, 293
Sperm motility, 273
Sperm motility gene, 195
Sperm motility inhibitory factor, 41
Sperm-oocyte interaction, 75,273
Spermatids, 49,119,127,195
Spermatocytes, 49,195
Spermatocytes, 195
Spermatocytogenesis, 41
Spermatogenesis, 127,139,195,251,257
Spermatogenic cycle, 41,127
Spermatogonia, 41,49,195
Spermatozoa, 41,49,63,75,99,195,251,257,273,293
Spermatozoon, 41
Spermiogenesis, 41
Sry, 17
SRY, 17
Stem cell factor, 49
Steroid hormones, 257
Steroidogenesis, 257
Steroidogenic cells, 179
Steroids, 157,189,207
Stromal cells, 167
Strontium, 273
Subhuman primates, 179
Substance P, 119
Subtraction hybridization, 49,127
Subzonal insemination (see also SUZI), 293
Subzonal microinjection, 251,293
Sulphasalazine, 251
Sulphated glycoprotein-2 (SGP-2), 127
Superovulation, 225,227,273,293
SUZI, 293
SV40, 189,195
SV40-DHFR transgene, 195
'Swim-up' technique, 273
Symplastic spermatids (sys), 195

T

αT3-1 Pituitary cell line, 189
Tamoxifen, 251,257
Teratospermia, 273
Teratozoospermia, 293
Terminal differentiation, 179
Testicular artery, 119
Testicular function, 119,139
Testicular microcirculation, 119
Testicular tubules, 49
Testicular tumours, 257
Testis, 1,5,17,31,41,49,63,119,127,139,195,237,251,257,273,293
Testis cord, 1
Testis-determining gene (*Tda-1*), 17
Testolactone, 251
Testosterone, 1,41,49,119,127,237,257
Testosterone buciclate, 257
Testosterone enanthate, 257
Testosterone esters, 127
TGF-α (see also Transforming Growth Factor-α), 139
TGF-β (see also Transforming Growth Factor-β), 49,119,139,217
Theca, 1,145,149,157,167
Theca cells, 1,145,149,157,167
Thecal/interstitial cells, 145
Threonine kinase, 49,99
Threonine phosphorylation, 99
Thymidine, 159
Thymidine kinase, 195,207
Thyrotroph, 195
TIMP, type 1 (TIMP-1), 167
Tissue plasminogen activator, 151
Toxigenes, 189
Transcription factor, 1,17
Transdermal testosterone, 257
Transferrin, 41,139
Transforming Growth Factor-α (see also TGF-α), 139
Transforming Growth Factor-β (see also TGF-β), 49,119,139,217
Transgenes, 17,22,24
Transgenic animals, 22,24
Transgenic mice, 207
Transgenics, 22,23,24
Transition protein-2 (TP-2), 127
Transplantation, 237
Trisomies, 225
Tubular complexes, 49
Tumor Necrosis Factor-α, 169
Tumoroginesis, 237
Tumour cells, 189
Tumours, 189
Tunica albuginea, 169